Education and Training in Dementia Care

Reconsidering Dementia Series Editors: Keith Oliver and Dawn Brooker

Other titles in this series:
Dementia and Psychotherapy Reconsidered
Richard Cheston

Education and Training in Dementia Care

A person-centred approach

Claire Surr, Sarah Jane Smith, and Isabelle Latham

Open University Press

Open University Press
McGraw Hill
Unit 4
Foundation Park
Roxborough Way
Maidenhead
SL6 3UD

email: emea_uk_ireland@mheducation.com
world wide web: www.mheducation.co.uk

Commissioning Editor: Sam Crowe
Editorial Assistant: Hannah Jones
Production Manager: Ali Davis
Marketing Manager: Bryony Waters
Cover Design: Adam Renvoize
Cover Art: Keith Oliver
Logo Design: Julia Heron

A catalogue record of this book is available from the British Library

ISBN-13: 9780335251124
ISBN-10: 0335251129
eISBN: 9780335251131

Library of Congress Cataloging-in-Publication Data
CIP data applied for

Typeset by Transforma Pvt. Ltd., Chennai, India

Printed in Great Britain by Bell and Bain Ltd, Glasgow

Praise Page

"'Education and Training in Dementia Care' gets to the heart of this important viewpoint by describing and evaluating methods that focus on whether the training approaches will impact on learners' knowledge, skills, and attitudes. It is this that will move health and social dementia care forward to where it must be in order to utilise training in the very best way to improve the lived experience of dementia."
Jackie Pool, Dementia Care Champion, QCS Ltd

"Focusing on involving people living with dementia as so-called "experts-by-experience" in the training and education of dementia care is one of the book's greatest strengths. Another is the authors' state-of-the-art proposals for numerous training and education methods sat in distinct dementia care-settings and supported with easy-to-understand didactic thoughts and theory descriptions. Something that sets the book apart from others in the field and, to a greater extent, enables the book to support those who are to train and educate care staff in dementia care. A relevant, innovative, and important book that can underpin better education and training in dementia care."
Associate Professor, Cand. Cur., Jesper Bøgmose,
Faculty of Health, University College Copenhagen, Denmark

"My grand expectations for this book were fulfilled beyond measure. It contains innovative ideas to challenge current dementia education; then drive forward the development of education and training focused on the involvement of and benefits to those directly affected by dementia. From the contemporary glossary of terms to the excellent summaries of each chapter, it is an accessible and inclusive read. Its person-centred, theory and practice-based approaches to learning make it an essential book for everyone involved in the delivery, review and commissioning of dementia education."
Dr Anna Jack-Waugh, Senior Lecturer in Dementia,
Senior Fellow HEA, Alzheimer Scotland Centre for Policy,
and Practice, the University of the West of Scotland, UK

"This book is a must read for those wanting to understand, design and improve our approach to workforce knowledge in dementia care. It provides the reader with an evidence base that is rarely put to paper and provides a much deeper understanding of the various approaches. At its core is what it means to work in a person centred way and how we can support the workforce to learn and develop. This book it timely as societies and governments begin to realise that we need to do more to

accelerate our approach in supporting people with dementia and their families."

Paul Edwards, Director of Clinical Services, Dementia UK

"'Education and Training in Dementia Care' is an excellent exploration of the role of training and workforce development in achieving person centred practice.

We are encouraged to consider a diverse view of what constitutes 'dementia training', review the evidence provided by sector specific interventions and acknowledge the important principles and practice of training design. This is not just another book about training, it is a comprehensive summary of the barriers and facilitators of effective learning for all dementia care services and practitioners."

Hilary Woodhead, Executive Director NAPA
(National Activity Providers Association)

Titles in the series

Dementia and Psychotherapy, Richard Cheston

Education and Training in Dementia Care: A person-centred approach, Claire Surr, Sarah Jane Smith and Isabelle Latham

Forthcoming Titles

Reconsidering Ethics in Dementia Care, Julian Hughes

Reconsidering Leisure and Dementia, Christopher Russell, Jane Twigg and Karen Gray (eds)

Neighbourhoods and the Lived Experience of Dementia: Spaces, Places and People, John Keady (ed)

Talking with Dementia, Reconsidered, Keith Oliver, Reinhard Guss and Ruth Bartlett

Contents

About the authors

Claire Surr is Professor of Dementia Studies and Director of the Centre for Dementia Research at Leeds Beckett University. She has earned international recognition for her expertise in dementia education and training design, delivery, and evaluation. Claire was inspired to start a career in dementia research having been taught by the late Professor Tom Kitwood as an undergraduate and his subsequent support to commence a doctorate in the field. Claire has spent most of her career delivering dementia education and training to staff working across all sectors within the health and social care system and at all levels. She has designed programmes of dementia training for a number of care provider organisations. In 2014, she was awarded a prestigious Advance HE National Teaching Fellowship for her contribution to innovation in dementia education and training and, in 2016, a Principal Fellowship recognising her sustained record of leadership in the field. Claire led the 'What Works in Dementia Education and Training?' research study, which evaluated the most impactful approaches to the design, delivery, and implementation of dementia training. The study has gone on to provide the gold-standard criteria for dementia training in the UK and beyond.

Sarah Jane Smith is a Reader in Dementia Research at Leeds Beckett University. Sarah trained as a cognitive psychologist and her early research examined cognitive impairment in people living with Parkinson's disease. Sarah's core academic interest is understanding the types of everyday cognitive difficulties people living with dementia or memory impairment experience, and the non-pharmacological steps that can be taken to redress these difficulties. Since 2011, Sarah has worked solely in the field of dementia care, as a Lecturer and subsequently Senior Lecturer and Head of Education for the Centre for Applied Dementia Studies at Bradford prior to becoming a Reader in Dementia Research at Leeds Beckett. Sarah is interested in improving services at the point of assessment and diagnosis and has focused on developing education and training in this area. She has developed a national postgraduate programme for people working in memory assessment services. She has also designed and delivered training for care providers and charitable care organisations. Sarah was workstream lead on the 'What Works in Dementia Education and Training?' research study, conducting a national audit examining the content of education and training provision in England. Sarah is co-chair of the UK Higher Education Dementia Network.

Isabelle Latham is Researcher-in-Residence for Hallmark Care Homes, a UK-based care home provider, having spent the previous 10 years as Senior Lecturer at the Association for Dementia Studies, University of Worcester. There she led both research and education programmes with a particular focus on care homes, becoming well known for her practical and passionate approach. She has developed and implemented several dementia care interventions via research and developed educational materials and programmes based upon that real-world evidence, believing that translating research evidence into practical tools is a vital role for the researcher. Isabelle began her career as a care worker in care homes and it was this experience that instilled not only an interest in dementia care, but also a passion for supporting and celebrating the work of frontline care staff. A specialist focus on preventing abuse and safeguarding followed, working across multiple sectors. This generated an awareness of the multitude of influences on staff practice and the need to understand factors outside training in order to improve outcomes and achieve real change. Isabelle's doctorate explored this further in 2019 by examining how care workers learned to care for people living with dementia through their day-to-day work.

Foreword

The person-centred perspective was first described by Tom Kitwood in 1997 and while, as this book says, dementia training has come a long way in the last 25 years, it still has many mountains to climb if this training is to become nothing less than the gold standard throughout the world. Whilst one size doesn't fit all, the book you are about to read is intended to be a comprehensive guide to designing, delivering, implementing, and evaluating dementia care training across all health and social care services. It shows the value gained by including people affected by dementia at all these stages and I believe, as someone living with dementia, that this is the only winning formula.

The pandemic showed that if you throw money at clinical research, a vaccine could be developed within a year – imagine what would happen if the same amount of money went into social care, including dementia care training?

As someone who may be in need of social care in the near future, I have a vested interest to get the training right now and not still be having the same conversation in another 25 years. This book shows the way forward to achieve this.

Wendy Mitchell, author and living with dementia

The Reconsidering Dementia Series

The dementia field has developed rapidly in its scope and practice over the past 25 years. Many thousands of people are diagnosed with dementia each year. Worldwide, the trend is that people are being diagnosed at much earlier stages. In addition, families and friends increasingly provide support to those affected by dementia over a prolonged period. Many people, both those diagnosed with dementia and those who support them, have an appetite to understand their condition. Care professionals and civic society also need an in-depth and nuanced understanding of how to support people living with dementia within their communities over the long term.

The *Reconsidering Dementia* book series sets out to address this need. It takes its inspiration from the late Professor Tom Kitwood's seminal text *Dementia Reconsidered* published in 1997, which, at the time, revolutionised how dementia care was conceptualised. The book series editors worked together on the second edition of this book entitled *Dementia Reconsidered Revisited: The Person Still Comes First.* This 2019 publication was a reprint of the original text by Tom Kitwood alongside contemporary commentaries for each chapter written by current experts. Many topics in the field of dementia care, however, were simply unheard of in Kitwood's lifetime. The subsequent titles in this series are cutting-edge scholarly texts that challenge and engage readers to think deeply. They draw on theoretical understandings, contemporary research, and experience to critically reflect on their topic in great depth.

This does not mean, however, that they are not applicable to improving the care and support to those affected by dementia. As well as the scholarly text, all books have a 'So what?' thread that unpacks what this means for people living with dementia, their families, people working in dementia care, policy-makers, professionals, community activists, and so on. Too many books focus on an academic audience *or* a practitioner audience *or* a student audience *or* a lived experience audience. In this series, the aim is to try to address these perspectives in the round. The *Reconsidering Dementia* book series attempts to bring together the perspectives of professional practice, scholarship, and the lived experience as they pertain to the key topics in the field of dementia studies.

This book series is jointly commissioned and edited by Professor Dawn Brooker MBE and by Dr Keith Oliver. Dawn has been active in the field of dementia care since the 1980s as a clinician and an academic. She draws on her experience and international networks to bring together a series of books on the most pertinent issues in the field. Keith is one of the foremost international advocates for those living with dementia. He also brings an insightful perspective of his own and others' experience of what it means to live with dementia gained since his diagnosis of Alzheimer's Disease in 2010.

Series Editors: Dawn Brooker and Keith Oliver

Preface

One of the titles that Dawn and Keith wanted to commission early on was this book on *Education and Training in Dementia Care*. Every time an issue is identified as difficult in the field of dementia, training is recommended as a solution. The authors of this book have all undertaken in-depth research into the *how*, the *what*, and the *why* of training and education in the many contexts in which people affected by dementia find themselves. Their knowledge and passion for utilising training in the very best way to improve the lived experience of dementia comes through on every page. It will be a must-read text for all those involved in training and education about dementia worldwide.

We hope that you will enjoy reading this book as much as we have enjoyed the editorial process.

Additional thoughts from Keith Oliver

It has been an honour and a privilege for me as a person living with dementia to fulfil the role of co-editor for Claire, Izzie, and Sarah's book, and from their clear introduction to the book I was drawn in and hooked by their knowledge, experience, and combined style of writing. Since sharing my brain with Alzheimer's Disease, I have had many good days and weeks, but frustration and challenge is never far away, lurking in what I describe as the fog of my dementia. However, as a former headteacher and local authority education schools adviser, it is in my DNA to recognise the importance of meaningful staff development and training. In my former life, this led to benefits to all stakeholders – children, parents, colleagues, and the school community generally; now this recognition is equally important to me as I strive to be an Alzheimer's Society Ambassador or NHS Dementia Envoy. When reading and co-editing this book, whilst learning an enormous amount, I was always mindful of the range of strategies that those delivering training need to consider, and then adopt, whilst focusing upon the needs of those receiving the training who would then return to their place of work better skilled, better motivated, and even one hopes inspired to 'climb further mountains', because when you reach the summit the view is spectacular, and the rewards for trainers and those receiving the training can be immense.

Acknowledgements

Collectively, we would like to thank Dawn Brooker for her initial approach inviting us to write this first book in the series, and to Dawn and Keith Oliver as series editors, for reading drafts of the book and for their constructive feedback. Our gratitude also goes to Jo Crossland, Danielle Woods, Sara Humphrey, April Dobson, and Suzanne Mumford who read and provided feedback on drafts of the service-specific chapters. We would also like to thank the following people and organisations for contributing case studies to this book:

Kenny Chui, Jockey Club Centre for Positive Ageing managed by the Chinese University of Hong Kong
Charles Cross, Anglian Care
Jo Crossland, Avery Healthcare
April Dobson, Hallmark Care Homes
Joanna James, Imperial College Healthcare
Gayle Madden and Caroline Scates, Dementia UK
Suzanne Mumford, Care UK
Clementinah Rooke, University of Huddersfield and AaroHelm
Wessex Academic Health Sciences Network
Danielle Woods, Bradford Teaching Hospitals NHS Trust

We would also like to thank the many colleagues we have worked with over the years who have helped shape our knowledge and understanding of dementia education and training. Our understanding of the field and what makes good dementia education and training has undoubtedly been enriched by the opportunity we have had collectively, to work alongside so many talented and passionate educationalists and dementia education/training researchers. There are too many of you to name individually, but you know who you are, and we are grateful for everything we have learned working alongside you. We would also like to thank our employing organisations and colleagues for giving us the time and support to work on what has been an undertaking of which none of us had quite foreseen the magnitude: Leeds Beckett University and our colleagues Rachael Kelley, Laura Booi, and Nicky Taylor, The University of Worcester, as well as Hallmark Care Homes and our colleagues Faith Frost, Tracey Williamson, and April Dobson. Finally, we would like to thank our friends and family for their support when we have spent too many hours at our desks 'just finishing' this chapter or book-related task. To Sadie, Jake and David, Stewart and Edna, Nicola and Wendy.

Glossary of terms

The terminology used in both dementia care and education can be inconsistent and sometimes contentious. We have clarified the terminology we have used throughout this book in this glossary for consistency and transparency.

Acute care – care provided in hospital for brief, sudden, and severe illness.

Advanced care planning – planning ahead for health and care needs that may arise in the future, perhaps at a time when the person no longer has the capacity to express their wishes directly.

Antipsychotic medications – drugs that are used to treat severe agitation, distress, or aggression caused by psychotic symptoms such as hallucinations or delusions. These can have severe side-effects for older people that worsen with continued use. They have also been over-prescribed in the past to people living with dementia in response to distressed behaviours. Good practice guidelines promote prescription only in specific circumstances.

Asynchronous learning – methods of online delivery that are intended for the learner to complete alone, separately from other learners. These methods, such as reading an e-learning module or completing a quiz, are usually self-directed by the learner and completed at a time of their own choosing.

Blended learning – a form of training delivery that uses a combination of online and face-to-face methods, such as attending some in-person sessions, followed up with online exercises and discussion groups.

Caregiver – any family member, relative, or friend providing informal care and/or support to a person with dementia.

Care home – a setting that provides both accommodation and care for people unable to live independently. This might be nursing care or social care only. Across the world these settings are variously known as long-term care, nursing homes, residential care, aged care, or assisted living.

Coaching – a method of learning where one person (coach) supports another (coachee) to develop skills and enhance practice through one-to-one or group reflection, problem-solving, and goal-setting. It focuses on helping the coachee to learn for themselves rather than on the coach to teach.

Competencies – a particular set of qualities (skills, knowledge, and abilities) that are required for a particular role. Competencies are usually expressed (and assessed) in terms of behaviours that a person needs to be able to demonstrate.

Continuing professional development – learning activities that professionals and paraprofessionals engage in throughout their working lives in order to enhance their knowledge and abilities.

Dementia Care Mapping – a well-established formal observation method used in dementia care settings to evaluate, reflect on, and improve person-centred care. It requires formal training to implement.

Dementia care workforce – the group of professionals and paraprofessionals who provide formal, paid-for health and social care support of different types for people living with dementia across a wide variety of settings.

Distressed behaviours – actions, words, or behaviours exhibited by a person living with dementia that may be a sign of stress or distress, including shouting, crying, calling out, hitting, biting, pulling, restlessness, pacing, withdrawal, and apathy. Within person-centred care, distressed behaviours are seen as a way of communicating unmet needs by the person living with dementia. Older terminology for such behaviours (behavioural and psychological symptoms of dementia, or 'challenging behaviours') tended to pathologise the behaviour and ignore the role of the care environment in causing (and thus resolving) such behaviour.

e-learning – a form of training delivery that uses computer-based content to be completed asynchronously by learners, without the input of 'live' interaction with facilitators or other learners.

Education – a formal method of learning focused mainly on gaining theoretical knowledge, via expert input (using teachers and other resources). It typically takes place within a systematic programme (such as in school, or via a qualification process).

Evaluation – the process of measuring the success or outcomes of a programme or intervention.

Evidence-based practice – practice that is guided by an understanding of what is demonstrated to work best in particular circumstances (as opposed to habit or guesswork). Evidence is gained through a systematic approach to evaluating activity (such as research) and its reflective application to day-to-day situations.

Experiential methods – methods used in training that encourage learners to directly experience and discover for themselves by 'doing' rather than only listening or watching. Experiential methods promote the active involvement of learners, through learning activities such as group problem-solving and role-play.

Face-to-face delivery – training delivered in-person, with a group of learners and one or two facilitators.

Facilitator – a skilled person who designs and delivers training sessions and helps learners to take on board this new information and apply it to their job role. Often also referred to as a teacher, trainer, or educator.

Formal care – health and care services that have a direct financial cost, usually provided by public, private, or third sector organisations. The cost can be covered by the individual themselves, others, or with governmental assistance.

Formal learning – training or other activities that have been specifically organised (usually by an employer) to encourage learning about a particular topic or issue (e.g. a training course or formal instruction).

General practitioner – a medical doctor who provides general medical care to people in the community (via a general practice). General practitioners are often a person's first point of contact with health services and treat common medical conditions that can be managed within the community (primary care), and refer patients on to more specialised care (acute care) when required.

Homecare – formal care that is provided in a person's own home, in the form of scheduled visits or 'live-in' care. Sometimes known as domiciliary care.

Housing with care – a form of accommodation by which a person owns or rents their own property within a setting that also provides options for care and support. This can variously be referred to as sheltered accommodation, extra care housing, or assisted living, with different types and levels of support being available in different settings.

Informal care – care and support provided by a relative, friend, or neighbour that is unpaid, and thus there is no direct financial cost to the individual or an external funder.

Informal learning – events that result in learning but that were not specifically organised and designed for it (for example, a critical incident at work).

Learners – the participants of training or education.

Learning – the process of acquiring new understanding, knowledge, skills, attitudes, or behaviour. It can be an outcome of training and education but also everyday experience.

Mentoring – a relationship between two people with the aim of professional development. The mentor is usually an experienced person who shares experiences, skills, and advice with a less-experienced person.

Multi-disciplinary – an approach that brings together people from several different professions and perspectives. This can be to learn together or to provide input to someone's care and support.

National Health Service (NHS) the NHS is the provider of universal health care in the UK, free at the point of delivery and funded via taxation. This accounts for most hospital-based and primary health care, but not social care, provided in the UK.

National Institute for Health and Care Excellence (NICE) – a public body in England and Wales that is part of the government department responsible for health and social care. NICE issues guidance on clinical practice and social care.

Online (remote) methods of delivery – a form of training delivery that uses electronic means, with learners at a distance from one another. This can include both synchronous and asynchronous activity.

Paraprofessional – a member of the dementia workforce whose role does not require qualifications or registration prior to commencing and whose competence is gained primarily through hands-on experience and in-service training, such as care assistants, support workers, and care workers. We have adopted this term as we believe that other commonly used terms for this group (such as 'non-qualified', 'untrained', and 'non-professional' staff) are misleading.

People directly affected by dementia – a term that includes both people living with dementia and those who live with and/or provide informal care for them (such as a spouse or friend).

Person-centred care – care and support that enhances the personhood of a person living with dementia. In person-centred care, all relationships impacting on the person living with dementia should focus on valuing that person, recognising them as an individual, understanding their perspective, and creating supportive social environments for them and those important to them.

Personhood – the status of being a whole, individual person. Accepting and promoting that a person living with dementia is a whole person, worthy of the same rights as those without dementia, is the fundamental tenet of person-centred care.

Primary care – care provided in the community as a first point of contact with health care services, most often initially by a general practitioner. Primary care services may include access to a range of practitioners, including community nurses and occupational therapists.

Randomised controlled trial (RCT) a research design in which an intervention is trialled with two randomly assigned groups: one (the experimental group) receiving the intervention that is being tested, and the other (the control group) receiving an alternative intervention or conventional practice. The RCT is considered a robust research design that produces high-quality evidence.

Reflective practice – a process of consciously thinking about one's own or others' practice and taking a critical stance, with the intention of adapting and improving over time.

Remote delivery – see *Online (remote) methods of delivery*

Shadowing – the process by which a new or inexperienced person follows and observes an experienced person doing a job or task with the intention that they learn how it is done.

Simulation methods – a specific form of experiential learning in which learners are enabled to apply skills in a risk-free environment and learn through a process of practice, reflection, and feedback. For example, simulation methods can include using mannequins, acted scenarios, or role-play.

Synchronous learning – methods of online delivery that are designed for learners to complete together with other learners, often mimicking what may happen in a face-to-face training session. These methods usually take place at set times, and could be led by a facilitator, such as a discussion group using Zoom or Teams.

Tacit knowledge – knowledge that a person has gained through experience in their professional and personal life. It is often known as 'common sense' or 'know how' and can be hard for people to explain or describe.

The Care Certificate (TCC) a common induction framework in England for all paraprofessionals working across health and social care settings. Not dementia-specific, the TCC is designed to equip workers with introductory skills and knowledge required to provide basic care. It is implemented by employers and assessed within the workplace.

The Kirkpatrick Model – a four-level model for evaluating training that highlights the different outcomes that can be achieved from training. The four levels are: (1) learner's reaction, (2) learner's knowledge, (3) learner's behaviour, and (4) outcomes and results.

Third sector – an umbrella term that includes a range of different types of organisation that are neither in the public nor private (profit-making) sector. These include charities, voluntary organisations, and not for-profit organisations. In many countries, they contribute a large proportion of health and social care service providers.

Training – a formal method to enable learning that uses expert input (via a teacher, trainer, or facilitator) to develop people's skills and understanding of a particular topic or task. It most commonly relates to a specific role and has a focus on application of knowledge to practice.

Training needs analysis (TNA) a review of learning and development requirements in an organisation or setting based on an assessment of what skills are needed, what skills presently exist, and what skills are lacking. Ideally, a TNA will take place at an organisation, team, and individual level.

Virtual reality – a type of simulated, experiential method using computer technology that aims to be fully immersive. It aims to support learning about dementia by simulating what some of the symptoms and experiences of dementia may be like.

Workplace learning – learning that takes place within a workplace whilst engaged in the activities of doing work.

World Health Organisation (WHO) an agency of the United Nations, the WHO has a responsibility for international public health.

1 Introduction

'This book is predicated on the assumption that good quality training and education is embedded in a person-centred approach.'

This book seeks to provide an evidence-based, practical resource for people intending to develop, deliver, review or commission **education** and **training** for the dementia workforce. It is aimed at those working in health and social care services and private and **third sector** organisations who are responsible for, or interested in, training and development for their staff, as well as commissioners of training.

In the last 20 years, since Tom Kitwood first published his seminal text *Dementia Reconsidered* (1997), there have been significant advances in our understanding of how to interact with and provide care for people living with dementia together with their family and friends. The evidence base for how to provide care for people with dementia has grown significantly. Despite this, until recently there has been less evidence of how to provide training and education for the dementia workforce.

This book has developed from our collective passion, as authors, for dementia education, training and workforce development, and the work we have undertaken throughout our careers, to understand what makes good dementia training and how to implement this to impact positively on care for people living with dementia. All three authors have designed, delivered, and evaluated many dementia-specific education and training programmes for staff working across the full spectrum of dementia care services and roles. We have also undertaken formal, broader research on dementia workforce development and impactful approaches to their **learning** and development. We recognised that there was a gap in evidence-based information about how to design, deliver, implement, and evaluate dementia training. This book aims to fulfil this gap by drawing on a range of evidence from our own research and experience, as well as real-life examples from across the sector.

The content of this book is rooted in the person-centred perspective first described by Tom Kitwood (1997) and subsequently developed by proponents of **person-centred care**. The book comprises a range of practical information including up-to-date international research evidence, case studies, and vignettes. The book covers best-practice approaches to the design, delivery, and implementation of formal programmes of dementia training and education as well as considering the importance of informal routes and mechanisms for workforce development. The authors of this book have been extensively and closely involved in research concerning dementia education and training, with a particular interest in what 'good' dementia training looks like. To this end, the book looks at the practice context and setting conditions required for successful training outlining individual, service, and organisational level factors that those responsible for workforce development should consider. It addresses approaches to driving and transforming practice change through training and workforce development, including consideration of ways those responsible for training may assess and evidence its impact and fully integrate the lived experience of dementia throughout provision, alongside barriers and pitfalls such as organisational issues and complexities in the makeup of the workforce.

This book has two parts. Part 1 (Chapters 2–7) focuses on the broader theory underpinning approaches to dementia training and the application of this in different health and social care settings. It also outlines the evidence for the efficacy of different training approaches currently used in these settings.

Chapter 2, 'The design and delivery of formal dementia training and education', introduces the broader theory and research evidence around the design and delivery of formal education and training to adult **learners**. It considers how to involve **people directly affected by dementia** in training, the theoretical underpinnings of adult learning, and the evidence base underpinning some of the more commonly used methods such as **face-to-face delivery**, **experiential** and **simulation methods**, and in-practice learning approaches.

Chapter 3, 'Informal ways of learning', considers learning in the workplace, revealing possibilities for influencing practice that remain somewhat untapped. It covers the theory and practice of **informal learning** as an opportunity to improve person-centred care, in different dementia care settings.

Chapter 4, 'Learning and development in care homes', addresses the extensive literature on training that is provided to the dementia workforce in **care homes**. Care homes are recognised as a crucial part of the system of care available for people affected by dementia. However, they also present unique challenges. This chapter outlines the challenges of training in care home settings and gives examples of methods used successfully to provide training for this diverse workforce.

Chapter 5, 'Learning and development in primary care', covers the current challenges of providing dementia-specific training for practitioners based in **primary care**, who have long been identified as being ideally positioned to respond to the needs of people living with dementia but have tended to have had limited opportunities for dementia training. Some examples from practice are presented, which may be useful for those developing or delivering training in this setting.

Chapter 6, 'Learning and development in acute hospitals', describes training provided to the hospital workforce in order to deliver good quality person-centred hospital-based care to people with dementia. It explores the evidence on delivery of dementia training in acute hospital settings and provides guidance on best practice for those designing, delivering, and implementing dementia training in this setting.

Chapter 7, 'Learning and development in community settings', describes training that is provided for the workforce delivering care for people living with dementia and their **caregivers** in their own or family home or supported accommodation. With many people with dementia living in community settings, this chapter reviews the evidence base for training the workforce responsible for supporting individuals in formalised and non-formalised ways.

Part 2 (Chapters 8–10) focuses on the theory and evidence underpinning the implementation of effective training and education for the dementia workforce. This includes practical considerations related to the contextual issues associated with the successful implementation of learning in practice (e.g. individual learner, setting, and organisational factors). It also considers ways of evaluating the impact of training.

Chapter 8, 'The person at the centre of the learning experience', examines the individual learner level factors that are important for supportive and successful learning. In doing so, it addresses the implementation of formal training and informal learning for the purposes of delivering person-centred care.

Chapter 9, 'Training implementation and driving practice and culture change', explores the conditions necessary for formal and informal learning and development to be used as a driver for practice change to support delivery of person-centred dementia care. It considers the role of 'implementation science' and provides an overview of models for considering how to optimally implement practice change through programmes of work that include training.

Chapter 10, 'Measuring and evidencing the impact of training', outlines models and methods that may be useful to adopt when evaluating the impact of a programme of dementia training, education or other workforce development activities.

Chapter 11, 'The future for dementia training and education', provides a summary of the book as a whole and draws together the take-home messages and implications for research and practice.

Tying these strands together throughout the book will be integration of the lived experience of dementia into training and education, and the continued relevance and need for Kitwood's concepts of person-centred care.

The landscape of dementia care

Dementia care is an umbrella term for the care and support provided to people living with dementia in any setting or context. The settings and contexts in which care is provided vary according to *who* is providing the care and *where* the care is being provided. Care can be provided by a variety of people, including paid health care professionals or **paraprofessionals** (**formal care**), as well as family and friends (**informal care**). The **World Health Organisation** (WHO) estimates that informal caregivers spend around 5 hours a day providing care for people with dementia, and that 50 per cent of the cost of care is attributable to this. The nature of this care can have a significant impact on the people providing it, with often negative psychosocial and health-related impacts because of the burden. Whilst the negative impact on informal caregivers is universal, there is a disproportionate impact on women, who provide around 70 per cent of caregiver hours (WHO 2021).

Improved formal care provides the opportunity to reduce the impact – both financial and psychological – on informal caregivers. Formal dementia care refers to care that is provided by staff employed within settings such as hospital or residential care, or care provided in people's own homes or in other places in their communities.

This book will primarily focus on training in formal care settings for the dementia workforce. That is not to say that those delivering informal or unpaid care do not require skills, knowledge, or training to undertake their role. However, their training needs and the methods and mechanisms for providing this are commonly different from providers of formal paid care. Improved training for the dementia workforce has the potential to improve care outcomes for people living with dementia, as well as reduce the negative burden on the informal caregiver.

Person-centred care

Throughout this text we will refer to person-centred care as the gold standard of care for people living with dementia. This book assumes that the goal of training for the dementia workforce is ultimately the delivery of good quality person-centred care. It is useful to recognise where this term comes from, what it means in practice, and the role that it occupies when we think about good dementia care practice.

The term person-centred care is as used in the context of dementia derived from the concept of **personhood** – first ascribed to people living with dementia by Kitwood (1997). In *Dementia Reconsidered*, Kitwood defined personhood as 'a standing or status that is bestowed upon one human being, by others, in the context of relationship or social being' (1997, p. 8). He argued that despite the impact that dementia can have on a person's cognitive function, there is no resultant degradation of the individual as a person (i.e. their personhood remains intact). Kitwood suggested that personhood is constructed by an individual's interaction and relationship with other people and argued it was only lost if others failed to acknowledge it. When he first wrote about this, Kitwood's account that personhood was maintained by people living with dementia flew in the face of the predominant biomedical views of the condition, which positioned individuals living with dementia as experiencing a loss of self, due to the disease process. Kitwood acknowledged that whilst the disease processes can impact the experience of a person, personhood is not tied to this experience. He also highlighted the need for those caring for people living with dementia to have knowledge about and empathy with those with the condition to support and maintain personhood.

The impact this definition of personhood has had on the delivery of care for people living with dementia is significant. Kitwood's model implied that the ways in which care is delivered can either enhance or undermine personhood. Social interactions and environments that undermine personhood, either intentionally or unintentionally, are described as 'malignant social psychology'. For example, Kitwood described the practice of talking in the presence of a person as if they were not there as a type of malignant social psychology he called *ignoring*. Overall, Kitwood described 17 ways in which personhood could be undermined by social environments and interactions.

On the other hand, he described ways of interacting that enhance personhood called 'positive person work'. For example, Kitwood described the process of *recognition*, either by recognising a person by simply using their preferred name or by careful active listening as a means of endorsing someone's personhood.

Further examples of positive person work and malignant social psychology are described in the *Dementia Reconsidered* text. Through raising awareness of positive person work and training the dementia workforce to adopt positive person practices, the delivery of *person-centred care* (care that supports personhood) is facilitated.

In his earlier work (1995), as well as in *Dementia Reconsidered* (1997), Kitwood recognised the role of organisational cultures in influencing outcomes for people living with dementia. Organisational culture is not a new concept or an understudied one, but it is complex, which perhaps explains its continued complicating presence alongside efforts to improve practice. He emphasised the need to transform to a 'new' culture to support the personhood of people living with dementia. Importantly, he described the habits of practice and ways of working that formed the basis of the current culture, which undermined person-centred practice (Brooker and Latham 2016; Kitwood 1997). In so doing he highlighted a key factor contributing to organisational culture's pervasive influence. Non-person-centred practice is not as simple as deliberately poor or harmful actions (i.e. malignant social psychology) carried out by individuals. Instead, it most often occurs through habitual and unquestioned day-to-day interactions, shaped unknowingly by the decision-making and problem-solving of many different actors in any organisation. Improving that practice therefore requires an understanding of these hidden processes and unknown actors. Organisational culture is complex to define and control because it is not one easily observable and identifiable thing; it is *everything* that occurs within an organisation. These issues are explored more fully in Chapter 8.

Kitwood's theories of person-centred care were subsequently expanded into a four-part definition designed to be accessible to the **dementia care workforce** (Brooker 2004; Brooker and Latham 2016; NICE 2018). The definition uses a VIPS acronym (as in 'very important persons') as a useful aid to remembering the key principles of person-centred care as espoused by Kitwood.

> **V: V**alue people with dementia and those who care for them, promoting their citizenship rights and entitlements regardless of age or cognitive ability.
>
> **I:** Recognise people's **I**ndividual lives, appreciating that all people with dementia have a unique history and personality, physical and mental health, and social and economic resources, and these will affect their response to neurological impairment.

P: Look at the world from the **P**erspective of the person with dementia, recognising that each person's experience has its own psychological validity, that people with dementia act from this perspective, and that empathy with this perspective has its own therapeutic potential.

S: Recognise that all human life, including that of people with dementia, is grounded in relationships, and that people with dementia require an enriched and supportive **S**ocial environment which both compensates for their impairment and fosters opportunities for personal growth.

Inherent to achieving person-centred care is a need for good quality relationships between those providing care, the person living with dementia, and their family and friends. In some applications of person-centred care, the relational can be overlooked, resulting in services that provide individualised care but ignore the more complex emotional and social components that are essential for supporting personhood (Nolan et al. 2004; Venturato et al. 2011). For example, a patient can have an individualised plan of care that meets their individual health needs, but if the hospital does not simultaneously enable staff to communicate in ways that make the patient feel safe or recognise their spouse's role in maintaining their sense of self, then they are not providing person-centred care.

Relationship-centred care is a recognised approach that has developed in response to this issue, with the aim of emphasising the importance of relationships to providing good quality care. Relationship-centred care notes the interdependent nature of relationships between the person living with dementia, their family and friends, and those who provide care. Efforts to support the personhood of a person living with dementia will be undermined if those important to them and those who are providing their care and support are not also emotionally and physically supported (Brown Wilson et al. 2013; Dewar and Nolan 2013; Nolan et al. 2006; Soklaridis et al. 2016). For proponents of relationship-centred care, without this holistic approach to relationships, achievement of the goal of person-centred care (maintained personhood) is not possible. Models such as the Senses Framework have been developed to help service providers consider their care provision from a relationship-centred perspective (Nolan et al. 2006). When we refer to person-centred care in this book, we consider relationships, and enhancement of them, as an essential component.

More recently, the person-centred philosophical stance has also developed in ways that present social citizenship and rights-based models of dementia which place emphasis on the voice and the human rights of the person living with dementia. People living with dementia report feeling marginalised in and by society (ADI 2019). Social citizenship approaches assume that it is the responsibility of society to ensure that people with dementia are not excluded because of their cognitive changes or disability. Bartlett (2022) frames this as a cognitive accessibility issue, such that inclusive social citizenship relies on access to systems, products, services, and environments despite cognitive disability. In other words, society (including its systems, services, and environments) should be structured in ways that are accessible to people with or without cognitive impairment. This might include adapting physical spaces, such as the use of signage, as well as making changes to social interactions, such as not speaking too quickly.

A rights-based approach is best represented by the work of people living with dementia and the growing number of people with dementia who are self-advocating and speaking up publicly through dementia advocacy groups. Dementia Alliance International is an international dementia advocacy group whose core beliefs (presented in Box 1.1) reflect a human rights-based approach.

Kate Swaffer, Dementia Alliance International Chair, has detailed a shift in dialogue from medicalised approaches to dementia towards human rights-based approaches and understanding and recognising dementia as a disability (Swaffer 2018). In a 2018 article, Swaffer describes the importance of international guidance and policy, such as the WHO Global Disabilities Action plan, to ensure that people living with dementia are recognised both locally and internationally in policy and law (Swaffer 2018).

Box 1.1 Dementia Alliance International core beliefs

- People living with dementia deserve quality of life and appropriate support to live their pre-diagnosis lives.
- Everyone has the possibility of having value every day of their lives, no matter what stage of the disease they are at.
- Well-being (quality of life) with dementia is possible.
- People with dementia must be included in all decisions affecting them: 'nothing about us, without us'.
- People with dementia are role models for each other and should learn from each other.
- People with dementia and the wider community must focus on what people with the disease *can* do rather than on what they *cannot* do, through all stages of the disease.
- Language must not devalue people with dementia.
- People with dementia still have capacity.

In the context of this book, we will consider person-centred care in its broadest sense, as care that supports an individual's personhood, recognises the importance of their relationships, and places them at the centre of the care they receive. We incorporate principles of citizenship that have grown from human rights movements by reiterating the importance of involving people affected by dementia as partners in the development, delivery, and **evaluation** of dementia education and training.

Dementia training for the formal dementia care workforce

The dementia care workforce refers to anyone providing formalised dementia care across health and social care services, including medical and health care professionals as well as a range of role titles (care assistants, care workers, well-being workers, support workers, etc.) that exist nationally and internationally for social care workers and paraprofessionals. Paraprofessionals are members of the dementia workforce who may not have a professional registration (such as a nurse or social worker will have). A range of terminology exists to refer to paraprofessionals. However, using terms such as 'non-qualified', 'untrained' or 'non-professional' for this group is misleading since, as this book outlines, paraprofessionals are in receipt of a range of training and are often highly skilled and knowledgeable.

The breadth of professionals and paraprofessionals included in the dementia workforce is matched only by the array of training courses, frameworks, and recommendations that exist for these roles. However, this can complicate the creation of guidance for a workforce that can, for some roles, lack national professional bodies, universally recognised qualifications, clear career pathways, and tends to be viewed in generic rather than specialist terms.

Standards and frameworks for dementia training

Over the last decade, developments internationally have seen an increased profile of dementia training, and advocacy for clearer and mandated training requirements for the workforce – both professional and paraprofessional. However, these still vary substantially across the world, relying most often on aspiration rather than government or regulatory instruction.

In general, the implementation of training standards is managed within country-specific health care systems and governing structures. However, in recognition of the importance of driving up global standards of dementia education and training, Alzheimer's Disease International (ADI) launched an accreditation process through which any global training provider can apply to earn ADI accreditation, which indicates that training has reached the ADI standards (ADI n.d.). The standards assess the design and delivery methods of training programmes as well as the presence of essential dementia-specific content. This type of global initiative speaks to the importance of using agreed benchmarking to drive up and ensure the quality of training – but still relies on the motivation of training providers to demonstrate the quality of their provision, rather than being a mandated activity.

Examples of country-specific activities illustrate the significant variation in the adaption of frameworks and standards globally. In Australia, there are no minimum standards or mandatory requirements for dementia training for the care home workforce (McCabe 2019). Nonetheless, the development of Dementia Training Australia (a nationwide government-funded consortium), the revision of the aged-care quality standards against which services are registered (Aged Care Quality and Safety Commission 2018), and a workforce strategy calling for the re-framing of qualifications and skills frameworks to include dementia and person-centred care (Aged Care Workforce Strategy Taskforce 2018), suggest movement in this direction.

In the USA, requirements for training vary greatly by state for both personal care assistants and long-term care facilities. A survey of state standards showed 28 of 50 states had no laws requiring dementia training in nursing homes and eight had none for assisted living facilities, with 14 states only requiring it within specialist memory care facilities (Burke and Orlowski 2015a). Thirteen states had laws related to dementia training for personal care assistants (regulating this through licensing of individuals rather than facilities). These set minimum standards and curriculum content, including addressing basic dementia awareness, communication, social and psychological needs, behaviour, and working with families (Burke and Orlowski 2015b). The Alzheimer's Association issued best-practice recommendations for long-term care, including guidance for a thorough induction and training programme for new staff and ongoing training built around the principles of person-centred dementia care (Fazio et al. 2018; Gilster et al. 2018), although this remains aspirational for some states.

In some countries at least, dementia-specific training standards have advanced significantly in the last 20 years with the development of frameworks to help guide the content and standards of training. Academics from the UK Higher Education for Dementia Network (HEDN), who are individuals with an interest in university dementia education, published one of the earliest curricula for pre-qualifying dementia education (Pulsford et al. 2007), updated in 2014. Scotland became the first of the UK nations to publish a national framework for dementia education and training content (NHS Education for Scotland and the Scottish Social Services Council 2011), with England (Skills for Health 2018), Wales (Care Council for Wales 2016), and Northern Ireland (Health and Social Care Board 2016) following suit. Now those providing dementia education or training for the dementia care workforce across the UK are expected to ensure this is aligned with the relevant framework for their home nation.

These UK frameworks have also been incorporated into national guidelines on dementia. In England, the **National Institute for Health and Care Excellence (NICE)** has recommended that all staff within care and support providers should receive training in person-centred care for people living with dementia. NICE specifies that those with direct care responsibilities should receive additional face-to-face training (including opportunities for feedback and case-specific discussion) on specific issues such as communication, responding to **distressed behaviours**, and approaches for those with severe dementia (NICE 2018). Whilst not mandatory, NICE guidelines hold significant weight in health and care service commissioning, particularly for regulated services such as hospitals and care homes. The NICE Guideline in the UK has been informed by:

- evidence about what kind of training approaches may be best for the dementia workforce based on the 'What Works' study (Sass et al. 2019; Smith et al. 2019; Surr et al. 2017a, 2020);
- the Dementia Training Standards Framework (Skills for Health 2018), which describes subjects and learning outcomes that training should address;
- and the Scottish Promoting Excellence framework (NHS Education for Scotland and the Scottish Social Services Council 2011), which describes values important for the dementia workforce.

In doing so, the NICE Guideline moves beyond general descriptions of person-centred care to specific issues of care; considering both induction and ongoing **continuing professional development**; and addressing matters of training delivery methods as well as content. For example, it is recommended to use face-to-face training with opportunities for follow-up.

One benefit of training frameworks is that they provide a standardised, comprehensive overview of what those providing different services should know and be able to do if they are to provide good quality care to people living with dementia. On the other hand, the comprehensive nature of such frameworks can also provide a barrier to implementation in time- and resource-poor services. To address this, some frameworks suggest tailoring the knowledge and **competencies** to specific job roles. In England, for example, the Dementia Training Standards Framework has been divided into three tiers. Tier 1 comprises a single topic – 'dementia awareness' – and should be achieved by all staff working in all roles across health and social care. This includes staff in non-clinical roles such as administration, catering, cleaning, and transport. Tier 2 is for those who have regular contact with people with dementia in their role and includes 11 additional core topics (e.g. 'person-centred dementia care', 'health and well-being in dementia care', 'end-of-life dementia care'). Tier 3 is for those working in managerial and leadership roles and includes additional learning outcomes across the core topics at Tiers 1 and 2, plus two additional topics ('research and **evidence-based practice**' and 'leadership in transforming dementia care').

However, the Dementia Training Standards Framework still includes a significant amount of content, which would not be feasible for most health and social care providers to cover in relevant depth in their provision for all staff. Not all staff working in roles with direct contact with people living with dementia require the same degree of knowledge across all the subject areas either. For example, someone working in memory assessment and diagnostics services would not need the same in-depth knowledge of end-of-life dementia care as someone working in a care home or acute hospital setting. Likewise, care home staff might need a less in-depth knowledge of dementia risk reduction and prevention, which might be more essential for staff working in primary care services.

Training needs analysis

It may be advantageous for organisations to take ownership of how national frameworks or standards are applied within their organisation through conducting a **training needs analysis (TNA)** for different roles across their organisation. This aims to aligns their training strategy and implementation plan with wider organisational goals, quality assurance mechanisms and the professional requirements of staff groups and individual staff members. This would include identifying the priority subject areas and learning outcomes for a particular job role. This could be coupled with development of individual learning needs assessment for each staff member as part of induction or annual performance review processes, to enable prioritisation of training identified as essential for their role. Tailoring training to the specific setting, role, and prior educational experience of staff has been consistently identified as more effective than a one-size-fits-all approach when evaluating dementia education and training within different service settings (Cunningham et al. 2020). Thus, there is strong evidence to support the case for conducting an organisational TNA based on existing training frameworks and using this to inform development of an organisational training strategy. This can then be implemented through tailored training provision that is designed specifically for the organisation and its staff.

A further limitation of using off-the-shelf frameworks is that the training is only as robust as the framework itself. This relies upon the integrity of the process for the development of the frameworks, and the expertise that has fed into them. This book is predicated on the assumption that good quality training and education is embedded in a person-centred approach. Therefore, the degree to which a particular framework reflects this philosophy will affect how well it will enhance development of a dementia training programme. For example, one might need to review the degree to which the standards are designed to maintain the personhood of an individual with dementia (Kitwood 1997), promote relationships, or endorse the rights of people living with dementia.

Elsewhere in this book, the importance of including people directly affected by dementia in the development of training is considered (Chapter 2). The extent to which the development of the framework or standards has involved people directly affected by dementia may provide a further test for how appropriate the framework is to shape a dementia curriculum. For example, the development of the Dementia Training Standards Framework in England was guided by an expert group that included people directly affected by dementia.

This book endorses the use of these standardised frameworks where they pass the test of promoting curricula that reflect person-centred values and philosophy. However, despite such frameworks being in existence, it is a limitation that we do not understand the extent to which they are applied in the real world. For example, Smith et al. (2019) conducted a UK-wide audit that highlighted the variability in the degree and nature of training across the UK using the English Dementia Training Standards Framework as a benchmark. The audit suggested that some topics and subjects were underrepresented, such as research and evidence-based practice, pharmacological interventions, equality and diversity, and end-of-life care (Smith et al. 2019).

Types of education and training

Non-dementia-specific mandatory training

Alongside dementia-specific training frameworks and guidance, the dementia workforce is often subject to other training requirements. This may include mandatory training to support the physical and health needs of individuals or related to issues such as risk or legislation. This can take the form of training provided at induction or on an ongoing basis. For the paraprofessional workforce, this type of training can be particularly significant due to their lack of pre-qualifications and the vast variation in job roles and types of employing organisation they may engage with across their careers. Within the four nations of the UK, for example, substantial work has been done to create standardised induction frameworks for adult social and health care workers across different roles and settings, including care workers for people living with dementia. The content specifics differ somewhat in each devolved nation but are broadly comparable, particularly in their implications for dementia-specific care. In England, Wales and Northern Ireland, the induction framework is standardised via regulation, whereas in Scotland induction is only recommended (Care Council for Wales 2016; Northern Ireland Health and Social Care Board 2016; Skills for Health 2018). In Scotland, however, care workers are registered within 6 months of commencing work, a requirement of which is to be working towards a named qualification (NHS Education for Scotland and the Scottish Social Services Council 2011).

In England, this induction framework is **The Care Certificate (TCC)** standards introduced in 2015: a set of 15 generic standards relevant across health and social care designed to equip workers with introductory skills and knowledge required to provide basic care. It is implemented by employers and assessed within a workplace through observation of practice and review of knowledge (Health Education England 2014). Whilst not technically mandatory, the regulator requires all registered care services to provide an induction for new staff that meets TCC Standards within 12 weeks of taking post (Care Quality Commission 2015; Thomson et al. 2018). This is designed to aid consistency of induction processes so that staff do not have to retake induction training if they move roles. However, an evaluation of TCC found that whilst implementation was high across all services, social care services were significantly less likely to have implemented it than health care services. In addition, considerable variation was found in employers' methods of implementation, and this led to uncertainty over quality and devaluation of TCC. For example, 10 per cent of organisations surveyed used only **online (remote) methods of delivery**. The features associated with effective implementation included blended, practical, and participatory approaches to training and the provision of peer support and **mentoring** (Thomson et al. 2018).

Continuing professional development

Continuing professional development (CPD) describes training that is provided over and above the education required for qualification and registration for professionals, or beyond mandatory training for paraprofessionals. Specific CPD opportunities for professionals and paraprofessionals are covered in the relevant chapters of this book. However, it is worth noting that CPD opportunities for both professionals and paraprofessionals vary internationally and are highly dependent upon the employing organisation and the regulatory environment.

CPD can be assessed or not. Non-assessed CPD opportunities might include, for example, attending meetings or workshops that are dementia specific. Examples of assessed CPD might relate to further education or higher education provided after professional registration – which should be distinguished from higher education designed to enable professional registration described in the following section.

Higher education for professional registration

In most countries, formal higher education is required to enable health care professionals to register within their specialist domains. For example, degree-level qualifications are required to register as a doctor, nurse or allied health professional in the UK and many other countries. It is not within the scope of this book to discuss in detail the delivery of dementia education in pre-registration programmes delivered within higher education. In Chapters 4–7, relevant research that may include pre-registration higher education is discussed, in the context of the setting in which learners are training to work. We do not, however, discuss pre-registration higher education exclusively in each chapter, except in summary here.

It is well established in the literature that dementia education in pre-registration qualifications is suboptimal (Scott et al. 2019; Tullo and Gordon 2013; Williams and Daley 2021). This means those qualifying as health professionals may lack the required depth or breadth of dementia knowledge and skills to deliver person-centred care. This then places a reliance on health and social care provider organisations to support development of the requisite knowledge and skills via CPD training, which as we have already identified can be limited due to time and resources. As identified in a review of pre-qualifying dementia education, a key issue in pre-registration education is the multiple ways and means of delivering education and lack of heterogeneity of content (Alushi et al. 2015). This is because different institutions may use different theoretical models and practical approaches to implement their curricula, so this is a pervasive issue when comparing any set of programmes (not just in the context of dementia training). This makes it hard to establish what dementia-specific content should be included and how best to deliver it, which is further complicated by limited evaluation of these approaches.

To this end, Williams and Daley (2021) conducted a scoping review of novel approaches to delivering dementia-specific education in pre-registration programmes, investigating the effect of the programmes on knowledge and attitudes towards dementia. Their review identified 27 studies from the USA, UK, Korea, and Australia. The programmes were targeted to medics and nurses, sometimes in combination with other health care students. The review grouped the studies based on the main method of delivering dementia education. Five of the studies adopted a long-term experiential approach. This approach is based on the traditional placement model, but all the studies described a novel component that built on this, for example, long-term placements that focus on one individual and their family (Banerjee 2015). All placements were of more than 6 months' duration and were designed to build a relationship between people with dementia and the student. The second approach was the use of activities centred around the person with dementia. Eleven studies adopted this approach, which involved students directly interacting with people with dementia through cultural or social activities, such as storytelling. Five of the studies adopted an interprofessional education approach, involving two or more distinct groups of health care students interacting with each other (and sometimes with people with dementia too) to discuss key issues and improve their dementia knowledge and attitudes. Three studies adopted what was called an 'immersive conference style' involving direct interaction with people with dementia in a conference style format. Finally, three studies used simulation – the use of devices to mimic sensory or cognitive impairment such as wearing goggles and thick gloves to mimic visual impairment and reduced dexterity. One of the studies employed simulation through video **virtual reality**, the idea being that the experience will induce empathy for what it is to live with dementia and promote understanding. This review provides a helpful overview of the kind of methods being used in practice in pre-registration programmes, some of which are returned to in later chapters of this book.

Summary

As this chapter has introduced, one of the challenges is the diversity in where training is being provided and who the training is being delivered to. We have not touched on the methods and practice of training and education in this chapter. However, we acknowledge that the approaches adopted in training are incredibly varied and so will be discussed throughout this book. It is not the endeavour of this text to make one-size-fits-all recommendations for how to design, develop, and deliver dementia training. Rather, we review the evidence on sector-specific interventions before going into some of the principles and practices of training design. We have also worked with collaborators to come up with case examples from different sectors of how some of the challenges in the field are being met and to provide potential ideas for practice. The case studies illustrate themes within each chapter. Some of them implement evaluated approaches, while others demonstrate innovation in, as yet unevaluated, areas. We also hope that this book serves to raise, and answer, some questions you may have about the methods appropriate for adoption in your own dementia training practice.

Part 1

Theories and research underpinning dementia education and training and their application in health and social care services

2 The design and delivery of formal dementia training and education

'The most effective training programmes combine a range of methods appropriate to what is being taught so that theory, practical application, and reflection on and consolidation of learning can take place.'

This chapter introduces some of the broader theory and research evidence around the design and delivery of formal dementia training to adult learners within the dementia workforce. It opens by discussing the importance of involving people directly affected by dementia in the design and delivery of dementia training. This will be a recurring consideration throughout the chapter and the book as a whole. It will then present an overview of foundational theories of adult learning, which provide a theoretical basis that can assist in the design of dementia training. It considers the evidence for, and potential limitations of, the models when applied to training on dementia. The chapter then moves to consider the evidence base for some of the more commonly used methods of delivering training to this workforce. This includes face-to-face delivery, experiential and simulation methods, and in-practice learning approaches.

Involving people directly affected by dementia in training

Involving people directly affected by dementia – often know as experts-by-experience (EBEs) – in the design and delivery of dementia training is a relatively recent development. Students, lecturers, and EBEs all value the input of EBEs to the education of health care professionals and EBE involvement is well established in areas such as mental health nursing (Horgan et al. 2020; Scammell et al. 2016) and social work education (Goossen and Austin 2017).

Involvement of those directly affected by dementia in research is more well established (Di Lorito et al. 2020; Flavin and Sinclair 2019; Goeman et al. 2019; Gove et al. 2018; Iliffe et al. 2013). However, evaluation and discussion of direct involvement in training is less well documented and published examples of that involvement are rare. One reason for more limited examples of involvement of people living with dementia, is the suggestion that the cognitive nature of dementia makes it more difficult to directly involve people with the condition in training than may be the case for other health conditions or disabilities. Subsequently, this may be used as a rationale for not exploring possibilities for active and ongoing involvement. However, there are now a growing number of examples of creative and innovative ways that people living with dementia have been directly and indirectly involved in delivering dementia training (Kenny et al. 2016). The few evaluated and published studies that do exist include:

- programmes offering students time-limited placements with people directly affected by dementia (Banerjee et al. 2017);
- producing audio- or video-recordings used across multiple deliveries of a training programme and/or directly including people with dementia in discussion activities during training sessions (Dodds 2003); and
- facilitated implementation of learning alongside people living with dementia, using arts-based approaches (Guzmán et al. 2017a).

Evidence from published studies indicates that positive exposure to people living with dementia leads to positive outcomes for learners. For example, regular home visits to a family affected by dementia over a period of time (2 years in this instance), alongside more formal education can facilitate compassion and positive attitudes towards working with people with the condition among medical students (Bickford et al. 2019). Likewise, positive psychology **coaching**, alongside theatre- and film-based activities involving care home staff alongside residents living with dementia, has been reported to lead to increased communication between staff and residents and improved person-centred attitudes in staff (Guzmán et al. 2017a). This type of activity is, therefore, worth doing because it enhances the learning experience. Involvement also brings benefits for those directly affected by dementia, including helping individuals to feel they are making a difference, enjoying contact with learners and providing an opportunity to share their experiences (Cashin et al. 2019; Guzmán et al. 2017a). This indicates the need to find ways to broaden the diversity of people affected by dementia who take part in training programmes and to develop inclusive practices to support involvement of those with moderate to severe dementia.

These published examples demonstrate the many reasons why involvement is important. People directly affected by dementia have a valuable insight into living with the condition that arguably cannot be gleaned from other sources, and which should form an essential component of the knowledge base provided by dementia training. This is needed to underpin the value of understanding individual experiences and perspectives and using this to deliver person-centred care. There are also many good practices in this area that have not been published and so are not currently in the public domain. Where we have identified such examples, we have, where possible, included them as case examples in relevant chapters. Box 2.1 provides a range of examples we are aware of or have used in our own training delivery.

Box 2.1 Examples of ways to include the experiences of those directly affected by dementia in training

Direct methods

- People living with dementia, family members, and informal caregivers delivering talks to learners.
- Learners having formal placements or spending time with people directly affected by dementia in service or home settings.
- Co-learning with/from people directly affected by dementia, such as during intergenerational activities or during artistic/creative sessions.

Digital resources

- Video- and audio-recordings made by or with people directly affected by dementia talking about their experiences.

Indirect methods

- Poems, books, and blogs written by people directly affected by dementia.
- Plays, exhibitions, and other artistic productions and representations of the experiences of people directly affected by dementia.
- Working with groups of people directly affected by dementia to gather stories of their experiences that can be used as case studies and examples within training.

When involving people living with dementia directly in dementia training, doing so in meaningful, inclusive, and supportive ways is imperative. A number of organisations have produced information and guidance on good, meaningful and inclusive involvement (DEEP n.d.; Dementia Alliance International et al. 2019). Involvement should always include payment or other recompense for the person's time and any out-of-pocket expenses incurred, and may include training or development opportunities for the person living with dementia to prepare them for the role.

Engaging directly with people affected by dementia as the experts is thus a moral, ethical, and theoretical as well as a logical decision in dementia training. From a theoretical perspective, involvement breaks down the 'us' and 'them' barriers that Kitwood (1997) described as important in establishing a 'new culture' of dementia care. Kitwood proposed that rather than seeing the ultimate source of knowledge as doctors and brain scientists, we should really be listening to the 'skilled and insightful practitioners of care'. In the critical commentary of Kitwood's new culture of person-centred dementia care in the book *Dementia Reconsidered Revisited*, one of this book's authors (Surr 2019) proposed a new *inclusive culture*. In this culture, people directly affected by dementia are recognised as the experts who possess the most reliable and valid knowledge about dementia and dementia care. They are also seen as full and equal citizens with a valuable contribution to make to society.

A critique of current engagement activity is that the demographic of people living with dementia who are involved in training, or dementia advocacy more broadly, does not reflect the diversity of people living with dementia (Burton et al. 2019; Ludwin and Capstick 2015; Parveen et al. 2018). For example, it does not often include representation from seldom heard or minority groups or those who are living in long-term care settings. It is important to recognise that not all people living with dementia are older (over 65), physically frail, living in a care home, or have a degree of dementia that means they are unable to manage many aspects of day-to-day living. The campaigning work by people living with dementia as individuals or through organisations such as Dementia Alliance International, and in the UK the Three Nations Dementia Working Group and the Dementia Empowerment and Engagement Project (DEEP), has led to a more widespread recognition of the diversity of people living with dementia and the talents and expertise people with dementia have to offer. Many people living with dementia who are members of these groups have contributed to the delivery of dementia training through direct and indirect methods. However, while this engagement has reflected a significant recent step forward in the field, providing an essential and valuable contribution to hearing and including the direct voice of people living with dementia in training, we must acknowledge this is the voice of only a subsection of those with the condition. Finding ways to engage, include, and gather the perspectives and voices of a broader spectrum of people directly affected by dementia must be an immediate and ongoing priority for those involved in dementia training. It is a challenge we encourage readers of this book to embrace when they design and deliver dementia training.

Case example: Employing a trainer living with dementia

To help staff understand the lived experience of dementia, a large health care provider secured funding to employ a person living with dementia to teach on their dementia study day. The sessions were held in the afternoon as this was easier for the trainer living with dementia. The trainer living with dementia joined in the afternoon sessions as a co-presenter and then ran a session herself, where she shared her experiences and invited learners to ask anything they wanted about dementia or what they had learned during the day. The trainer living with dementia also presented to other teams in the Trust, highlighting the importance of hearing the voice of the person living with dementia and challenging stigma.

The role had a big impact at different levels. It was impactful as a training programme for learners, but also the process of securing funding and recruiting a person living with dementia into a post provided essential learning for the health care provider. For example, the provider had to consider unconscious bias within approval and recruitment processes and equality and support for people with cognitive impairment to work in the organisation.

The book will now move on to consider broader theories and evidence for the design and delivery of dementia training. It includes examples of where inclusion of the voice of people directly affected by dementia can be applied.

Theories of adult learning

For a century, adult learning and education has been recognised as a specific field of practice. Early work in the field indicated that adults learn differently from children in a number of ways (Merriam 2001). There are a wide array of adult learning theories that can be grouped into several broad categories (Taylor and Hamdy 2013):

- *Instrumental learning theories* – focus on individual experience in the learning process, including behavioural, cognitive, and experiential processes.
- *Humanist theories* – are learner-centred and promote an individual's development, growth, and motivation.
- *Transformative theories* – explore how critical reflection can be used to challenge assumptions and beliefs.
- *Social learning theories* – see learning and thinking as social activities that are influenced by the context (tools available) and setting or community in which they occur.
- *Motivational models* – see motivation and reflection as critical to adult learning. Motivation is seen to relate to expectations of learning success and the value or impact of that success.
- *Reflective models* – focus on how the act of reflection leads to action and change.

Here we outline key foundational theories that have important theoretical and practical implications for the design and delivery of dementia training across all health and social care contexts: *andragogy, self-directed learning, **experiential** learning, transformative learning, and reflective learning.*

Andragogy

Andragogy, defined as 'The art and science of how adults learn', was first proposed by Knowles (1970). Andragogy falls under humanist theories, in that it takes a learner-centred position, recognising the specific qualities and needs of adult learners as core to facilitating effective learning. Knowles contrasted andragogy to pedagogy (the education of children), stating adult learners differ from children in several ways:

1 Adults need to know what they will be learning and why this is important.
2 Adults are problem- rather than subject-centred and need to see immediacy of application of learning.
3 Adult learners have a need to be helped to be self-directed throughout the learning process.
4 Adult learners bring a wealth of experience with them to the learning environment, which the **facilitator** should draw and build upon.
5 Adults will not learn until they are ready and motivated to do so, and these motivations tend to be internal rather than external.
6 Adults may come to the learning environment with inhibitions, behaviours, and beliefs about learning which may need to be overcome.

Andragogy is not without debate. For example, it has been criticised for providing an approach to teaching and a set of assumptions about adults as learners, rather than provision of a theory of adult learning processes (St. Clair 2002). It has also been criticised for underestimating the complexity and ways of learning within children's education (Darbyshire 1993). Despite this, however, andragogy has placed a focus on learner-centredness within the adult learning context. This position aligns well with Kitwood's notion of person-centred care and the positioning of the person living with dementia at the centre of care and the importance of recognising individual needs and perspectives.

Self-directed learning

Self-directed learning theory builds on the humanist principles of adult learners' need for self-direction identified within andragogy. It focuses on a learner's need to take control of their own learning, including what is learned and how (Merriam 2018). What a facilitator can do in a formal classroom setting to foster self-direction and learner control is also a key consideration. Self-directed learning theory recognises that learners vary in their readiness for autonomous learning according to the specific training context and a range of individual factors (e.g. educational level, creativity, learning style) (Merriam 2001).

Garrison (1997) argues that self-directed learning is comprised of three overlapping dimensions:

- *Self-management* – the extent to which the learner engages socially and behaviourally with the tasks associated with learning.
- *Self-monitoring* – the extent to which the learner integrates their learning into their current worldview and meets their learning goals.
- *Motivation* – the learner's perception of the value and potential benefits of their learning goals and activities.

Therefore, a facilitator must consider how all these factors may be addressed in training design and delivery. The theory also emphasises the need for considering preparatory work with learners to understand and work with their personal motivations.

Criticisms have been made of self-directed learning theory, particularly that it focuses primarily on individual dimensions of learning, without adequate consideration of the wider context of the learner (Brookfield 1984). Workplace or societal culture may exert a big influence, for example. Nevertheless, self-directed learning theory, like andragogy, recognises the importance of placing the learner at the centre of the learning process and the need to support the learner to have control over their own learning.

Experiential learning

Experiential learning falls under instrumental learning theories, but recognises learning is a process in which reflection and assimilation are core components. Kolb (1984) is probably one of the best-known experiential learning theorists. He proposed that adults learn best through discovery and experience. However, successful learning requires more than just 'doing' and his experiential learning cycle (see Figure 2.1) outlines a process for learning that includes doing, reflecting, learning, and applying learning. He argued learners can step into the process at any point and learn successfully. However, they must progress through the whole process to do so.

Kolb's model of learning styles (1985) suggests that individuals naturally prefer different phases of the learning cycle. For example (Kolb and Kolb 2008), those with a *diverging style* prefer working with concrete examples and enjoy generating ideas in groups. Those with an *assimilating style* like to put a wide range of information into a logical and concise format; they enjoy reading,

Figure 2.1 The experiential learning cycle and learning styles (developed from Kolb 1984)

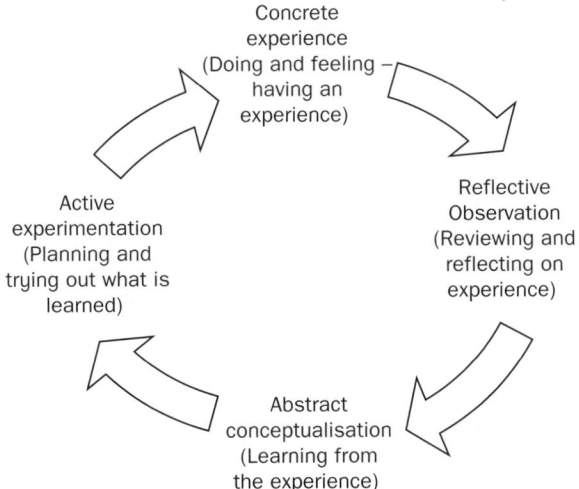

lectures, models, and having time to think things through. Individuals with a *converging style* have strengths in providing practical applications for ideas and theories; they enjoy experimentation and practical activities. Individuals who have an *accommodating learning style* learn primarily from 'hands-on' doing but may turn to others for information to inform their problem-solving; they enjoy working with others to set goals and complete tasks.

It is clear, however, that most individuals do not fit neatly into one of these learning styles and may have different learning preferences in different situations. The idea of learning styles, however, can provide a useful starting point for facilitators in ensuring their training design employs learning activities that cover the range of styles. For example, a facilitator might provide content on the theory of person-centred care in a lecture format, which they might follow with a case study discussion in small groups and then a care planning activity. Learners might then be asked to conduct some in-practice activities applying their learning after the educational session. It can also be useful for learners to consider their preferred methods of learning, particularly in planning their own development opportunities.

Transformative learning

Transformative learning originates in the work of Mezirow (1978). It describes the process of a person's critical self-reflection to consider and reconsider their beliefs and experiences. Through this process, learners challenge assumptions by which their experiences are interpreted, leading to an altered 'frame of reference' or way of seeing the world (Mezirow 1997). A frame of reference includes meaning schemas and meaning perspectives (Howie and Bagnall 2013). *Meaning schemas* are beliefs about how something should be done, or how to view particular groups or oneself. So, in the context of dementia care, it may include approaches to delivering care and taking a person-centred perspective on people living with dementia. *Meaning perspectives* are more concrete or fundamental assumptions into which experiences are assimilated, or which frame the new experiences; a way of framing the world. They can include things such as values, beliefs, or goals.

Transformative learning is triggered by 'disorientating dilemmas', which are experiences that do not fit with a learner's current beliefs about the world (Merriam 2018). This forces them to reconsider their beliefs through a process of critical reflection, to assimilate this new experience into their existing worldview.

Mezirow outlined 10 phases of transformative learning (see Figure 2.2), which include a process of supported critical reflection, exploration, planning, skills acquisition, implementation, and integration of learning. This process is one that is structured and actively facilitated and does not happen naturally or by chance. The *critical* component of reflection is particularly important in the process. This is where reflection not only includes a personal assessment of the

Figure 2.2 Mezirow's 10 phases of transformative learning (based on Kitchenham 2008)

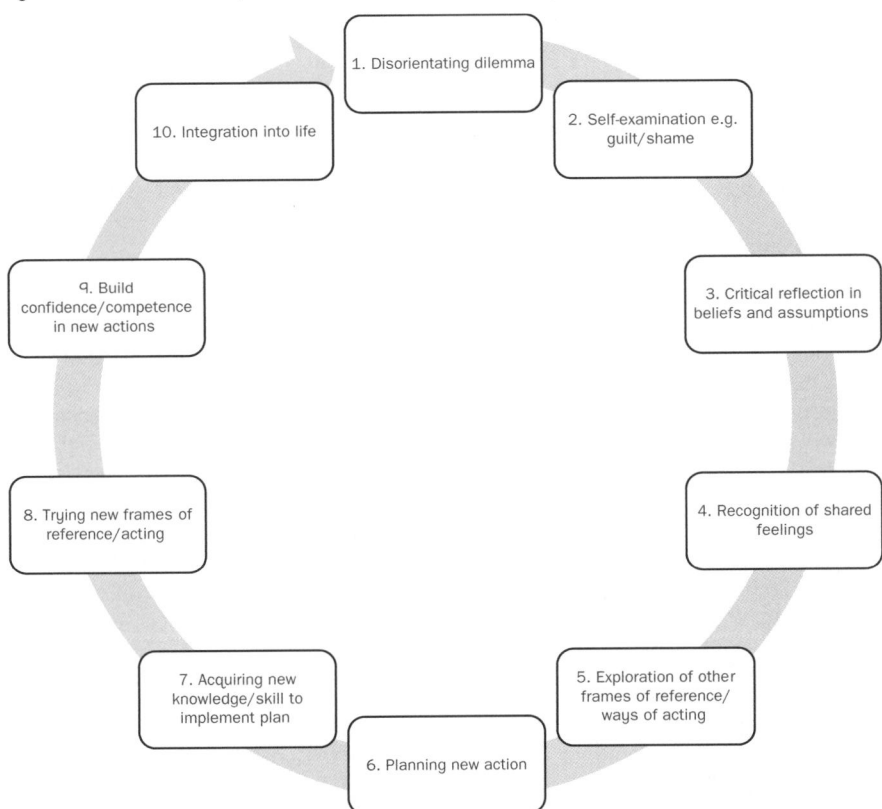

nature and consequences of our actions, but also of the origins or circumstances that led to them. It includes considering:

- content (what could be done differently based on my past actions, and existing knowledge and experience?);
- process (what new factors might inform me on how to do things differently?); and
- premise (what values and beliefs are underpinning my actions and how could I see things differently?) (Kitchenham 2008).

From this follows a process of reframing.

A core component of transformative learning is the dialogue (self-reflective and external with others) through which transformation occurs. Thus, learning experiences must facilitate such opportunities for successful learning to occur. Similarly, opportunities to practise and then implement new learning are deemed critical to integration into a learner's viewpoint. An example of how the phases of transformative learning may be applied in dementia training is presented in Box 2.2.

Box 2.2 An example of application of Mezirow's 10 phases of transformative learning to dementia training

This example relates to dementia awareness training provided to staff who have had limited previous exposure to dementia training and who work in general rather than dementia specialist roles or settings. It is written as if all learners progress through the transformative learning process during the training session. However, we acknowledge this is unlikely to be the case when applying this process in a real training context.

Phase 1: Disorientating dilemma

Learners are shown a video of people with moderate to severe dementia expressing what it is like to live with the condition. The approaches used to do this include joint interviews with informal caregivers and taking time to let the person communicate even though they may have difficulties expressing themselves. The people living with dementia give clear and powerful insights into their experiences, to say how dementia makes them feel and to share views on how they want to be treated by others.

The facilitator asks people about their initial thoughts of the video: learners in the group express surprise that people with more advanced dementia can communicate in this way and that they have such insight into their dementia and experiences.

Phase 2: Self-examination

The facilitator asks learners to spend some time individually reflecting on their thoughts and feelings related to the video and how it relates to their past experiences of, and contact with, people living with dementia. They are asked to focus on whether the way they have communicated with and supported people living with dementia reflects what people say they want and need.

Learners note that often their practices have not reflected what people living with dementia say they want or need and that they feel sad or guilty that their approaches may have made people living with dementia feel distressed or not cared for.

Phase 3: Critical reflection on assumptions

The facilitator acknowledges that people may feel sad, upset, or guilty. They ask them to discuss with another learner: (1) a specific approach or care instance from their own practice which they now feel they should have approached differently; (2) why they used the approach or acted in the way they did at the time.

Learners identify that the way they have viewed and treated people living with dementia in the past has not acknowledged that people have insight and awareness into their condition and are able to meaningfully express themselves. They discuss how their knowledge about people living with dementia has largely come from things colleagues have said, the media, or family and friends. This has generally been very negative and led them to assume people living with dementia were unable to communicate their wants, needs, and choices and were often distressed or aggressive because of their condition. There was nothing they or others could do about this.

Phase 4: Recognition of shared experiences

The facilitator asks the pairs to share some of the general points from the discussion related to the type of care instances and approaches taken and their thoughts on the underlying reasons for this.

The learners see there are many commonalities in their approaches and also why people feel they have acted in this way.

Phase 5: Exploration of other options and frames of reference

The facilitator gives a short presentation about person-centred dementia care, with a particular focus on Kitwood's (2019) work. They talk about seeing the person first and the dementia as one part of who a person is, emphasising the need to think about someone's life history, personality, health, and the social context they find themselves in. They talk about a focus on meeting people's psychological needs, the use of positive person work and approaches to good communication with someone living with dementia.

Phase 6: Planning a new course of action

The facilitator asks the group to split into smaller groups of four to five and gives each group a written case study. The case study is based on the setting in which the participants work and gives details of a care scenario when a person living with dementia is not understood by staff. It details examples of care approaches that align with those that participants have shared in the previous exercise. The scenario results in the person living with dementia becoming increasingly distressed. The scenario also gives some life history and other information about the person with dementia.

Learners are asked to identify different approaches staff could take that draw on their knowledge of the person and of person-centred approaches to care. They are also asked to identify what further information staff might need about the person and what additional knowledge and skills staff in the scenario might need to deliver person-centred care. The groups are then asked to share their ideas.

The facilitator asks learners to reflect on what they have learnt in the session and to identify one approach to care they will take away from the session to apply in their own practice.

Phase 7: Acquiring new knowledge and skills to support implementation of one's plan

Each learner is allocated an in-practice mentor who is a more experienced member of staff, who will support their ongoing learning and development. Learners meet regularly with their mentor to discuss their learning and where they feel they have additional development or support needs. Approaches to meeting these learning needs are identified and put into place; for example, working alongside their mentor, attending additional training, or taking part in action learning sets. This runs alongside Phase 8.

Phase 8: Provisionally trying new frames of reference, ways of acting and relating

The learners spend time putting their learning into practice in their day-to-day role, initially focusing on the approach to care they identified at the end of the formal training session and then moving onto new approaches identified through discussion with their mentor.

Phase 9: Building confidence and competence

The learner meets regularly with their mentor to reflect on their practice and receive ongoing support and feedback. This continues until the learner feels confident in delivery of person-centred care in their role.

Phase 10: Reintegration into one's life and worldview

Once the learner feels confident in their understanding of person-centred care and its application in their role, they may then take on the role of mentor to new learners.

There are critiques of Mezirow's theory, including whether the type of critical reflection Mezirow indicates is possible for all learners and in every learning process, as well as the definition and nature of 'transformative'. For Mezirow, transformation is seen as a positive, enlightened state driven by a personal desire to see the world in a different way, underpinned by learning (Howie and Bagnall 2013). However, as will be explored further in Chapter 3, learning for those working in dementia care takes place in both formal and informal contexts. Informal contexts may provide opportunities for experiencing disorientating dilemmas, but not for the facilitated, deep, critical reflection Mezirow advocates, or in fact circumstances that support reflection that is likely to lead to positive enlightenment. Indeed, informal mechanisms for learning can be extremely powerful in influencing frames of reference, but in both positive and negative ways. They can reinforce stigmatic views and approaches to care that are not person-centred, just as they can be highly effective in supportive positive practices.

Reflective learning

Reflective practice is a widely used concept in health and social care education, particularly in qualification programmes for health professionals such as nurses and associated roles. Reflective learning is grounded in Schön's (1983, 1987) work on 'reflection-in' (reflecting on an experience while experiencing it) and 'reflection-on' (reflecting on an experience afterwards) action set within a context of feedback (from others or from the outcome of the experience). The concept of reflection as a critical process within education dates back to the work of Dewey in the 1930s. Dewey identified two types of experiential process within learning – trial and error – which he considered lower-order and higher-order reflection, which he argued led to a learning loop (Redmond 1997). It is this loop which Schön developed in his later work around the practice and education of professionals.

Schön described practical implicit knowledge that underpins actions as 'knowing-in-action' or **tacit knowledge**. This is knowledge learned through many past experiences, but which cannot easily be explained. Building on this Schön identified that when surprising results (either good or bad) occur in the application of such knowledge, an opportunity is provided to reflect on that action, which up until that point has been spontaneous or automatic. This reflection can be at the time (reflection-in-action) or afterwards (reflection-on-action) and represents a skilled learning process beyond trial-and-error methods (Redmond 1997).

Schön argued that professionals who employed a reflective framework to their practice would be more responsive to those they were supporting/caring for and more capable of appreciating each individual's situation. Thus, professionals would be enabled to adopt more equal positioning within relationships (Redmond 1997). This clearly aligns well with a person-centred approach to dementia care, where power imbalances between people living with dementia and those who support them can occur easily, where the voice of the person living with dementia is at risk of not being prioritised, and where positioning of the individual and their experiences as the central point for care provision is essential. However, it is likely that the mechanisms of reflective practice, tacit knowledge, and reflection-in and -on action, are more complex than Schön's model suggests. Schön's model assumes that reflection, by definition, leads to positive learning and improved practice. As will be discussed in later chapters in this book (see Chapters 3, 4, 8, and 9), this may not always be the case. There are many individual and external factors that influence how events are perceived and thus the direction that any learning takes. For example, organisational culture or the influence of peers can impact how a particular situation is framed and determine what are considered positive – or desirable – alternative actions if that situation is experienced again. This will be explored further in Chapter 3 in relation to informal learning.

In dementia training, reflective practice might be used as an activity within a formal training session, or it might be applied as the focus of formal or informal supervision or mentorship meetings. The process can also be used as part of action learning sets, which are meetings arranged with the specific intention of solving workplace problems. There are many different reflective frameworks or models that can be used to guide reflective practice. Common models include Gibbs' (1988) reflective learning cycle (see Figure 2.3) and Johns' (1995) model for reflective learning (see Box 2.3).

Common components of the many models include describing the situation to be reflected on, exploring feelings and reactions to the situation, considering alternative viewpoints and courses of action, drawing conclusions about what has been learned, and considering how one might act differently in the future.

Figure 2.3 Reflective learning cycle based on Gibbs (1988)

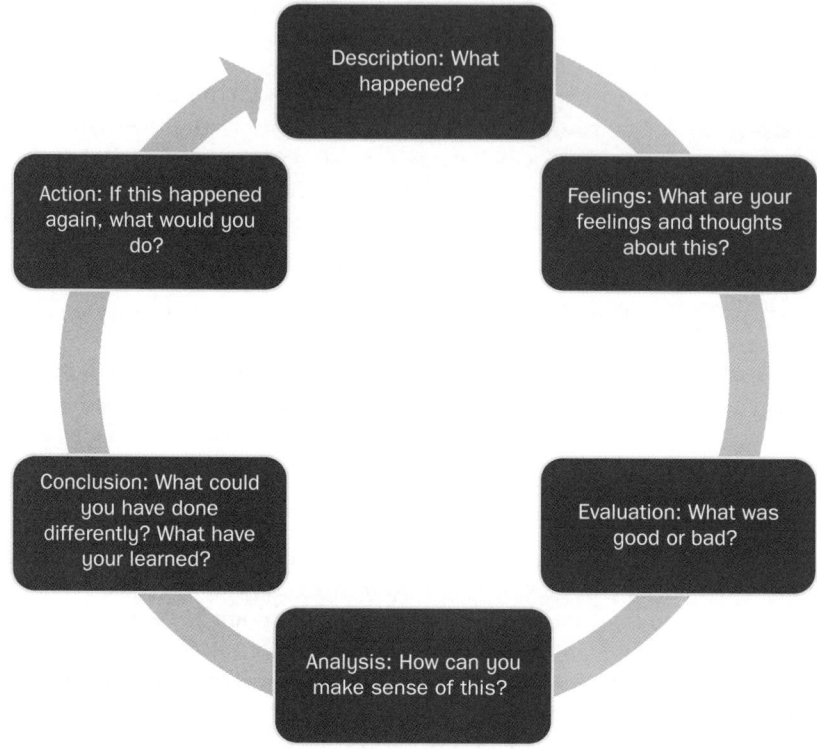

Box 2.3 Model for structured reflection based on Johns (2017)

- Make space in your mind for reflection.
- Describe the experience.
- Consider what is significant and should be paid attention to.
- How did I respond and why?
- How effective was this (think about outcomes for me and for others)?
- What made me respond like this?
- If this happened again, how might I respond that would be more success-ful/effective?
- How might a different response affect the outcomes?
- What influencing factors need to change and how, for me to respond differently?
- What do I think I have learned?
- How can theory or ideas inform and deepen my learning?
- How does exploring this with others change my views or add to my learning?
- Thinking about the same situation – how do I now feel?

As identified earlier, critiques of reflective practice highlight how many models fail to acknowledge or address the broader social context and associated ethical frameworks in which individuals are located. Rather, reflective practice is understood simply as a subjective, internal process that occurs in the head of the learner (Zukas et al. 2010). These are clearly important factors to consider in applying reflective practice to support implementation of person-centred dementia care. It means that those responsible for delivering dementia training need to consider how the reflective cycle or process can be facilitated to occur within and after a training session. This will include provision of relevant theoretical and knowledge content, opportunity for individual reflection, discussion and reflection with peers, and guided consideration of implementation and action planning. It will also be important to consider ongoing reflection outside of the formal training context, which is often a neglected dimension. How can this be both encouraged and utilised to elicit practice change? This could be through mentorship or supervision, and in day-to-day activities. This will be considered further in Chapter 3, which focuses on informal learning.

Adult learning theories indicate that the design of dementia training, specifically the process and methods of delivery, play a crucial role in whether and how those attending learn. To a lesser extent, the design of training also affects if and how learners then apply this learning within their practice. However, application of learning into practice is a somewhat neglected dimension of learning theories, which may be seen primarily as theories of the process of learning, rather than of knowledge application. They may have much to offer us in considering how **formal learning** opportunities are designed and delivered, but may be less helpful in identifying mechanisms, barriers, and enablers to transfer into behaviour and practice change. Implementation of learning will be considered in depth in Chapter 10.

Regarding utilisation of learning theory to support the design and delivery of dementia training, it is likely that a multi-model approach is required, which considers the most appropriate components of these different models to use in specific situations and for specific learners and learning activities. Core components from across these models that we would recommend those responsible for the design of dementia training consider are presented in Box 2.4.

Box 2.4 Implications of adult learning theories for the design of dementia training

Learner needs and motivation

- Ensure the content of training is inclusive to learners with a range of prior life and work experience, recognising learners do not all have equal ability or capacity to learn.
- Ensure that learners' individual learning and support needs are assessed and met within personal development planning and as part of training design and delivery.

- Learners should be guided to be self-directed in identifying their own learning needs, setting their own learning goals, and choosing appropriate strategies for meeting these needs and goals.
- Recognise that learners will have varying levels of skill in the areas needed to be a successful self-directed learner and so need to be guided and assisted through the process.
- Recognise that adult learners have specific needs and motivation for learning which is embedded in relevance, application, and benefit to them and their work role.

Learning outcomes and content

- Ensure training content and learning objectives are relevant to the learner's role and applicable to their practice.
- Provide learners with the learning objectives at the start of a training programme and reinforce what is being learned and why throughout.

Learning activities

- Delivery methods should prioritise variety in order to address individual learner needs and styles and to provide a layering of approaches to learning about specific content.
- Learners should be encouraged to share and apply their existing expertise to the learning process.
- Design learning activities that will challenge learner values and beliefs, which may be incompatible with a person-centred approach to dementia care.
- Support learners to identify alternative viewpoints and new ideas and facilitate them, through a range of learning activities, to engage in reflection and critical thinking that questions their assumptions and beliefs in a safe but challenging way.
- Include practical learning activities that support learners to gain new skills and apply learning to practice through adopting new ways of acting and relating and the assimilation of new ideas into learners' worldview.
- Create a safe learning environment that becomes a peer community of learners who are undergoing a transformative learning experience, with whom ideas can be shared and which supports critical dialogue and reflection.

Facilitator skills and qualities

- The facilitator's role includes providing feedback on learning and achievement; encouraging self-evaluation, planning, goal-setting, implementation, and monitoring; providing a supportive learning environment to stimulate development; and gradual transfer of responsibility for learning from the facilitator to the learner.

This chapter will next discuss a range of delivery methods that may be adopted, their strengths and limitations in the context of adult learning theory, and current evidence around their effectiveness in the context of dementia training.

Methods of training delivery

There are a range of methods that can be used to deliver or facilitate learning. While they are explored individually here, in reality, programmes of dementia training are best delivered using a combination of these methods. Methods should be selected based on offering a variety of experiences for learners, to suit those with different preferred learning styles, and based on the method(s) that are best suited to delivery of different content. Often a layering approach is desirable with content covered using a range of methods, such as a short talk or lecture to cover theory or information-based content, an interactive activity or simulation, followed by reflection and discussion.

The components of impactful dementia training

Two of the authors of this book (Claire Surr and Sarah Smith) carried out a large study in the UK which explored the components of impactful dementia education and training across the health and social care workforce (the 'What Works?' study). This involved:

- carrying out a large review of published research on dementia education and training (Surr et al. 2017a);
- auditing current dementia training content against the Dementia Training Standards Framework for England through a national survey (Smith et al. 2019);
- surveying staff who had completed dementia training programmes reported in the audit to ask about the experiences of the training and applying it in practice and its impact on their knowledge and confidence (Parveen et al. 2021);
- in-depth case studies in ten health and social care provider organisations whose training, as reported in the audit, showed evidence of good practice (in terms of content, delivery methods, and implementation) (Sass et al. 2019; Surr et al. 2018c, 2019b).

Using data from all these sources, we developed a set of criteria that the evidence suggested leads to more impactful dementia training. We have written this as an audit tool (Surr et al. 2017b), with a supporting manual, that can be used by training providers and commissioners to design, deliver, and audit their dementia training provision. Criteria that apply to all training programmes are presented in Boxes 2.5, 2.6, and 2.7. Those that apply to specific methods of training delivery are discussed in the relevant section. The tool and manual can be downloaded from the study website (Leeds Beckett University n.d.). While the study was conducted in the UK, its findings will have relevance for dementia training in other high-income countries.

Box 2.5 Components of impactful dementia education and training – general features applicable to all training programmes

Design, content, and materials

- Training has been designed for/tailored to the specific service setting and job role of learners who will attend.
- Training maps onto the intended, relevant Dementia Training Standards or Framework subject area(s) and associated learning outcomes.
- Training content covers all learning outcomes in a depth that is relevant to the tier and learners' job roles.
- Training includes interactive learning activities.
- Training includes group discussion.
- Training includes knowledge-based/theoretical content.
- Training includes use of written, video, or in-person case examples/vignettes/scenarios as a basis for discussion.
- Training includes learning activities that involve the application of what is learnt in a practice-based situation.
- Training includes the introduction of structured tools, methods, or approaches to care delivery.
- Training materials are clear and easy to follow (e.g. they are jargon free, clearly laid out, consider educational background of learners).
- Training materials are succinctly written, are an appropriate length for their mode and purpose, and can be completed in the allocated time.
- Learners can bring their own practice examples and problems for discussion.
- Training includes opportunities for learners to engage in practice-based problem-solving.
- Consideration has been given to the full costs of developing and delivering training and the potential benefits.

Training design, content, and materials warrant careful consideration. Any training programme or individual learning session needs to be designed with the above principles in mind. This will likely mean tailoring programmes and sessions to the group of learners, particularly where the roles and skill-mix of a group may change each delivery. The inclusion of practical, interactive exercises and activities and time for discussion is paramount.

Case example: Interactive and engaging dementia training activities – the escape room

A large health care provider has a long-running knowledge exchange programme with an academic institution. As part of this, they use an escape room training experience within their dementia study days. Escape room training is based on a social or leisure activity where people are locked in a room and have to solve a series of puzzles to escape. When used in a training context, the problem-solving activities focus on developing skills, knowledge, and teamwork to help 'save' a service user or patient.

The dementia escape room training employed by this health care provider explores humanity, bias, empathy, and pain in a safe space, through asking those taking part to make decisions about safety, care, and living in society. The methodology is therefore an escape room with a conscience.

The escape room involves a live 60-minute workshop, where those taking part have to make decisions about how to free a character who might be considered as vulnerable, followed by a 60-minute reflective debrief. It aims to challenge participants to identify and unpack unconscious bias, develop reflective practice, and collaborate within a team to save the life of the central character. This is a timed experience and the consequences of every decision made by participants are seen instantly. The session can ideally happen live but is also available via Zoom.

The provider has found the escape room experience to be a contemporary, exciting, and fun workshop, but to also unravel values and to call upon those who take part to think deeply about and reflect on their actions.

Training costs

The costs of developing and delivering dementia training (including the costs of backfilling staff time to attend training, or paying for attendance outside of contracted hours) are often a neglected dimension for consideration. If a care organisation is purchasing external training, it can be much easier to understand what the cost per learner trained is. However, for internally developed and delivered provision, this can be harder to estimate. Costs are an important consideration in services which must prioritise resources. They are also important to consider in relation to potential benefits and impacts of training programmes. For example, a training programme may appear to be high cost, because it is delivered by an external provider, over 3 days to thirty learners, and requires them to also undertake practice-based activities between sessions. However, if the outcome of that programme is that learners can better understand and communicate with people with dementia and this reduces agitation levels and incidents of distress including aggression, then this may result in cost savings to the organisation. They may see reduced staff stress and sickness levels and lower staff turnover. It may be that the financial savings made as a result, plus the increased quality of life of residents are equal to, or greater than, the initial investment. On the other hand, an organisation may provide every staff member with a self-directed **e-learning** programme, which takes 30 minutes to complete and involves learners reading through various screens of information before a short multiple-choice test at the end. This may at first seem relatively low cost as it only involves initial purchase of the access plus 30 minutes of paid staff time per learner. However, if that programme has little or no impact on staff knowledge or practice, then that is a wasted investment of financial and human resources.

It is always important, therefore, to consider training outcomes in the context of investment, to assess what the return on investment is. In Chapter 10 we discuss methods for evaluating dementia training in detail, which may contribute to a return-on-investment assessment.

Training length and depth

Deciding on the length of a training programme and the content to be covered is often challenging. There can be a temptation to try to cover as much content as possible in the available time for training, in the belief that it is better to be comprehensive. However, a review of 153 studies that had evaluated dementia education and training programmes (Surr et al. 2017a), and a study of individuals who had undertaken dementia training from organisations across the UK (Parveen et al. 2021), found this was not the case. The training programmes most likely to lead to positive impacts on learners' knowledge, attitudes, confidence, and behaviours and to lead to improved outcomes for people directly affected or staff, were those which were longer (at least one day in total) and more in-depth/focused on one topic. This research also identified that where longer programmes were divided into shorter individual sessions, maybe running over several weeks, these individual sessions were more likely to be impactful if they were at least of 2 hours' duration.

Box 2.6 Components of impactful dementia education and training – general features applicable to all training programmes

Training length
- Training is at least 8+ hours in total although training of at least 3.5 hours was also beneficial compared with training programmes of shorter duration.
- Individual training sessions are of at least 2 hours' duration.

Practical issues
- Learners are provided with detailed information about the format of and commitment(s) the training involves ahead of attendance.
- Training can be delivered flexibly to meet the needs of an individual group or service (e.g. content can be adapted to the group; flexibility of delivery in one or multiple sessions; not required to be delivered to set script).

We recognise the challenge that this poses for organisations who may have many staff to train and limited resources and time in which to do this, often alongside high staff turnover. It requires a delicate balancing act between feasibility and providing training under circumstances where it is most likely to have an impact. This is where a training needs analysis (see Chapter 1) is important at organisational level and for individual staff members. A training needs analysis can help organisations identify priority areas for dementia training, based on feedback from people directly affected by dementia, from staff, and from other service indicators. Likewise, while undertaking refresher training is important for retaining and reinvigorating skills and knowledge, it may be more important for a staff member to attend a training programme that is relevant to what they perceive their current learning needs are (see also Chapters 1 and 8) than to have a one-size-fits-all approach. Training becomes a tick-box exercise where covering topics is seen as more important than the impact of learning. Offering separate, in-depth training sessions on core topics and individualised training prioritisation for staff members will likely provide a more impactful approach.

Facilitator qualities

The qualities of a 'good teacher' have been explored extensively in the literature (Gibson et al. 2019; Mikkonen et al. 2018; Singh et al. 2013; Sutkin et al. 2008). This body of work indicates that teacher/facilitator qualities fall into several key areas: (1) personal attributes; (2) teaching skills, knowledge, and the ability to create a supportive learning environment; (3) subject knowledge; (4) communication skills; and (5) enthusiasm. In research on dementia training conducted by the authors of this book (Surr et al. 2017a, 2018c, 2019b), the personal attributes of the facilitator were extremely important for training impact. Facilitators needed to be experienced in both training facilitation and in working with people living with dementia if they were to be seen as credible to learners and thus able to facilitate flexible and responsive training. There is a risk that clinicians who are undoubtedly good role models and who may be very good at facilitating in-practice learning, may be given training responsibilities for delivery of face-to-face training without adequate experience or preparation for the role. This can be a barrier to supporting effective learning (Surr et al. 2018c).

Box 2.7 Components of impactful dementia education and training – facilitator qualities

- Facilitator is experienced in the delivery/facilitation of training.
- Facilitator is knowledgeable about the subject area and/or has clinical experience of working with people with dementia.
- Facilitator creates a safe environment for discussion and asking of questions.
- Facilitator adapts the training to meet the needs, issues, and concerns of a learner group.

For some individuals, support to develop these skills via a train-the-trainer approach can be helpful, although not everyone who is a good clinician will necessarily make a good training facilitator. Therefore, careful selection of appropriate individuals to take on facilitator roles is necessary, as is understanding and meeting their development needs. The potential impact of any programme of dementia training can only be achieved through effective facilitation coupled with knowledge of dementia.

Face-to-face, synchronous learning

Face-to-face, **synchronous delivery**, including group work and discussion, is consistently reported to provide the most effective and learner-preferred delivery method for dementia training across the range of health and social care settings and roles (Cunningham et al. 2020; Surr et al. 2017a). Face-to-face learning offers the opportunity to employ a range of activities and methods to deliver content that are aligned with adult learning theory, and which encompass some of the methods below (e.g. experiential learning/simulation). A strong message that comes from the evidence around face-to-face learning is that learners prefer interactive content with the opportunity to engage in discussion with peers. Face-to-face delivery also permits greater flexibility of delivery, allowing the facilitator to adapt content and discussion to the needs of the group, in the moment. It also provides an opportunity to challenge beliefs, facilitate critical reflection, provide additional theory or knowledge, or to adapt delivery methods to those the group best responds to. However, face-to-face delivery also presents challenges, often of a practical nature, including learners being pulled from training programmes to work (especially if training is on-site) and challenges with arranging venues, transport, and making childcare or other arrangements if travelling to another location.

Didactic content (delivery of lecture-based content that is predominantly talking or presenting slides to an audience) should be kept to a minimum. It is widely cited in educational practice that learners can only concentrate for 15–20 minutes in a lecture. While there is a lack of robust evidence for this claim and research seems to indicate that attention in fact goes up and down for learners across a traditional 50-minute lecture (Bradbury 2016), it remains good practice to vary teaching methods across any training session. For example, providing theoretical content in a short lecture and then reinforcing this and promoting learning about its application in practice, via a practical exercise or activity, followed by reflection and discussion.

It is important to recognise that there are many forms that face-to-face, synchronous training can take. These include in-person, small group learning through to large group lectures. Some of these forms, such as small-group face-to-face, lend themselves better to some of the other methods discussed below (e.g. experiential learning or simulation), to facilitating peer-to-peer discussion, and others to more traditional didactic lectures. The COVID-19 pandemic has led to many organisations adopting videoconferencing software to deliver virtual, synchronous learning in an attempt to mimic some of the benefits of face-to-face methods via online methods.

This more widespread use of technology means many more people feel comfortable using technology for learning and recognise the range of benefits it can offer. These include efficiency of delivery, ease of access, the ability to bring together diverse groups of learners, and reduced financial and human costs associated with travel (Sharp et al. 2021). It seems likely that given some of these benefits, we will see videoconferencing continuing to play an ongoing role in dementia training for the dementia workforce. This may be to a greater or lesser extent. It will be important for training facilitators to consider whether the subject area and methods most appropriate to deliver it are suitable for online methods.

Case example: Converting best-practice-designed, in-person training to an online format

Like many care providers, a large organisation with over 60 care homes and retirement living facilities had to respond to the COVID-19 pandemic by ceasing all in-person training. They rapidly converted their training to an online format so that staff could continue to receive dementia training.

Their dementia training is part of a comprehensive evidence-based approach to developing and delivering high-quality care for residents living with dementia across the organisation. It is comprised of a five-stage pathway that provides a programme of learning for all members of staff, from basic awareness for every staff member (Stage 1) to an advanced leadership programme for senior managers (Stage 5). The bespoke training pathway has been designed to draw on a range of approaches to adult learning and best practice in dementia education design and delivery as discussed in this chapter. Therefore, face-to-face delivery by skilled specialist facilitators, including opportunities for peer-to-peer discussions, formed a vital component of the programme. It is underpinned by a range of additional resources available to staff in each home, including written case studies, podcasts, and pre-recorded short films that provide the basis for additional group sessions and discussions within each home.

Due to restrictions on visiting care homes during the COVID-19 pandemic, all dementia training materials were adapted in Spring 2020 from original half- or full-day face-to-face taught modules to enable training to continue via the live-streaming video platform Microsoft Teams. Key adaptations to support the translation of the core components of interaction and discussion to the online environment included:

- Reviewing and in some instances simplifying existing case studies. Although these worked well during face-to-face learning to help to transfer knowledge to practical situations, it quickly became apparent that during online training, staff found it more difficult to engage in detailed group discussions.

> • Separating the training modules into shorter sessions, with full-day face-to-face modules being delivered as three 2-hour online sessions and half-day modules being delivered as two 1½-hour sessions with short comfort breaks built in. This helped learners to remain engaged by making sure they were not required to spend prolonged periods of time focusing on a computer screen, as well as making it easier for managers to release staff from their shift duties.
>
> Whilst not without challenges, working with smaller groups and finding different ways of engaging learners in discussions has meant that staff training and opportunities for learning has been able to continue online, whilst still adopting best practice in educational design and delivery, and staff have continued to develop their dementia care knowledge and practice.

There is also a need to tailor delivery approaches to suit the online environment, with approaches used during in-person delivery often not directly transferable to online, synchronous delivery (Howe et al. 2021). Facilitators will also need to consider who the training is aimed at and whether online learning may further disadvantage some learners, who may already experience educational and technological inequalities (Allen et al. 2020). Therefore, not all face-to-face methods are equal in their ability to support delivery of training online.

Use of face-to-face approaches can provide a clear route to the involvement of people directly affected by dementia in dementia training. Inviting people living with dementia to give a talk, or to take part in a question-and-answer session with a group of learners, can provide an accessible route to participation for some people living with dementia and has the benefits of providing direct, real contact between them and the learners, which is likely to be the most impactful method of engagement. However, not all people directly affected by dementia are able or willing to participate in this way and such approaches do incur additional resources to manage the logistics as well as additional financial costs. Therefore, it may be necessary to consider other non-direct methods of involvement. For example, people directly affected by dementia might be asked to make a video that can be played during training sessions to prompt discussion. There are also a range of existing videos made by dementia organisations. If using external resources, it is important to check their quality and messaging first. People directly affected by dementia can also be involved in supporting the design of training, including providing advice and feedback on content, activities, and exercises.

Asynchronous e-learning and self-directed learning

Organisations often choose to use **asynchronous learning** methods like e-learning or self-study booklets as a resource-efficient method of delivering dementia training to a large number of learners. However, reviews of research across a range of service settings present a consistent picture that e-learning that is asynchronous or self-directed (e.g. working individually through an e-learning 'module' or programme or completing a workbook), whether with or without additional group work, is disliked by learners, often poorly completed, and results in high dropout rates (Cunningham et al. 2020; Surr et al. 2019b). This is particularly reported in care home settings (Keenan et al. 2020) where a lack of access to IT equipment, and a lack of confidence and competence in using IT on the part of some learners, can create particular barriers. Few studies have compared asynchronous e-learning in dementia care to other methods in terms of its impact. However, those that have found no benefits of asynchronous e-learning alone compared with receiving no dementia training at all, on outcomes such as staff attitudes to caring for people living with dementia. Combining interactive, multi-media e-learning with support from an external dementia specialist (a **blended learning** approach), however, led to positive impacts on staff attitudes to delivery of person-centred care compared with the e-learning alone (McDermid et al. 2018).

Recognising this challenge with acceptability and uptake of e-learning, and its poor performance when used as a stand-alone, self-directed method of delivery, Moehead et al. (2020) undertook a review of published studies to identify the key features of effective and functional online learning. They identified 14 features (see Table 2.1). These features encompass those identified in the 'What Works?' study (Surr et al. 2017b) regarding online learning, and indicate the need for successful online leaning to adopt many of the key features of synchronous, face-to-face learning, such as group learning, active skilled facilitation, interactive activities including interaction with peers, and careful consideration of multi-modal content. The online site for accessing learning must be user-friendly, easy to navigate, and have technological support available to tackle problems rapidly. Thus, effective online learning is more than 'e-learning' that is delivered in part or entirely synchronously. Ongoing resources not dissimilar to face-to-face learning are required to facilitate it well. E-learning and online methods can, however, provide a useful way to engage geographically spread individuals in flexible learning that can be undertaken at times and in ways to suit their job and personal circumstances. It also offers the opportunity to include the voices of people directly affected by dementia through participating online and by the use of video- and audio-clips of people talking about their experiences, for example. People directly affected by dementia might also be involved in creating content such as case studies and reflective questions to include in e-learning programmes.

There is strong evidence, therefore, to indicate that asynchronous, self-directed study via e-learning is not an effective approach to delivery of dementia training, when used as a stand-alone approach. However, online methods and e-learning can have a role to play in dementia training if delivered synchronously or as part of a blended learning approach, including opportunities for direct discussion and interaction with facilitators and other learners.

Table 2.1   Key features of effective online learning based on Moehead et al. (2020) and DeSouza et al. (2020)

Online learning feature	How this may be applied to the design and delivery of online learning programmes
Self-directed and self-paced	Programme allows learners to engage at a time, location, and pace that suits them.
Individualised, taking into account learner's background and learning needs	Content is relevant to learners regardless of their role and experience. Learners are able to choose online learning content that meets their needs from an available catalogue.
Interactive	Online learning should include interaction with facilitators and other learners through forum discussions (asynchronous) and live (synchronous) audio/video chat.
Multi-modal	Online content includes a variety of modes, including video, written resources/literature, quizzes, case studies, virtual experience, and interaction with facilitators and other learners.
Flexible	Materials can be used flexibility (e.g. face-to-face, online or a blended approach of the two) and learners are able to access content flexibly so they do not miss learning if they are unable to attend synchronous activities.
Accessible	There are no barriers to access – learners have 24-hour access to the site and have free access to the internet and a suitable device on which to undertake learning activities.
Consistency, repetition, and reinforcement	Content is up to date, quality assured, evidence-based, and able to be used consistently by facilitators. Learning is reinforced in various ways, such as video, reading, and quizzes. Formal or informal assessment of learning should be included so learners and facilitators can track progress. Learners may be required to achieve a consistent percentage mark on assessed activities in order to progress to the next learning component.
Cost-effective and good value for money for learner and organisation/system	There is equitable access for all learners no matter their location and meets their learning needs. The learning produces a more knowledgeable and skilled workforce.
Gathers learner feedback via various mechanisms	Learners are regularly asked for feedback on the programme and their satisfaction with the learning experience.
Enables equitable engagement	Learning is open to all, and all learners have equal access to their peers and facilitator input.
Facilitated	Learning is facilitated by an expert who supports and encourages learners. They can be contacted by learners at any time. Technological/IT support is available for technical issues and troubleshooting.
Nurtures critical thinking and reflection	Content is designed to encourage critical thinking and reflection through activities and discussion with peers and facilitators. Learners are encouraged to discuss practical applications, barriers, and facilitators to practise implementation.

(continued)

Table 2.1 *(continued)*

Online learning feature	How this may be applied to the design and delivery of online learning programmes
Establishes a learning community	Learners are supported to remain in touch once the programme ends (e.g. via a social media network, forums, and newsletters).
Can be translated into practice	Learning activities encourage learners to develop and implement quality improvement activities in their workplace during and after the programme.

Experiential learning and simulation

Simulation is defined as the creation of a risk-free environment in which learners can master skills they need for clinical practice, involving stages of deliberate practice, reflection, and feedback (Maran and Glavin 2003). Simulation, therefore, follows an experiential learning cycle. However, simulated experiences aim to directly mirror a real-world scenario. Experiential learning, on the other hand, may involve a range of 'active' approaches to learning which may or may not reflect the real world. Therefore, simulation is a specific form of experiential learning. The value of simulated learning for training the wider health and social care workforce is well established, with it reported to lead to increased knowledge, and feelings of confidence and competence (Cant and Cooper 2017; Hanshaw and Dickerson 2020).

It is important for a facilitator to consider if and how they can assess what learners have learnt, and how this translates into practice. This might be through formal mechanisms such as assessments or more informal approaches within training sessions or the workplace. A useful model to consider in this context is Miller's framework for assessing clinical competence (Miller 1990). This includes four levels (Figure 2.4). The 'knows' level relates to knowledge about the topic. 'Knows how' refers to competence in knowing how to use the knowledge. 'Shows how' is the ability to perform the action, and finally 'does' relates to action or the application of knowledge in day-to-day practice. Miller argued that clinical education should include consideration of how all levels of the pyramid may be assessed within learning programmes.

Simulation offers many opportunities for assessing different levels of the pyramid within a training session. There are a range of methods or approaches used to facilitate simulation that range from low- and medium-fidelity modalities – that is, simulations that seem least real to the learner (e.g. paper-based or computer-based scenarios, role-play, or manikins/parts of manikins without feedback mechanisms) – to high-fidelity realistic modalities (e.g. virtual reality, computer-based manikins that provide interactive feedback as simulated patients) (Maran and Glavin 2003).

The benefit of low- and medium-fidelity simulation modalities is that they are relatively easy and low cost to implement. For example, facilitators

Figure 2.4 Miller's (1990) framework for clinical assessment

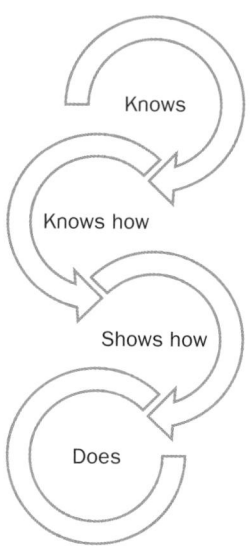

reported that a UK-based, flexible, simulation-based dementia training programme for acute hospital staff that used role-play and experiential exercises
enriched and improved their training, was enjoyable for staff, and supported
them to apply learning into practice (Heward et al. 2021a). However, they do
not offer the same real-life experience that the higher-cost and more resource-
intensive high-fidelity modalities can provide. Thus, they may not be able to
provide an insight into the 'shows how' level of Miller's pyramid. Studies comparing high- and low-fidelity simulations, however, have found varying results,
with low-fidelity simulations sometimes performing similar to or better than
high-fidelity ones in terms of knowledge and skills acquisition (Massoth et al.
2019). Overall, the level of fidelity that is likely to provide the greatest learning
benefits will depend on the type of task and level of learner. Therefore, afford-
able and practical low- and medium-fidelity simulations can offer high-quality,
impactful learning experiences.

Experiential learning and simulation are becoming increasingly recognised
as a potentially useful method for delivery of dementia training programmes.
They are being used in particular to bring out emotional and empathic responses
in learners and facilitate them to recognise the personhood of those with
dementia. Examples that have been evaluated and published include low-
fidelity programmes (Haugland and Reime 2018; Heward et al. 2021b; Naughton
et al. 2018) that include activities such as role-play, video, and written case
scenarios and interactive group activities that encourage discussion and reflection on what it might be like to experiences symptoms of dementia in the context
of the experiential learning cycle. Medium-fidelity programmes (Beville 2002;
Gilmartin-Thomas et al. 2018; Kimzey et al. 2021) often aim to simulate what it
might feel like to live with dementia through props aimed to distort the senses,

including special gloves, glasses, and shoe inserts. Learners are then asked to complete a series of tasks in a specialist environment designed to confuse. High-fidelity programmes have included simulated people living with dementia using actors and scenarios involving multiple health and social care disciplines (Katwa et al. 2020; O'Brien et al. 2018).

Experiential learning and simulation offer a range of opportunities for involving people directly affected by dementia in training. Direct methods include simulating the role of 'a patient' so that learners can practise their skills in assessment or interventions. Appropriate training and support are necessary for this type of simulation with opportunity for preparatory and/or debriefing sessions. Indirect involvement could include helping to design and develop simulation scenarios and experiential learning activities based on their experiences.

Evaluations of all simulated programmes indicate benefits of this type of approach over standard didactic or traditional 'lecture'-based training methods. This approach is particularly valuable for increasing staff empathy and understanding of people living with dementia, facilitating ongoing reflection and challenging them to reconsider current care approaches, including slowing down and having greater patience (Meyer et al. 2022; Peng et al. 2020; Slater et al. 2017; Surr et al. 2019b). Low-fidelity programmes are also well evaluated with learners and have been found to increase confidence, skills, and knowledge (Haugland and Reime 2018; Heward et al. 2021b; Naughton et al. 2018). However, engaging in tasks like role-play may be challenging initially and perceived as unpleasant. To optimise impact they may need to be used several times within programmes of training, offering opportunities for learners to change roles and grow in confidence using the method (Haugland and Reime 2018).

Some medium-fidelity programmes (virtual dementia simulations) have received criticism for the following: lacking authenticity and an evidence base; not providing an opportunity for adequate, structured debriefing as is essential for the experiential learning cycle; causing learner distress; and increasing fear and anxiety about developing dementia (Farina et al. 2021; Merizzi 2018; Slater et al. 2017). Due to their standardised, generic content, they may lack relevance to realistic scenarios as experienced in the day-to-day work of some learners (Gilmartin-Thomas et al. 2018). It is therefore recommended that particular commercial versions of such training (usually delivered as a stand-alone 2-hour training session) are used with caution and only within a wider programme of dementia training and implementation (Merizzi 2018; Slater et al. 2017; Surr et al. 2017a).

High-fidelity simulations evaluate well with learners and have demonstrated impacts on knowledge, confidence, and behaviour change in practice (Katwa et al. 2020; O'Brien et al. 2018). However, they often require ongoing resources that may be unsustainable in delivery of training in the longer term.

As technology advances so will opportunities for simulated learning, for example through techniques such as virtual reality (Hirt and Beer 2020). Such approaches may offer potential opportunities for engaging in safe, realistic scenarios that may help to improve learner knowledge and skills in supporting people living with dementia. They are also likely to become cheaper and more accessible over time. However, research indicates that effective simulated learning can also be delivered using well-designed and well-facilitated, low-fidelity, low-cost and low-resource methods, which are accessible to all and practical to implement.

Case example: The use of virtual reality to deliver experiential learning opportunities to homecare staff

An established **homecare** company identified that there has been a chronic underfunding and underdevelopment of social care training, particularly in homecare services. This has often led to the use of basic e-learning solutions, which focus on descriptive and informative training without an emphasis on real-world techniques and best practice that is useable for a trainee. The homecare provider partnered with a virtual reality (VR) training company, whose VR technology is able to develop real-world training scenarios and capture learners' reaction time, intuition, and knowledge when responding to them in the virtual world. This information can be displayed for the individual or at an organisational level and used to understand individual learning and skills, as well as to identify organisation-wide learning, development, and skills needs. Through this partnership a virtual reality training course was developed that gave practical advice and knowledge through the presented VR scenarios and showed best practice with the aim of empowering trainees with greater knowledge, skills, and confidence in their practical application when delivering care.

An academic with expertise in dementia training worked with the homecare company to develop the VR scenarios and the training script. The intended learning outcomes are drawn from a national training standards framework. The VR training is made up of five scenarios of engagements between a person living with dementia and two members of a care team. The scenarios take place in a bedroom, bathroom, living room, and kitchen to provide different settings in which the learner might work when supporting someone living with dementia in their own home. The scenarios have different interactive features such as identifying person-centred and non-person-centred care practices they observe, identifying individual, social, and environmental issues that might negatively impact a person living with dementia, and choosing from different care approaches to a situation. In the latter of these the VR technology permits the learner to watch the different outcomes unfold to reflect on the potential usefulness and impact of different approaches.

Once the training is completed, learners are asked to reflect on the situations and the key questions/information presented during the training. The VR training is also supported by a downloadable information document that provides the learner with factual and information-based content on dementia care to accompany the training.

The 'What Works?' study (Surr et al. 2017a, 2017b) identified a number of good practice criteria to inform safe and impactful experiential or simulated learning. These are summarised in Box 2.8.

Box 2.8 Good practice criteria for experiential learning and simulation

1 Simulation/experiential learning or role-play should be part of a broader range of training methods that include theory/knowledge-based content, reflection, and discussion.

2 Learners need an opportunity to build trust and rapport with a facilitator and other learners ahead of the use of simulation/role-play/experiential learning activities.

3 Simulation/experiential learning must include time for learner preparation ahead of the simulation/experiential activity/role-play.

4 Simulation/experiential learning must include adequate time for formal debriefing of the activity, reflection, and generation of specific learning (e.g. for people to discuss how they are feeling, what worked well, what they could have done differently).

5 Simulation/experiential learning should include the opportunity for wider discussion of emergent issues and thus for the implications of the simulation/experiential activity/role-play to be contextualised within wider theory and practice.

6 Simulation/experiential learning should include the opportunity for learners to engage in positive or best practice simulation/experiential learning activities where they are able to identify, experience, and apply desired practice(s) and not just poor practice to be avoided.

7 Provision must be made for immediate and ongoing support of learners who may become distressed during simulation/experiential learning activities.

8 At least one of the facilitators of simulation/experiential learning should have prior experience in use of such techniques.

9 Simulation/experiential learning scenarios must be piloted/tested and refined ahead of use within formal training delivery.

Practice-based learning, mentorship, and supervision

Practice-based, in-service, or work-based learning (sometimes also called on-the-job training) includes informal learning that occurs in day-to-day work with people living with dementia, as well as more structured approaches to learning in practice settings. Informal learning is covered in more detail in Chapter 3. Formal approaches often used to support practice-based learning include **shadowing** (working alongside a more experienced colleague); being observed in day-to-day practice and receiving feedback, mentoring, or coaching; or participating in a placement in a service setting other than the learner's usual workplace. However, the boundaries between formal and informal learning are often blurred. For example, unintended informal learning can occur during formal, practice-based learning opportunities, as the boundaries between the formal and informal are not set, if they exist at all.

Formal, practice-based learning is a cornerstone of education across all health and social care disciplines for the development of in-practice competencies, for example through clinical placement and shadowing as part of induction. However, the 'What Works?' study (Surr et al. 2017a, 2017b) identified that as a stand-alone approach to training, practice-based learning was not impactful and led to a number of challenges. These include: a lack of time (for both the learner and/or mentor) during day-to-day practice for the formal aspects of learning to take place; the service setting not providing the right opportunities and experiences to facilitate learning; and mentors/supervisors lacking the appropriate skills or knowledge to provide an appropriate learning experience. A summary of good practice criteria for practice-based learning based on the 'What Works?' study (Surr et al. 2017b) and from reviews of evidence more broadly on practice-based learning in health and social care education (Pollard et al. 2007; Williams 2010) is provided in Box 2.9.

Box 2.9 Practice-based learning good practice criteria

1 Practice-based learning should build on theory/knowledge-based learning (for example, that gained through face-to-face training sessions).
2 It should draw on the principles of experiential learning, including ensuring opportunities for critical reflection on experience and the creation of new professional knowledge.
3 The mentor/facilitator and the learner must both be allocated dedicated time to support practice-based learning.
4 Practice-based learning needs to take place in care environments where there is an organisational learning culture (see Chapter 9).
5 Practice-based learning needs to take place in settings where practice is supportive to learning, offers opportunities for 'experiences' that can underpin learning, and where care is at least of adequate quality.
6 Practice-based learning should take place in care environments suitable for the planned learning activities.
7 Practice-based learning should be facilitated by an experienced mentor who is able to effectively support the learning of required skills.

Ensuring that the environment in which practice-based learning takes place is one that is suitable for supporting learning of the right nature is critical and requires a consideration of existing organisational culture, as discussed further in Chapter 9. Having a skilled mentor and role model(s) who can facilitate learning that reflects best practice should be the hallmark of good in-practice learning. This must also be accompanied by formal opportunities to engage with theory and knowledge-based content to underpin practical learning. Ensuring congruence between these two aspects requires careful consideration and implementation.

In-service learning offers many opportunities for learning from people directly affected by dementia and can help to identify staff training needs. This can include people living with dementia as well as family and friends giving their views on care approaches used, or asking for feedback on communication or how they feel about being cared for by the member of staff. There are also opportunities for observation of care interactions occurring between a staff member and people with more advanced dementia and using reflection in- and on-action to try to understand the person's experiences. This can be particularly helpful where the person living with dementia may be unable to verbalise their experiences. This could be undertaken informally or through using more formal observational methods such as **Dementia Care Mapping** (Bradford Dementia Group 2005) and the Person, Interactions, and Environment tool (PIE) (Godfrey et al. 2018).

Creative approaches

Recently, there has been a growth in creative approaches to dementia education and training, including the use of theatre, film, and other arts-based methods. Examples of arts-based methods used within training sessions include comic books to communicate information, music, film, TV documentaries, excepts from plays, storytelling, attending venues such as museums and art galleries, and creating poetry, drama, and art work (Greenwood 2015; Roberts and Noble 2015; Windle et al. 2020; Zeilig et al. 2015). There are also examples of the creation of dramatic or theatre performances that seek to act as educational experiences (Schneider 2017). In some approaches, art-based methods are undertaken by learners alongside people living with dementia. For example, evaluation of a UK-based training programme involving the co-creation of a theatre production between care home residents and staff suggested this may lead to improved communication between staff as learners and residents, and more positive learner attitudes towards residents (Guzmán et al. 2017a, 2017b). Similarly, a small-scale study in the US found the attitudes of medical students towards people living with dementia improved following a storytelling-based training programme with people living with dementia in nursing homes (George et al. 2013). While large-scale and robust evaluation of arts-based education and training in dementia care remains limited, art-based methods do indicate promise, particularly in areas such as learner engagement, improving attitudes, empathy-raising, and enhancing staff communication skills (Roberts and Noble 2015; Windle et al. 2020; Zeilig et al. 2015).

Summary

This chapter has provided an overview of some of the key theories of adult learning that are relevant to considering the way dementia training is designed and delivered. It has highlighted how these have often not been explicitly discussed but may provide a good foundation for the design of dementia training programmes and learning activities. The chapter has also provided an overview of the evidence base surrounding some of the common methods used in the delivery of dementia training. We have also provided some good practice guidelines to consider when employing different training methods. It has argued that the most effective programmes combine a range of methods appropriate to what is being taught so that theory, practical application, and reflection on and consolidation of learning can take place.

Implications for those delivering dementia training

Those leading and facilitating dementia training should:

- Draw on adult learning theories when designing or revising dementia training programmes and sessions, choosing and applying those that are most appropriate for the training content and learners.
- Carefully consider the methods used to deliver dementia training and the evidence around their effectiveness in different settings (see also Chapters 4–7), for delivery of different types of content and for training for different types of learners. This must also be balanced against the practicalities of delivery, including available resources. Often a combination of methods will prove to be most effective.
- Ensure the voice of people directly affected by dementia is present throughout the training programme, recognising this will be most effectively achieved through using a range of different approaches.

Implications for managers in dementia care settings and services

Managers in dementia care settings and services should:

- Ensure they ask those facilitating training about how they have designed the programme and whether it draws on adult learning theory and the current evidence regarding what works.

- Support staff to identify their learning needs and make provisions for these to be met in ways appropriate to each individual.
- Make provision for staff to have opportunities to learn in-practice and to implement learning into practice in supported ways, either formally or informally.
- Encourage staff to engage in reflective practice as part of formal supervision or mentorship arrangements and in informal ways, such as during handover, or in response to critical incidents or practice challenges.

Implications for staff providing care, services, or support to people living with dementia

Staff working in dementia care should:

- Reflect on their own learning needs and preferred ways of meeting these, either individually or with support, and discuss this with their manager to develop an individualised programme of learning.
- Recognise there is not just one way to learn. They should try to understand their own preferred methods of learning and share these with those responsible for their training provision, to ensure as far as possible these are met.
- Actively engage in training sessions to maximise opportunities for learning.

Implications for those directly affected by dementia

- The voices of people directly affected by dementia should be embedded throughout training programmes and sessions.
- Those directly affected by dementia can provide face-to-face or online learning opportunities as mentors and trainers.
- There are many audio and visual materials and indirect methods (such as use of case studies developed with people affected by dementia) that can be employed as part of the education process to challenge assumptions and teach new skills.
- There is a lack of diversity of voices and experiences in existing published examples of involvement of people affected by dementia in dementia training and within audio, video, and other indirect resources. This needs to be addressed to ensure that the diversity of those directly affected by dementia is reflected in training materials.

3 Informal ways of learning

'Many in the dementia care field share the concern that much of what they teach is undermined when a learner returns to their workplace.'

As the previous chapter showed, training and education are well established, if complex, routes to improving the quality of care and support provided for people living with dementia in a wide range of services; routes that have been increasingly acknowledged internationally over the last decade and affirmed in governmental policy and regulation. However, there is a danger that formal training and education are seen as synonymous with learning to the exclusion of less obvious harder to evidence, but no less promising, paths to influencing practice.

Considering the wider lens of learning, and particularly learning in the workplace, reveals possibilities for influencing practice that remain significantly untapped in both quality improvement efforts and research within dementia care at the current time. This chapter explores relevant theory and research about informal learning methods and their relevance and potential for improving person-centred dementia care, as well as examining their relationship with more traditional training and education. It ends with an example of what can be revealed by innovative research that explores this broader understanding of learning within a dementia care setting.

The distinction between training and learning

Training and learning are often considered synonymous because discussions of learning often take place alongside consideration of how learning should be facilitated through formal training. However, this is problematic because it sees learning through a narrow lens and fails to address that learning is also occurring at other times, outside of formal training activities. However, if we ask, 'could learning occur without a person intending it?' and 'might learning happen whilst a person is doing something that is not part of training?', then the answer to these questions is definitely, 'yes'. Learning happens all the time for all of us in many different contexts.

Therefore, it is important to consider the full range of opportunities that might exist to influence that learning within a workplace, not only so that they can be used to influence person-centred care, but also to understand the effect that may have on practice and on the outcomes of formal training. Indeed, many in the dementia care field share the concern that much of what they teach is undermined when a learner returns to their workplace. What use is investing in comprehensive, evidence-based training if it is diluted or contradicted by learning that occurs through other means in the workplace? This is a common occurrence in all areas of life: after all, not many of us drive in the exact way we were taught to in order to pass our driving tests. It is normal for people to adjust formal learning in the face of 'real-world' experiences, and not always for the better.

Considering learning beyond formal training provision broadens our thinking in four key ways. These have particular relevance when considering person-centred dementia care and how to influence development of practice:

1 Learning needs to be viewed in context: an individual and their experience meet in a particular place, at a particular time, in a particular set of circumstances and this means that any learning that occurs is influenced by the context within which that 'meeting' happens (Illeris 2003; Rogers 2003). As highlighted in Chapter 2, conventional learning theories often fail to address that this context can have both a positive and negative affect on what is learned.

2 Learning has a strong social element: it occurs in interaction with other people and thus is influenced by other people (Bandura 2018; Wenger 2009).

3 Learning is ongoing: it is not tied to a specific time or space. It can happen whenever an individual encounters anything that could prompt a change in their behaviour, understanding, or emotional capacity (Billett et al. 2006; Illeris 2003).

4 Learning can be both an intentional, purposeful process and one which occurs without planning, unintentionally or unconsciously (Reece and Walker 2007). Chapter 2 showed that conventional learning theories consider learning an active process but ignore the potential learning that might occur as a by-product of a person's engagement in other tasks or without awareness. This is known as incidental learning (Eraut 2007; Marsick et al. 2009).

Person-centred care in context: Learning is a social activity

Considering how to support and influence the delivery of person-centred care is perhaps the best example of how learning needs to be understood as an inherently social activity. Caregiving is a social activity because it is about interactions between people. In fact, the more person centred caregiving is, the more prominent the social aspect is, as interactions become genuine two-way collaborations rather than one-way channels of 'doing to'. Kitwood emphasised that maintaining personhood was the primary aim of person-centred care for people living with dementia and that this is achieved first and foremost through *relationship* (Brooker 2004, 2007; Kitwood 1997). Learning is therefore not simply about how I provide person-centred care; it is about how *I* provide person-centred care *with you* through our relationship. Moreover, within services, this social aspect is extended because support requires a team of people. This means the experience of the person living with dementia is a result of how that team functions together to provide support, not simply the result of each individual's understanding and actions. Again, this means that learning is no longer about how *I* learn to provide person-centred care but about how *we, as a team,* learn to provide person-centred care.

Therefore, the social aspects of learning are very important to consider. They have been researched internationally across different workplaces although usually outside of health and care settings. These investigations emphasise the influence of social context on how and what learning takes place. This social context occurs at two levels, which overlap and interact together:

- *Local level*: the day-to-day relationships and situations encountered in the workplace.
- *Organisational level*: the structure of the work, workplace, and organisational culture.

The role of organisational culture will be discussed in more depth in Chapter 8. However, at the local level, **workplace learning** research demonstrates that to carry out work, a person does not simply engage in particular tasks or roles, but also has to negotiate relationships, hierarchies, routines, and customs of a particular setting in order to do so. Therefore, learning any type of work cannot be separated from these activities, because work *is* these activities. This makes learning to work primarily a process located *within* the workplace, not external to it (Bandura 2018; Billett 2014b; Lave and Wenger 1991; Somerville 2006). Acknowledging this social view of learning, together with the social nature of person-centred care itself, has important implications for learning within dementia care in the following ways:

1 It suggests that relationships within the workplace may matter more in influencing what is learned than any formal 'teaching' of what should be learned. Therefore, training about person-centred care will be less influential on practice than the practicalities of 'doing' care that are communicated, encouraged, or prevented by others in the workplace.

2 It suggests that learning to work successfully is about more than the ability to expertly perform specific tasks. Instead, it is about a broader ability to function within a particular workplace community. Therefore, learning to deliver person-centred care requires more than being taught what person-centred care looks like, but must also address how to negotiate, shape, and participate effectively in a particular workplace community.

3 Uniquely to caregiving situations, people living with dementia themselves form part of this workplace community and thus could be influential on the learning that takes place in the right circumstances.

Box 3.1 Communities of practice and the social view of learning

An important concept to the social view of learning is that of 'communities of practice'. A 'community of practice' exists whenever practitioners share similar roles and engage with each other as part of day-to-day action. In this view of learning, workers do not gain knowledge and skills predominantly via instruction and observation but instead through a more complex process of participating in the community (Lave and Wenger 1991). Learning through this route is therefore ongoing, evolving, informal, and highly influenced by existing members and relations within the community.

Thinking about the communities of practice relevant to our workplaces can create opportunities to influence informal ways of learning by being aware of and getting involved with what goes on within a particular community.

Over time, the concept of communities of practice has grown and been adopted into some formal approaches to learning, especially with the growth of social media and technology, for example, by forming an online community of practice following a training programme, or around certain practice issues. This can enable interactions within a community to be influenced towards certain standards via moderated discussions, information-sharing, and common values in the group. Essentially, it is a way to insert some formal influence over the informal dynamics of a community of practice.

This demonstrates that aspects of informal learning can be 'formalised' when their dynamics and significance are understood. Therefore, when wishing to influence dementia care practice, one needs to actively consider the communities of practice that exist in that workplace and how they might be shaped towards appropriate practice (Fuller et al. 2005; Illeris 2003; Lave and Wenger 1991; Wenger 2009).

What is 'informal' learning and why is it important?

There is a stark contrast between the focus within dementia care on formal training and the workplace learning research that emphasises the dominance of informal ways of learning. However, this is not unique to dementia care. It is estimated that informal learning accounts for up to 80 per cent of workplace learning, contrasted with 80 per cent of organisational learning budgets typically invested in formal training. Informal learning is thus characterised as a 'powerful yet taken-for-granted resource … deployed only by default' (Marsick et al. 2009, p. 593). One reason for investigating informal routes of learning is that such learning takes place in many unplanned, day-to-day, and incidental ways and is embedded within the accepted culture of a workplace, and, as such, is validated by what works within that setting (Rogers 2003). Therefore, it is (if unattended to) a potential route of learning poor practice. As Rogers succinctly puts it, 'everyone is engaged with learning. They may not be learning what we want them to learn, but they are all learning' (2003, p. 10). This suggests that it should be an essential component of any effort to improve care quality. Simply because informal learning is not purposefully arranged does not mean that it cannot be changed. With awareness, individuals and organisations can influence and use such events to their advantage.

There are many definitions of informal learning, meaning it can be challenging to translate such ideas into the solution-focused field of dementia care quality and practice improvement. Distinctions are sometimes made between formal and informal events by location of the activity (classroom or workplace) or sponsor (employer or employee) but these can create a false barrier between different learning opportunities (Eraut 2007; Malcolm et al. 2003; Manuti et al. 2015). More comprehensive classifications of learning have recognised there is a continuum on which different types of learning opportunities sit, allowing for overlap and interaction between them. These classifications suggest a better approach is to distinguish between learning opportunities on the basis of whether the event is specifically intended for learning or not (Kyndt et al. 2016; Rogers 2003). Rogers (2003) describes formal events ('learning-conscious learning') as being at one end of a spectrum and unintentional, accidental learning events at the other. Opportunities for learning in which the learner is primarily concerned with something else, such as completing a task ('task-conscious learning'), but learn as a by-product of those experiences, exist between these two poles. Figure 3.1 illustrates this spectrum.

Thinking of types of learning in this way allows for the ongoing and overlapping nature of learning during work. It better illustrates the potential for contradiction between different sources of learning and the possibilities of actively influencing learning taking place at different points on the spectrum. It also shows the risk of focusing exclusively on formal learning, without awareness and attention to the nature and impact of other sources.

Figure 3.1 The continuum of learning (based on Rogers 2003)

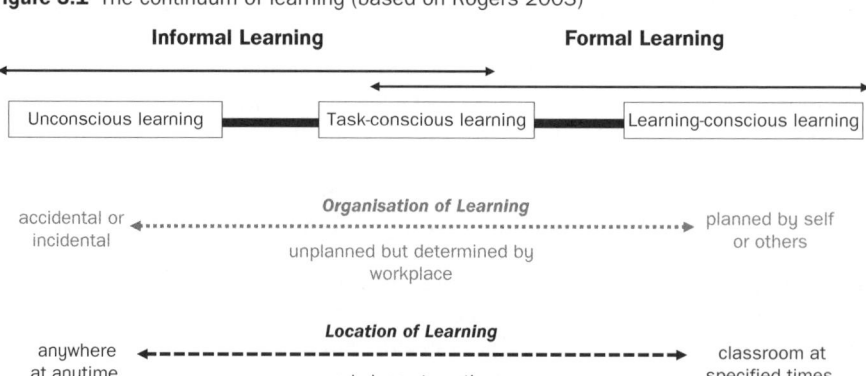

For example, a care worker may take part in formal learning through a dementia training course, but they may also seek their own self-directed learning about a particular person or situation by discussing it with colleagues. Both are learning-conscious learning but may produce different (and maybe conflicting) outcomes. Further to this, in undertaking their daily work, the worker may also encounter a 'best' way of completing tasks (task-conscious learning), but the nature of this will be highly workplace dependent, perhaps actively contradicting training by valuing getting tasks done quickly above meeting a person's preferences. Unexpected problems or crises such as a person being unwell, or unavailable resources, will also provide opportunities for learning which may influence future decision-making and task completion, for better or worse. Accidental and unconscious learning could occur throughout all these activities, as a worker may absorb understandings through hearing certain language used, participating in social interactions with colleagues, or inferring meaning from feedback and rewards. Without actively identifying and considering these different mechanisms within any setting, it is impossible to affect, reinforce, or reverse the learning that takes place.

This chapter will now examine some of the key mechanisms through which these informal types of learning have been shown to take place and discuss their possible relevance for person-centred dementia care.

Types of informal learning

The different ways that informal learning takes place through work have been theoretically and practically explored within adult and workplace learning research. However, their investigation within dementia care specifically, or the health and social care sector more generally – particularly on a large, systematic scale – is limited. This is because of how complex such issues can be to explore and also the tendency to conflate learning exclusively with training within dementia care. This means that it is not simple to identify specific approaches to activating informal learning that have resulted in positive outcomes for dementia care practice. What it is possible to do, however, is to bring together the findings from a diverse international field and consider the potential this evidence has for improving learning in dementia care and make the case for expanding our thinking about learning away from an exclusive focus on training. This is in the hope that innovative practitioners will be able to use these ideas and begin to build a body of practice and research evidence of their usefulness to dementia care. The following subsections discuss the key types of informal learning, their theory and evidence base, and the implications for person-centred dementia care.

Learning by being there: Socialisation

Socialisation into the workplace is a persistent and influential type of informal learning at work, and one that is rarely explicitly recognised in activities

such as training. It is broader than learning the tasks associated with a particular role and involves learning the intricacies of how to carry out practice
within a particular workplace via day-to-day interactions with others
(Rogers 2003). It emphasises and overlaps with the social aspects of learning
theory discussed previously. It occurs through observation, imitation, and
listening, and is prompted simply by 'being there', rather than specific activities (Billett 2014a). It is more than simple copying, as it involves taking in a
range of sensory, non-verbal, and embodied messages that can be hard to
articulate (Chan 2015).

Billett (2006) suggests that the norms and practices of a particular workplace or work role create a curriculum for workers to learn the work, by
structuring what experiences are available in day-to-day practice. This has
unintended consequences for what is learned because workplace patterns may
not coincide with ideal or expected practice. For example, a health care assistant's learning through socialisation is determined by the activities they encounter on the hospital ward in which they work. If the normal ways of working on
this ward emphasise completing physical tasks above communicating with
patients, then this is how the assistant's 'curriculum' will be shaped; this is how
their work will be explained at the beginning and end of the shift; it is what will
structure their workday; and it is what will be recorded, monitored, and talked
about amongst colleagues. Thus, the health care assistant becomes socialised
through day-to-day interactions into work as completing physical tasks and,
significantly, misses out on opportunities to explore their work as communicating with patients.

It therefore becomes very important to understand the specific ways in
which socialisation learning occurs and to consider how it can be influenced if
one is interested in directing learning towards certain standards of practice.
A few research studies have investigated socialisation learning within international health care and social work settings, shedding some light on how
influential it is likely to be in dementia care settings. Three key aspects appear
significant: interactions, communication, and interpersonal relationships.

Interactions

Hunter et al. (2008) investigated how Australian neonatal nurses learned within
their workplace and discovered that a key feature was learning the 'ethos' of
the workplace – 'how we do things here'. Formally learned knowledge from
training was often superseded by new workplace knowledge as the worker
interacted with colleagues and incorporated prevailing beliefs, values, and
practices. Ajjawi and Higgs (2008) found that physiotherapists in Australia
modelled their clinical reasoning on that of others in the workplace, and thus
workplace shaped the behaviours a person learned. Investigating social work
practice in Sweden, Avby (2015) identified that practitioners learned by making
sense of what they experienced alongside others. In one of the few studies
examining learning by care workers in care homes, an English study showed
that care workers learned daily by observing others' practice and receiving

advice from others. However, these processes were only sometimes formally organised (such as through induction or management guidance) and more commonly determined by who was available and acceptable to the worker at the time the new learning was needed (Latham 2020).

This socialisation process implicates the role of organisational culture in influencing the learning of practice. This will be discussed further in Chapter 8. However, from a practical point of view, socialisation learning suggests that the range of colleagues a person has contact with, and the quality of insight they provide into work practices influences the learning that can take place. Therefore, paying attention to the colleagues a worker is interacting with is an important component of influencing learning in the workplace.

Communication

How people communicate with one another is also highly significant in passing on messages about work and workplace environments (Boud and Middleton 2003; Eraut 2007; Rooney et al. 2016). This communication helps determine the ways in which a worker may frame their understanding of work situations and the extent to which that understanding is open to reframing (Marsick et al. 2009). For example, in a study of management of a Swedish care home, it was identified that particular communication strategies helped to 'activate' workers (encourage their involvement and empowerment). These strategies included: invitations to join in problem-solving; helping to categorise issues (e.g. 'this is about time management'); and open agenda invitations for staff meetings. These communication strategies were successful because they positioned the workers as people who could and were expected to have solutions and knowledge about certain issues. This engaged staff in day-to-day decision-making, and they learned skills of involvement and pro-activity (Fejes and Nicholl 2011).

Language choice has also been shown to be important. Latham (2020) found that 'shorthand' used by English dementia care home workers (non-literal, unspecific explanations of actions such as 'I am going to do Mrs Jones') could result in less person-centred practice being learned, because it conflated person and task and offered few opportunities for discussion of what the practice actually entailed.

Interpersonal relationships

Finally, the interpersonal relationships between colleagues have been identified as significant in the socialisation learning that takes place, because they influence the choices (both conscious and unconscious) workers make about who to interact with and thus learn from. For example, in a Norwegian study, interpersonal relations between nurses were identified as a key workplace characteristic to influence learning because these relationships provided sources of specialist and experienced knowledge (Skar 2010). Newcomers in particular have been shown to seek out colleagues who they perceive as 'safe' from whom to learn, suggesting that how a worker comes across to others affects their influence over learning (Mornata and Cassar 2018). The understandings workers gain from developing relationships with clients also form part of learning that takes place, and in a study of frontline staff in mental health and learning disability services in both Sweden and England, this learning was significant for workers when negotiating the conflicts that emerged in their working practice (Kubiak and Sandberg 2011). Within care home dementia care, care workers chose which colleagues to learn from based on personal relationships and opinions on their practice. Most significantly, they also learned from residents themselves through personal feedback, with workers who had opportunities to interact with residents in a broad way (across different parts of the day, during different activities, etc.) showing more person-centred practices (Latham 2020).

In dementia care, the potential role of socialisation as a type of informal learning that can supersede formal training and act as a vehicle for transmitting organisational culture resonates strongly with the findings from many investigations of training interventions (as will be discussed in Part 2 of this book): namely, that whilst training interventions can show effect, this is often muted by the impact of forces within the workplace over time. This is socialisation learning in action. Moreover, in practice, the preference for 'shadowing' as a means to induct new staff in many health and care settings embeds socialisation learning opportunities firmly; practitioners will also tell how influential this experience is for them and others in shaping the worker they become. The issue is therefore not a matter of whether socialisation learning occurs in dementia care settings, but rather one of how to ensure its influence towards person-centred care.

Interactions, communication, and interpersonal relationships are key areas of influence and so Box 3.2 outlines some key practice recommendations to influence these areas towards learning person-centred care.

Box 3.2 Good practice recommendations

Socialisation for person-centred dementia care

Dementia care practitioners and educators can maximise the influence of this aspect of informal learning towards person-centred care by acting on the following recommendations:

- Ensure that staff are skilled in communication with each other as well as people living with dementia. Interpersonal skills and interactions of staff matter because relationships shape learning, so ask the following: how well do staff provide feedback, challenge others, or give instruction?
- Maximise the range of situations and people that staff encounter within their day-to-day work. This should enable them to gain a comprehensive perspective on the person living with dementia and how their work and that of others impacts their well-being.

- Identify the 'curriculum' that is offered by a typical worker's day-to-day encounters. Ensure that it provides a person-centred view of the work and enhances knowledge and relationships rather than being structured by task.
- Address the ways in which relationships with people living with dementia themselves can be enhanced within day-to-day socialisation. Actively introduce the person's perspective into routine events in the workplace.
- Consider the language used to describe work tasks and people and encourage language that affirms a person-centred outlook, and empowers workers.
- Socialisation is particularly significant for new workers. Pay special attention to the quality of interactions, communication, and relationships facilitated at this stage of work.

Learning by doing: Problem-solving, reflection, and feedback

Intertwined with socialisation-type learning but focused more on the key tasks of the work rather than social interactions, is the learning that takes place by simply doing the tasks, decision-making, and problem-solving the job involves. Carrying out a job requires more than robotic repetition of actions. Instead, it requires a worker to master organisational processes that shape how decisions are made and to respond to atypical events (Boud and Middleton 2003). For example, Dutch nurses have been found to make a distinction between 'nursing' and 'being a nurse doing the job', with the latter being a broader experience that includes coping skills (Berings et al. 2008). Learning by doing is ongoing and highly influential in determining practice, with both routine and unusual situations providing opportunities for a worker to reinforce existing learning or learn something new. Pool et al. (2015) identified that in the Netherlands, nurses' continuing professional development was most often triggered by their daily work, especially when encountering new tasks. Autonomy in decision-making and problem-solving is positively associated with this type of learning, particularly for established workers, notably in a study of Japanese nurses (Billett 2015; Takase et al. 2018).

In a longitudinal UK study of three professions including nursing, 'doing work' was shown to be an ongoing process of assessing situations in context, deciding on what action is needed, and then monitoring oneself and the situation whilst carrying out the course of action. Learning about how to do the work occurred as a by-product of engaging in these ongoing problem-solving and reflective activities (Eraut 2007). Paré and Le Maistre (2006) described this as engaging in the 'rough and tumble' of practice when examining learning by new social workers in Canada. Within this process, more formal learning can be tested by applying it to day-to-day decisions. In addition, critical or unusual events are important in triggering learning, especially for experienced workers (Manuti et al. 2015), because they require problem-solving that has not been utilised before.

Learning by doing therefore implicitly suggests the presence of the reflection-in-action (Gibbs 1988; Schön 1992) and experiential learning (Kolb 1984; Wilkinson 2017) as discussed in Chapter 2. However, informal learning emphasises that these processes, occurring as they do in the midst of doing work, are imperfect. They are highly dependent on the individual and context and often happen in incomplete ways, without conscious awareness. In busy, stressful, and complex work (such as dementia care), actions and inactions have multiple and unpredictable consequences. Therefore, it is not safe to assume that a reflective or experiential cycle will naturally be triggered or 'completed' (a worker may be interrupted at any point in the cycle to engage in more 'doing'). Or that the information drawn on within the process is comprehensive (a worker has only a partial, biased picture of action and consequence). For example, in an English study within two dementia care homes, learning by doing was a consistent, daily feature of workers' learning and it was most strongly influenced by seeing successful results to decisions and actions. However, the care home context strongly affected what was considered 'successful'. A similar situation can therefore prompt similar reflection but result in more or less person-centred outcomes depending on context (Latham 2020).

Moreover, and of particular relevance to dementia care, 'doing work' is often not about holistically completing a task from start to finish, but instead about performing parts of a larger process during a particular period of time (Eraut 2004). For example, a care worker carries out an action with a particular person living with dementia, making decisions and solving any problems that arise before passing the person's needs onto others at the end of a work period, or when they cross into others' areas of responsibility. In these conditions, an 'ideal' reflective cycle would therefore need to be a group rather than individual process, requiring an understanding of how the parts and the whole fit together.

Reflection and feedback

As was discussed in Chapter 2, learning through reflection is a process by which meaning is made of experience by individuals, resulting in an outcome of changed perspective, new insight or recharged, revised, or rejected knowledge that can be applied to future experiences (Gibbs 1988; Johns 2017; Schön 1992). Learning by doing highlights that this has the potential to occur continually in the process of doing work, but also that there are many opportunities for the reflective process to be stalled or misdirected towards non-person-centred learning outcomes. Therefore, considering what can be learned from existing research into reflection is important.

Reflection has been shown to be a frequent and diverse way in which people learn informally within different professions and internationally, although most studies have focused on trainees or new practitioners (Berings et al. 2008; Fowler 2008; Meirink et al. 2009; Skaalvik et al. 2012). Within health and social care, Kyndt et al. (2016) identified that the opportunities for reflection were significant routes of informal learning for nurses in Belgium. In a study of

Swedish social workers' use of reflection, it was shown to be especially useful when complex decision-making, working with uncertainty and/or flexibility were required (Ryding et al. 2018).

Effective reflection is connected with workplace opportunities for feedback (Kyndt et al. 2016), with feedback intending to prompt reflection by a worker to consider a situation and guide future action (Sparr et al. 2017). Feedback, and opportunities to integrate it into reflective practice, is thus a significant way that leadership and the work environment can shape and influence informal learning, and encourage transfer of knowledge from formal education and training (Takase et al. 2018; Yen et al. 2016). Feedback and reflection are both significantly associated with self-reported competence for nurses in Japan, with feedback being particularly relevant for those with more experience (Takase et al. 2015). Both are also identified as a necessary characteristic in workplace learning for nurses in Japan (Takase et al. 2018).

A few specific practices have been shown to prompt reflection in health and social care settings, such as receiving recognition for actions, responses from service users, journal writing, group debriefs, and critical incident appraisals (in which specific notable incidents are formally reviewed to assess how behaviours related to outcomes) (Hetzner et al. 2015; Kubiak and Sandberg 2011; Latham 2020; Liveng 2010; Wilkinson 2017). Nonetheless, for paraprofessional workers in particular, opportunities and spaces for reflective practice whilst essential for learning are not always present (Kubiak and Sandberg 2011).

Impactful training does acknowledge the importance of reflection by relating cases, problems, and discussion to workers' own practice settings, and using reflective discussions (Surr and Gates 2017; Surr et al. 2017a). The effectiveness of such training methods is likely because they help connect the formal training to this aspect of informal learning. However, there is a notable lack of interventions that address how to affect learning by doing in-situ reflection (rather than via the classroom) in the dementia care setting. Opportunities for positive learning experiences are lost by not capitalising on the problem-solving, decision-making, and feedback opportunities that occur every day. Several steps could be taken to improve the use of 'learning by doing', and particularly reflection, in dementia care and these are outlined in Box 3.3.

Box 3.3 Good practice recommendations

Learning by doing for person-centred dementia care

Dementia care practitioners and educators can maximise the influence of this aspect of informal learning towards person-centred care by acting on the following recommendations:

- Recognise that person-centred dementia care embraces the unpredictability that can come with cognitive challenges. Therefore, reflection-based in-work learning is particularly well-suited to this type of practice and thus should be maximised.

- Do not assume that reflective practice is understood or happens automatically. Better explain the components of reflective practice for dementia care practitioners and embed it within training, particularly for paraprofessional staff.
- Discover and actively discuss the common problems/decisions that occur within daily work. This will help identify points within daily work where focused, formalised reflective learning within the workplace should take place.
- Actively enable workers to develop understanding and experience of how different roles contribute to a person's experience, interact with each other, and thus help or hinder person-centred care.
- Create the time and space within daily work to provide opportunities for reflective activity. Encourage and formalise these opportunities through facilitation and direction.
- Skill and empower specific staff to facilitate reflective practice in others.
- Consider how feedback from people living with dementia themselves is used as a trigger for reflection on everyday practice. Facilitate this and embed it within reflective activities.
- Consider how to maximise feedback from people living with dementia who cannot communicate verbally, such as through the use of observation (e.g. DCM feedback) and enabling staff to effectively interpret behaviour.

Case example: An organisational approach to informal learning

A large care provider organisation with over 20 care homes has an organisation-wide dementia care strategy built around the Senses Framework. The Senses Framework promotes 'relationship-centred care', an approach not dissimilar to person-centred care. It emphasises the critical importance of relationships between staff, families, and people living with dementia to achieving positive outcomes (Nolan et al. 2006).

Whilst training for staff has been part of this strategy for a while, a decision was made to embed this within a revised structure for the organisation's dementia care teams. This new structure recognised that the most impactful influences on care practice were daily influences in the workplace and so aims to positively shape these. Each of the organisation's dementia care communities has a dementia care manager, whose role is to provide coaching and support for dementia care teams in the home alongside responsibilities for staff training and resident care coordination. The role is supernumerary to the care team in order to protect it from being engulfed by day-to-day tasks and thus enable the manager to have an overarching view of care practice and to emphasise the importance of such daily coaching and support.

The dementia care managers are supported by regional dementia care practitioners, who provide specialist advice and support to a portfolio of care homes. These roles are overseen by an organisational head of dementia care and wellbeing, who is also responsible for evaluating the impact of this staff structure. At the time of writing, whilst recruitment in some regions was slower than planned and the COVID-19 pandemic created challenges for all care homes, the organisation has seen an improvement in dementia care provision in most care homes as measured by their own audits and CQC inspection outcomes.

Learning by trial and error and negative knowledge

Embedded within the process of learning by doing is the role played by actively trialling different approaches and generating negative knowledge (knowledge about what *not* to do). To learn from reflecting or problem-solving, a worker needs to be able to gain knowledge about what does not work as well as what does. In a Brazilian study across professions, learners engaging in trial-and-error learning informally at work was positively associated with professional development (Haemer et al. 2017). Teunissen (2015) showed that health care professionals in the Netherlands experience a range of different actions in their practice which they then employ in other situations to see if they do or do not work.

In a study of error-related knowledge by nurses in German nursing homes, negative knowledge was used by nurses when making decisions and to avoid mistakes. Negative knowledge could relate to procedures (what not to do), mis-conceptions (common misunderstandings), and personal deficits (limitations to ability). However, the 'effort-cost' (adverse impacts on the nurse themselves) meant that nurses only selectively engaged in processes that were designed to help them learn such negative knowledge, such as critical incident procedures (Gartmeier et al. 2010). This type of learning can be affected by tendencies to cover up errors, the strain of negative emotions, and workers' perception of their working environment as safe and trusted. These aspects contribute to an organisation's 'error culture' and the extent to which it is learning oriented (i.e. errors are seen as unavoidable and as learning opportunities) or blame oriented (i.e. errors are seen as unacceptable and staff members are judged or blamed for errors made) (Leicher and Mulder 2016; Leicher et al. 2013). Fur-thermore, the extent to which a worker and others will learn from an error is intertwined with whether organisations encourage activities such as reflection and seeking advice, and if discussing and learning from errors is openly embraced (Rausch et al. 2017).

In a study of two English care homes, workers showed that a significant feature of their day-to-day learning was to engage in 'trial and error'. This involved trying out different strategies and options with the intention of achiev-ing a particular outcome. In particular, with people living with dementia, this was seen by workers as an inevitable and necessary way of learning because situations and people could change significantly from moment to moment. What worked one day would not necessarily work the next (Latham 2020). This suggests that, at least in some situations, good practice could be less about knowing the right practice in advance and more about understanding appropriate boundaries and process to follow to ascertain the right outcome for a person or situation. Trial and error may be an essential component of person-centred dementia care.

Within dementia care training, the impactful nature of content that allows discussion of real-life issues and relates directly to practice has been noted (Surr and Gates 2017; Surr et al. 2017a). The effectiveness of these methods may relate to their connection and usefulness within trial-and-error learning. However, recognising the importance of trial-and-error learning to dementia care suggests that more work is needed to influence these informal processes as well as to acknowledge them within training. In particular, dementia care training will need to better explore and support the sophisticated decision-making involved in trial-and-error learning as applied within dementia care. This will both build the confidence of care workers to engage in it and counteract perceptions of a haphazard and unskilled process.

Box 3.4 Recommendations for good practice

Learning by trial-and-error for person-centred dementia care

Dementia care practitioners and educators can maximise the influence of this aspect of informal learning towards person-centred care by acting on the following recommendations:

- Explicitly acknowledge in both training and day-to-day work that meeting the needs of individuals requires an openness to trial and error (within boundaries of safe and rights-based practice) accompanied by reflective practice.
- Where trial and error is used, make sure to explicitly discuss the outcome to be achieved. Is everyone interpreting it the same? Does it support person-centred experiences or is it focused on achieving tasks or workplace outcomes?
- Normalise care plans that provide a range of different strategies and options to support individuals in common situations rather than seeking a single or vague course of action.
- Create an open and supportive environment that encourages and enables trial-and-error approaches (e.g. daily opportunities to share discoveries, admit failure, ask advice, receive feedback from others).
- Ensure frequent praise and celebration of successful strategies as well as questioning of less successful strategies.
- Embed reflective opportunities as outlined previously and use them to establish how different options might be trialled in certain situations, or the boundaries of acceptable and safe trial and error.
- When errors are made that need to be prevented in future, use processes such as critical incident reflection across the whole team and in ways that are focused on learning and future-action rather than blame and punishment.

Learning by using tacit knowledge

Tacit knowledge is a resource applied within informal learning processes, often without conscious awareness. It is knowledge that is personal, difficult to artic-ulate, and highly subjective, described as 'know-how', 'common sense', or 'tricks of the trade' (Collis and Winnips 2002). Whilst it can be rooted in work experience, professional practice and training (Johns 2017), it also relates to much broader interpersonal, emotional, and mental frameworks through which people process their experiences (Marsick et al. 2009). These are often unre-lated to work.

Exploring learning by workers in English care homes, Latham (2020) identi-fied that life experiences as well as previous work experiences formed a 'per-sonal resource' for workers to draw on within day-to-day decision-making. In a study of Swedish social workers, tacit knowledge was one way in which they made sense of case-work, contributing to a process of 'muddling-through' (Avby 2015). It has also been identified as a significant component to practical judgements in other professions (Hager 2000).

Again, as with other ways of informal learning, tacit knowledge cannot be assumed to be a 'positive' resource within the learning process. A person's 'tricks of the trade' may not be person-centred. Eraut (2004) highlights that tacit knowledge is most often used when a person does not have the time, will-ingness, or ability to identify better strategies (commonplace when a person is overworked or alienated) precisely because it is so readily and 'internally' available. This highlights another area where awareness of and potential 'for-malisation' of informal learning could be useful within dementia care. Identify-ing the content and source of tacit knowledge used in very good or very poor practice will enable it to be shared or corrected within the workplace. For example, Fuller et al. (2007) investigated a variety of work settings and identi-fied that where workplace relations encouraged autonomous decision-making by workers but also high levels of practical involvement by managers, this helped individuals' tacit knowledge to be explicitly recognised and then shared across teams (Fuller et al. 2007). Box 3.5 provides some recommendations for good practice in dementia care settings, based on the current understandings of the use of tacit knowledge in informal learning processes.

Box 3.5 Recommendations for good practice

Learning by using tacit knowledge for person-centred dementia care
Dementia care practitioners and educators can maximise the influence of this aspect of informal learning towards person-centred care by acting on the fol-lowing recommendations:

- When examples of very good care or exceptional dementia care workers are identified, take time to explore with individuals their thought process leading to the action. This will help to bring an unconscious process into awareness and provide the language to share it across the team.

- When poor practice occurs, take time to explore the thought processes that led to the action. This will provide the opportunity to expose tacit knowledge that is being applied incorrectly (e.g. someone draws a parallel between disciplining their child and caring for a patient living with dementia).
- Skill senior staff with the ability to encourage reflection and coach understanding of these incidents from others alongside more conventional supervision and management skills.
- Ensure that reflective activities (as recommended previously) explicitly draw out the thought processes and tacit knowledge that workers may have applied.

The interconnections between informal and formal learning

In Figure 3.1 we showed the continuum of different types of learning, highlighting that formal and informal learning overlap rather than being separate phenomena. In discussing the different types of informal learning, we have shown the potential for interaction between formal efforts to influence learning and those informal processes that occur in the workplace on a day-to-day basis. However, we have also illustrated that these interactions are not currently well understood within dementia care workplaces and require conscious awareness and effort to make best use of them towards person-centred care. In this section, we share the findings from an original study by one of the authors of this book (Isabelle Latham) that illustrates the insights gained from exploring learning through the eyes of workers themselves and the potential created when we examine how learning happens within the real world of practice. This study explored the learning of care workers in two care homes in England for people living with dementia, using observations of care and in-depth interviews with staff over 13 months. Whilst the implications of this study for training and learning in care homes are explored in depth in Chapter 4, the findings are shared here to illustrate the ways in which various types of formal and informal learning interact within the care home workplace to create a 'system' of learning to care. Understanding the holistic system that operates within any setting is the key to making best use of learning opportunities and directing them towards person-centred care. We begin by illustrating the system as a whole, before describing each element in detail.

In the system of learning to care shown in Figure 3.2, there are three interconnected elements that were significant to the learning experienced by care workers in both care homes in the study. However, the process often produced different care practices on the ground, with some more person centred than others. This shows that it is the interaction of all the different parts of the learning process with the context of the care home that influences practice rather than any one factor being dominant.

Figure 3.2 The system of learning to care (based on Latham 2020)

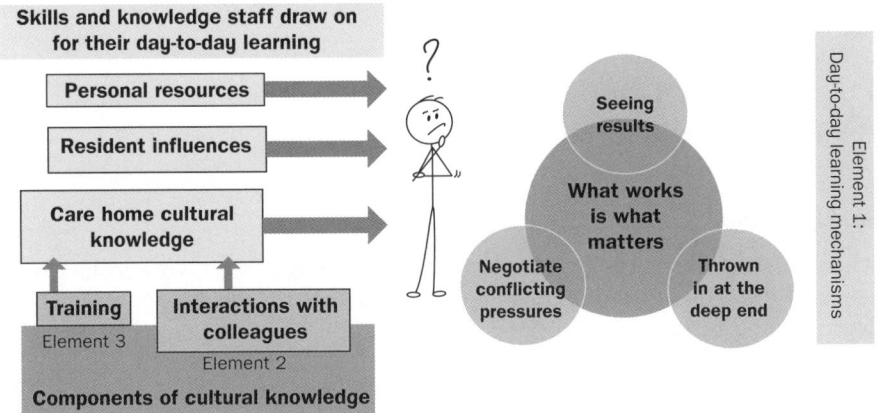

The System of Learning to Care

Element 1 (*What works is what matters*) explains the main way that learning occurs. It shows the mechanisms through which care workers apply, refine, reinforce, or reject their learning whilst doing their daily work. This encompasses much of the informal learning by doing and trial and error described earlier in this chapter. During this process, care workers draw on three sources of knowledge in increasing order of importance: their own personal resources, resident influences, and care home cultural knowledge. Within these three sources, the informal processes discussed earlier of learning by being there (socialisation), learning by doing and using tacit knowledge, as well as formal learning are implicated. Care home cultural knowledge (the biggest source drawn on by the care workers in their day-to-day learning) was made up of a further two elements of learning through *Interactions with colleagues* (Element 2) and formal learning through *Training* (Element 3).

When taken together, this system illustrates three significant things about how care workers learn to care for people living with dementia: First, informal day-to-day interactions account for a large proportion of their learning. Second, more formal learning, such as training or management instruction, is used within these day-to-day interactions rather than directly influencing practice. Finally, the overall 'culture' of the care home plays a highly influential role in learning, and thus the outcomes of practice, through these day-to-day interactions. Each element making up the system will now be described in detail.

Element 1: What works is what matters

The most frequent and influential type of learning experienced by care workers occurs as they encounter work activities on a moment-to-moment basis and see whether a particular action achieves a successful outcome in a particular circumstance. If a successful outcome is achieved, the practice is likely to be repeated in similar situations and passed onto their colleagues. This 'what works is what matters' type learning could result in different care practices being performed because what was determined as a successful outcome (what 'worked') was dependent on three contributing factors:

- seeing results;
- negotiating conflicting pressures; and
- being thrown in at the deep end.

Seeing results

When workers interacted with residents, they learnt what worked based on seeing if a particular practice achieved a satisfactory result or not. This was determined through:

- *Results for residents* – when an action taken achieved what it intended to (such as initiating personal care, movement, eating, or conversation) whilst simultaneously achieving behavioural/emotional outcomes for the resident (such as avoiding negative emotions or promoting positive expressions). For example, care workers often subtly varied how they responded to residents living with dementia who asked after family members, sometimes telling the literal truth and other times sidestepping depending on what avoided negative emotions for the individual resident. Learning through seeing results for residents produced care outcomes that were generally in line with person-centred care.
- *Fulfilling expectations* – where a successful outcome was determined by the extent to which the practice achieved its intended aim (such as initiating personal care) whilst also demonstrating the worker had carried out an expected part of their job (such as being in a certain place or acting in a particular way), regardless of how person-centred the outcome to a resident. For example, in one care home it was common to hear care workers described as 'very busy' and 'always on their feet', which reinforced choosing practices that resulted in 'being busy' over anything else.
- *Trial and error* – where a worker tried out different things in response to a situation and learned through both success and failure. This type of learning was particularly important as care workers recognised that the needs of residents with dementia could change rapidly, meaning that a solution could be found one day that would not be successful the next.

The relative importance of these was influenced by the workplace and the organisation of work roles and tasks, meaning significant differences could be seen in the outcomes of learning in different homes.

Negotiating conflicting pressures

A fundamental part of care involved encountering frequent and inevitable situations in which workers were pulled in opposing directions. They occurred where care worker knowledge ('what I am supposed to do'), care worker reality ('what I can practically do'), and care worker values ('what I want to do') clashed. Learning that occurred here was an acceptance that it is not possible to resolve the issue equally and that a decision must be made as to how to achieve an outcome that was acceptable. This depended upon the degree to which time, staff, and facilities enabled all resident needs/wants to be met and how staff interpreted what was expected of them. In both cases, where there was flexibility in how staff could manage their time, their role, and the resources they could draw on, they were more able to find person-centred solutions even under pressure. However, without such flexibility person-centredness was compromised because there were less solutions available to consider.

Being thrown in at the deep end

Care workers in the study described being placed in unfamiliar situations for which they felt unprepared and saw this as an inevitable and inescapable part of the job, related to the nature of care work and dementia care. While this was more likely to occur earlier in their employment, it was also seen as a frequent and inescapable occurrence in dementia care work. In these situations, they learned through their success or failure and developed a more sophisticated response for the next time a similar situation occurred. Being willing and able to 'get stuck in' was seen as a key skill and a major component of learning, with no substitute.

Drawing on skills, knowledge, and experience

When engaging in informal day-to-day 'what works is what matters' learning, care workers drew on three sources of knowledge and experience that had increasing levels of influence over practice outcomes:

- personal resources;
- resident influences; and
- cultural knowledge.

These sources were a bridge between day-to-day learning mechanisms and the influences of the wider team and learning from formal training. Importantly, the influence of these sources on practice was primarily indirect: a specific skill, knowledge, or experience only influenced learning if it 'worked'. If it didn't 'work', it was ignored.

Personal resources

Personal resources tended to influence an overall approach rather than a specific situation or decision, and occurred through the worker applying aspects of themselves to the situations they encountered. This included their own previous work and life experiences, including where they had dealt with a similar situation before or learned a particular way 'to be' and personal values, which steered them towards options with which they felt most comfortable.

Resident influences

Learning occurred here whenever a worker adopted a particular practice because of their relationship, interactions with or knowledge of an individual resident. Such a practice was repeated, drawn on, or shared if it was seen to be successful in achieving a desired outcome. Care workers gained this knowledge in two ways:

1. Learning *from* residents through personal feedback (e.g. via verbal and physical responses or as a feeling of connection) and knowledge about their choices and preferences. Actions that enhanced the worker–resident relationship (from the perspective of the worker) were more likely to be utilised repeatedly, shared with other workers, and applied across the resident group. Learning from residents generally contributed towards person-centred outcomes.
2. Learning *about* residents, where information about a resident came from a source other than direct interaction (e.g. formally through care plans or from other staff and family members). This type of knowledge was less influential than information learnt directly from residents themselves, because it was not as successful at solving day-to-day dilemmas as knowledge gained from residents themselves.

Care home cultural knowledge

Cultural knowledge is much more influential to learning and to determining the likelihood of person-centred practice than the previous aspects. It is formed of two additional areas of learning: interactions with colleagues and formal training.

Element 2: Interactions with colleagues

Learning occurred every day through relationships and communication with colleagues at all levels. Whether a particular practice was learned or not depended on the type of interaction, its circumstances, existing relationships, and whether it provided a useful solution within the 'what works is what matters' process. There were four aspects of interactions that influenced learning:

- *Being formally shown and told,* where senior staff explicitly anticipated and encouraged learning to take place by instituting opportunities to show or tell care workers how practice should be carried out (e.g. through shadowing or senior instruction). However, it was often said to be a flawed process, affected by staffing issues and, depending on the organisation of teams and workloads, it could result in very different kinds of practice being learned.
- *Asking and being given advice,* where learning occurred through frequent, often casual interactions, prompted by seeking out the input of others or

being given advice unsolicited. These interactions could encourage person-centred practice through the wide range of people and situations available for these contacts. However, if care workers only interacted with a set team of the same colleagues around the same sorts of task every day (because of the way shift patterns and role boundaries were organised), then learning opportunities could be limited.

- *Observing others* was distinct from 'being shown' as it was unofficial and the worker chose who to learn from based on whether the observed practice was successful in achieving 'what works' and their own opinion of the worker. Therefore, personal relationships were important in influencing the learning that occurred. As with 'asking for advice', this appeared to result in more flexible practice and person-centred care when there was a broader range of people and situations for care workers to learn from.

- *Communication* in the homes sent implicit messages to be integrated into the 'what works is what matters' learning process by setting out expectations and boundaries of care work through written documents (care plans, memos, notices, etc.), management talk (phrases used to describe care work), and team talk (day-to-day conversation). Communication was also via shorthand, which occurred whenever a task or resident was communicated about in a non-literal way (e.g. 'I'm going to *do* Mr Jones' instead of 'I am going to help Mr Jones get out of bed'). To understand shorthand, a worker referred to previous experiences and understanding. Shorthand thus formed a powerful and influential way of learning throughout a team because it communicated meaning and values. Most importantly, shorthand seemed to work against person-centred practice unless it was regularly interspersed with more descriptive or literal language that made explicit what was represented by the shorthand.

Element 3: Training

The final area describing how care workers learn to care concerns formal training. It was not as significant in influencing practice as the previous two elements and its influence was as a component of cultural knowledge that workers drew on within the 'what works is what matters' process. There were three particular ways that training had an effect on practice in the study care homes:

- *Gatekeeper tasks* were specific tasks that required hands-on training, without which you could not act as a care worker. These 'gatekeeper tasks' involved moving people (applicable for all care workers) and medication administration (for senior staff only). However, learning gained through training could still be replaced by informal learning when the option of contradicting training advice 'worked' from the staff's member's perspective. This highlights that the effect of training on practice is dependent on that being reinforced by other mechanisms of learning.

- *Knowing the job, not care* reflected aspects of training that care workers identified were relevant to doing the job of care worker, but not to the act of caring itself. Training was therefore important in relation to being allowed to be a care worker, but not necessarily connected to the factors that made someone good at caring. Despite the use of different types of training, it was often viewed by both workers and management as something disconnected from the day-to-day realities of practice and therefore something to get past in order to focus on hands-on caring.

- *Application of training* was important for the potential impact of training on care home practice. The more sophisticated approach to training by management, such as care workers being paired together to attend sessions, training outcomes being revisited in supervision, and staff being encouraged to implement new ideas on return, tended to result in more person-centred practice in the home. However, this required active work by management, without which changes to practice were not guaranteed.

This study showed how interconnected different types of informal learning are with each other and with formal training. It is a complex system, in which different aspects interact within the care home itself to affect the type of practice that results. The same system of learning can produce very different practice depending on the care home in which it takes place. Therefore, interventions to influence the outcomes of learning must acknowledge that complexity and the role of context, otherwise they may be undermined by other parts of the system. This will be discussed further in Chapter 4 (in which we address training and learning in the care home sector specifically, making recommendations from this study) and Chapter 9 (in which we discuss the implications of organisational culture for training and education efforts).

Summary

Throughout this chapter, a broader view of learning has been introduced, highlighting the many ways learning can take place outside of conventional training. An argument has been made that the current focus of training and education in dementia care is too narrow and misses many valuable opportunities to influence practice towards person-centred care. The different types of informal learning have been discussed, highlighting research from a broad workplace learning field that may have relevance to dementia care as well as a unique study establishing the interrelation between formal and informal learning within a particular setting. Practice recommendations related to each type of informal learning have been given. It is hoped that this will help practitioners and researchers alike to see the potential available when opening up a view of learning beyond traditional training and education.

Implications for those delivering dementia training

Those leading and facilitating dementia training should:

- Acknowledge the influence of informal learning on practice and help learners to understand the mechanisms through which their and others' practice is influenced in the workplace and during day-to-day interactions and conversation.
- Include content to build skills that influence informal learning: reflective practice, providing effective feedback, problem-solving, trial and error, and drawing on tacit knowledge.
- Support organisations to understand learning beyond training. If a conventional training programme was accompanied by just one action in a service to meet the recommendations for each type of informal learning made in this chapter, the influence on practice would multiply.

Implications for managers in dementia care settings and services

Managers in dementia care settings and services should:

- Recognise the extensive influence of informal learning on practice and consider how the organisation of work tasks and teams in the workplace can structure the learning opportunities available to staff. Ensure this informal 'curriculum' is person centred in what it teaches.

- Create time and space for reflective practice on a regular basis. Skill and support senior staff to facilitate this throughout the team.
- Ensure that feedback given to staff is frequent and empowering and helps them to identify the specific knowledge and actions which contribute to person-centred practice.

Implications for staff providing care, services, or support to people living with dementia

Staff working in dementia care should:

- Think about the language used to talk about the work and people living with dementia. Remember that language transmits underlying meanings as well as literal descriptions and instructions.
- Create time and space to reflect on your own practice and encourage others to do so as well. Taking time to think about what went well/badly and why, creates the chance for learning to take place.
- Think about and maximise the way that residents' own feedback is used to reflect on practice. Creating a positive relationship with someone is the focus of person-centred care, so whether the relationship is working or not matters.

Implications for those directly affected by dementia

Those directly affected by dementia are integral to informal learning processes in dementia care. To maximise the benefit of this it is suggested that everyone should:

- Provide frequent opportunities for staff to build relationships with those directly affected by dementia whom they support.
- Maximise the person's perspective in feedback given to staff, whether this is from the person themselves directly or through means such as observation and interpretation of behaviour.
- Enable staff to see the 'big picture': how all roles and tasks in a setting contribute to the experience of the person living with dementia.
- Actively build mutual trust, respect, and good communication between family members and staff, to ensure their perspectives are integrated into feedback.

4 Learning and development in care homes

> 'There is a risk that care home dementia training is hard to navigate, resulting in wasted resources, contradictory initiatives, confusion and short termism.'

Care homes are unique care settings that, whilst differing across the world, form a crucial part of the system of care available for people living with dementia and their supporters, particularly once a person is unable to live independently and in-home support is no longer sufficient. Known internationally by a variety of terms (long-term care, aged care, nursing homes, residential care, etc.), they are charged with providing 24-hour care, most often over the last years of a person's life. Care homes support a diverse group of people with varied support needs whilst simultaneously aiming to provide a 'home-like' environment within a communal setting. The provision of specific medical services in addition to help with activities of daily living and social support within care homes varies according to national arrangements and registration of services (with some – nursing homes – providing in-house nursing care and others relying on health care from the community). Regardless, the international reality over the last two decades has been a drastic increase in the complexity of the care provided by care homes of all types, primarily because of the increase in dementia-related needs of their residents. In the UK, approximately 39 per cent of people living with (later-onset) dementia reside in care homes, constituting approximately 70 per cent of the care home population in 2013, a rise of 10 per cent from the previous decade (Matthews et al. 2013; Prince et al. 2014). Of those living with dementia in care homes in England, 80 per cent have severe dementia (Wittenberg et al. 2019a). Severe dementia is set to more than double in the general population by 2040 (Wittenberg et al. 2019b), meaning that care homes will continue to care for people with this high level of need.

The care home's dual function of providing both a home and increasingly complex care means that it occupies a crucial and unusual space in terms of providing person-centred care: a space where the person living with dementia, their neighbouring residents (both with and without dementia), the care home's workforce, those important to the person living with dementia, the local community, and the wider health care system all meet and need long-term coordination by the care home to achieve the best outcomes for individuals. This is a challenge not faced by any other service or workforce. Moreover, whilst workforce requirements and composition vary internationally, a large proportion of the workforce in care homes in the UK, and in many other countries, is made up of paraprofessional staff. Both these factors have implications for the achievement of person-centred care and the ways in which training and education can support this goal.

This chapter will first discuss the evidence related to the needs and opportunities of nurses and leaders within care homes, as distinct roles within the sector. It will then move to explore the range of evidence-based person-centred dementia training interventions available for staff in the sector before moving on to discuss the facilitators and barriers of successful training interventions. Unique research exploring the nature of informal learning for dementia care in care homes will also be illustrated, allowing discussion of the interconnection between formal and informal means of learning within this sector. Throughout, the implications for the involvement of people living with dementia and the consequences for person-centred care will be discussed.

Needs and opportunities for nurses and managers

In Chapter 1, we discussed the frameworks and qualification pathways in place for many health and social care roles involved in dementia care in the UK and across the world. Where these exist, there is generally overlap across sectors, even when training and research may be sector specific. Nevertheless, there is a growing understanding of the distinct nature of the nurse and/or manager role within a care home, setting it apart from counterparts in other sectors. Therefore, we will now address the training evidence base specifically related to these roles within care homes.

Nurses in care homes

In most countries, nurses form a part of the care home workforce. The specific roles and proportion of qualified nursing staff to paraprofessional staff in care homes is determined by governmental and regulatory requirements. This results in care homes staffed similarly to acute hospitals in some countries and in others staffed predominantly or exclusively by non-nursing staff. However, in a large proportion of care homes the interaction between the qualified and paraprofessional workforce is a significant feature, with implications for the design and implementation of training. Training of nurses is addressed in Chapter 6. However, there are some specific issues of relevance to the nurse workforce within care homes because nurses are often in positions that greatly influence care ethos and the ways in which paraprofessionals carry out practice. The Queen's Nursing Institute identifies 'teaching the unregulated workforce' as a key responsibility of the care home nurse (Queen's Nursing Institute 2021).

A survey of 350+ registered nurses in the UK showed that nursing degrees did not adequately prepare nurses for care home work (Cooper et al. 2017), primarily because they favour training placements within acute health care settings. Taken together with the lack of dementia specialism within pre-registration training in the UK as noted in Chapter 1, this suggests that education for continuing professional development (CPD) is a vital component of skilling nurses for dementia care within care homes. The Queen's Nursing Institute (2021) created the first set of educational recommendations for nurses new to the care home sector in England, designed to help registered nurses transition into the sector and support their competency-based revalidation (see Box 4.1). These standards are generic but contain specific criteria of relevance to dementia care. In addition, they foreground the responsibilities of the nurse in facilitating learning for others in the home. This is a promising, if small, development as it appears to recognise the dual role a care home nurse will play in leading person-centred care, providing dementia specialist skills but also facilitating learning – an aspect of practice requiring explicit expertise that has long been ignored.

Box 4.1 The Queen's Nursing Institute Standards of Education and Practice for Nurses New to Care Home Nursing 2021

These standards for England were developed by the Queen's Nursing Institute and Skills for Care in partnership with care home providers and commissioners. They were designed to support nurses' professional development and curriculum development within higher education.

The standards create a set of benchmarks that can be used to assess the skills and knowledge required by a registered nurse in a care home setting in the UK.

They are presented within four domains, with each domain consisting of several specific standards:

1 Clinical care (13 standards)
2 Leadership and management (14 standards)
3 Facilitation of learning (5 standards)
4 Evidence, research, and development (6 standards)

The standards are mostly generic so that they can be applied to a range of care specialisms. However, of particular note to dementia care are the following:

Standard 1.3: Demonstrate effective planning, implementation and evaluation of person-centred care, understanding the presenting connection between physical health issues and mental health problems.

Standard 1.8: Demonstrate an understanding of Kitwood's personhood model and person-centred care for people with dementia and other models which support person-centred care.

Of particular note to the issue of training is the inclusion of a specific domain related to the facilitation of learning:

Standard 3.1: Apply ... and assimilate the roles of Practice Supervisor and Practice Assessor within the Care Home nursing learning environment.

Standard 3.2: Use creative problem-solving to develop a positive teaching/learning environment that will enhance the development of nursing students, nurse associates and the wider care home team. Evaluate the impact of educational interventions for students, nurse associates, care workers, residents and families.

Standard 3.3: Demonstrate the values of compassionate nursing and support the ongoing development of these values in others.

Standard 3.4: Demonstrate non-judgemental and value-based care to promote a culture of openness and recognition of the duty of candour in which each resident is valued and all staff support and develop a shared purpose to deliver high-quality effective care.

Standard 3.5: Provide educational information to families enabling them to support the care you are providing within the Care Home. (Queen's Nursing Institute 2021)

Elsewhere in the world, state laws in the USA require dementia-specific training for licenced nurses in only two states, although certified nursing assistants (who assist with specified nursing tasks and undergo competency assessment) have stipulated requirements in 24 of 50 states, addressing dementia-specific communication, understanding behaviour and management techniques, and reducing the effects of cognitive impairment (Burke and Orlowski 2015b). As in the UK, this suggests a developing awareness of the need for specialist dementia skills, but a lack of consistency in application and an over-reliance on pre-registration training and individual nurses to identify and source their own CPD needs.

The need for further consideration of dementia-specific standards and requirements for care home nurses is emphasised by the few research studies exploring nurses' learning needs in various European countries. Dementia and person-centred care is identified as a learning need regardless of the specific type of service (Cooper et al. 2017) and within dementia-specific learning needs, managing challenging behaviour, supporting families, and managing pain are commonly identified topics (Attard et al. 2020; Bolt et al. 2020; Smythe et al. 2017). Staff shortages and lack of time are commonly cited barriers to CPD for nurses (Cooper et al. 2017; Smythe et al. 2017).

Managers and leaders in care homes

The training requirements and opportunities for management and leadership roles in care homes reflect the variation in service type and regulation across the world, with some requiring managers to be registered nurses in order to undertake the role. In England, similar to other UK nations, registered care home managers should hold or be working towards an appropriate qualification (Care Quality Commission 2015), which includes units on person-centred practice and (optional) units on 'leading and managing dementia care services'. In addition, mandatory units include exploration of learning culture and supporting team development (City and Guilds 2016). This is evidence of recognition of the specialist skills required to lead care homes both in dementia care and through facilitating others' learning, at least for those managers who opt for qualification through this route. However, the regulation of managers' ongoing fitness to practise does not include specific CPD requirements (Care Quality Commission 2015). In the USA, 15 of 50 states have laws requiring dementia-specific training for administrators of nursing homes and assisted living facilities, with most of these states regulating the training standards for assisted living facilities. All require CPD for administrators, although only some specify dementia-specific CPD hours (Burke and Orlowski 2015b).

The role of leadership in facilitating implementation of person-centred care practice will be discussed in more detail in Chapter 9, but it is notable that very little research has addressed the specific dementia education needs of care home managers or interventions for the group specifically, especially when compared to the volume of research into training interventions overall. Only one small-scale qualitative study examined a programme specifically for care home managers, although this was not dementia-specific. The My Home Life leadership programme enabled 15 manager participants from Northern Ireland care homes to develop skills and improve relationships with staff, families, and residents as intended (Ryan et al. 2018).

The lack of research in this area, together with the acknowledged importance of leadership to achieving person-centred care suggests a significant gap in understanding. Further exploration of dementia care learning needs of managers would be worthwhile to identify any specific interventions for this group and describe their distinct roles within the process of transferring learning from education and training into practice.

Formal education and training for care homes

We outlined the range and variation in dementia care training frameworks and qualifications that exist for those working in care homes in Chapter 1. In this section, we will address the current evidence base for training and education programmes for this sector.

The most notable thing about formal education across the care home sector is the sheer volume of training programmes and educational interventions that exist, alongside an almost permanent rhetoric on the need for more training. It is hard to find a research study or report addressing dementia care in care homes that does not contain a recommendation for increased training, regardless of the specific subject under discussion. This is a mixed blessing. Whilst it is an improvement on the lack of attention experienced by the sector just a few decades ago and demonstrates a welcome recognition of the skilled, complex work carried out by care homes, there is a risk that the field is hard to navigate for many practitioners and organisations, resulting in wasted resources, contradictory training initiatives, confusion, and short-termism. A number of strategies to address this from an organisational point of view are discussed in Chapter 9, where we discuss what organisational resources are required to ensure effective use of training, and in Chapter 10, where we address how organisations can effectively drive practice change.

In addition, within Chapter 2 we outlined the features of impactful dementia training delivery overall, based on a large-scale review of evaluated programmes (Surr et al. 2017a). These are summarised in Boxes 2.5–2.9, including an audit tool which can be used to assess the quality of training available (Surr et al. 2017b). This is highly relevant to the care home sector, especially given the range of unevaluated training programmes available to the sector. It provides a means through which an organisation or commissioner can review or plan a programme based on what is known to produce successful outcomes. This large-scale review included a collective case study of three care home provider organisations' experiences of dementia training to establish the features of impactful training specifically within this sector. The findings are summarised in Box 4.2 (Surr et al. 2019b).

Box 4.2 The features of effective and valued dementia training in care home organisations

Design and delivery
- Bespoke designed for the care home/organisation and tailored to the job role of leaners.
- Tailored to specific learners' needs.
- Delivered face to face, avoiding the use of self-study workbooks/paperwork.
- Delivered using interactive methods.
- Delivered by experienced facilitators.
- Opportunities provided to reflect on learning.

Positive impacts commonly included:
- *Staff*: improved empathy, knowledge, and recognition of individual needs.
- *Staff–resident interactions*: increased levels of activity, improved communication, less task-focused care, and increased resident well-being.

However, positive aspects of care and resident well-being were not consistently seen across all care homes and residents, even in care homes self-selecting for a positive experience and impact of training. This suggests that training does not provide a complete answer to issues of quality PCC care.

Building on this, we will now explore the evidence emerging from the latest international research on formal training initiatives in care home dementia care, identifying the issues of most significance within this sector specifically. Simply identifying the range of topics covered by published evaluated dementia care training interventions from the last 5 years reveals the breadth of specialism expected within care homes, unparalleled in other sectors. Table 4.1 lists these topics.

Table 4.1 Topics addressed by evaluated dementia-specific training programmes

Topic	Study references
Person-centred care and general dementia knowledge (comprehensive programmes sometimes linked to a particular focus)	**Focus on antipsychotic reduction:** • WHELD: Ballard et al. (2018, 2020), Fossey et al. (2019, 2020) • HALT: Aerts et al. (2019), Chenoweth et al. (2018), Jessop et al. (2017) • FITS into Practice: Brooker et al. (2015), Latham and Brooker (2017) **Focus on Dementia Care Mapping:** Griffiths et al. (2019), Surr et al. (2018b, 2019a, 2021) **No specific focus:** Dobbs et al. (2018), Gleason et al. (2019), Inker et al. (2020), McKay et al. (2021), Reinhardt et al. (2020), Rokstad et al. (2017), Scerri and Scerri (2019), Sheaff et al. (2018), Smythe et al. (2020), Yasuda and Sakakibara (2017)
Distress behaviour/ responding to challenging behaviours	Fukuda et al. (2018), Karlin et al. (2017), Keenan et al. (2020), Lichtwarck et al. (2019a, 2019b), Moniz-Cook et al. (2017)
Reducing restraint	Abraham et al. (2019), Dahl et al. (2018), Jacobsen et al. (2017), Kong et al. 2017), Testad et al. (2016)
Advance care planning	Goossens et al. (2019), Katwa et al. (2020), Sævareid et al. (2018, 2019)
End-of-life/palliative care	Di Giulio et al. (2019), Verreault et al. (2018)
Psychoeducation of staff	Barbosa et al. (2017), Elpers et al. (2017)
Pain assessment/treatment	Brunkert et al. (2019), Kutschar et al. (2020), Petyaeva et al. (2018)
Reviewing medication	Gerritsen et al. (2021)
Namaste care	Kaasalainen et al. (2019)
Validation therapy	Oliveira and Sousa (2020)
Oral health	Deutsch et al. (2017)
Activity (varied focus)	Clark et al. (2017), Hurley et al. (2020), Tompkins et al. (2020)
Compassionate Touch	Han et al. (2020)
Communication skills	Williams et al. (2017, 2020)
Theatre for culture change	Guzmán et al. (2017a, 2017b)

This again highlights the skill required by the care home organisation to effectively navigate the range of programmes on offer and expectations placed on them, regardless of the training frameworks and requirements that may exist within the country or region. In an international review of dementia-specific training for nursing home staff published from 2006 to 2015, Riesch et al. (2018) identified that whilst some training topics recommended by contemporaneous UK guidelines and US recommendations were addressed well within evaluated training, some topics were not, such as family dynamics, palliative care, and the roles of different professionals. In addition, the majority of training evidence available demonstrated an improvement in staff knowledge and attitudes (the lower Level 2 'Kirkpatrick' outcomes discussed in Chapter 11) but were more varied on other, more sophisticated measures.

This variation emphasises the need for a better understanding of how care homes can identify quality, impactful training, and a need for better coordination and communication by researchers to support translation of findings into the real world of care home dementia care: it takes more than a published study. Further reviews addressing specific types of dementia training conclude with the need for more thorough explanation of how interventions are applied in practice (Faraday et al. 2019; Keane et al. 2020).

The wide variety of educational interventions developed and evaluated internationally in the last 5 years demonstrates a continued desire for an educational 'solution' to achieving quality dementia care in care homes. However, the increasingly sophisticated nature of some interventions and the exploration of longer-term outcomes and experience of implementation help to shine a light on the likely complexity of this solution and the need for a much broader and coordinated outlook in the future. Bauer et al. (2018) reviewed international training interventions for impact on functional quality of life for people living with dementia and concluded that the most successful programmes included multifaceted components (e.g. management support, monitoring of practice, reviewed policy, implementation of specific tools) in addition to education. Therefore, one of the simplest ways to organise the variety of evaluated initiatives available is to separate those which use a 'training-only' approach (the intervention is the delivery of training *only* using various methods) from those which use a 'training-plus' approach (the intervention includes the delivery of training, but also other components that enable and reinforce learning and practice change within the workplace). These two categories will be discussed in turn, drawing out the significant lessons for the care home sector that add to the findings summarised in Box 4.2.

Training-only interventions

Evaluated training-only initiatives vary greatly according to topic focus, with some addressing specific needs and others focusing broadly on general dementia knowledge and person-centred care. Given our growing understanding about the impact of different training delivery methods, these will be addressed according to primary method of delivery.

Face-to-face training including experiential learning

Interventions using a training-only approach most often adopt face-to-face delivery methods with a range of staff from within the care home and with courses varying substantially in length. Training focused on a specific topic such as behaviours that challenge or end-of-life care (Di Giulio et al. 2019; Fukuda et al. 2018) is generally shorter in duration than training addressing person-centred care as a whole (Scerri and Scerri 2019; Yasuda and Sakakibara 2017), which lasts multiple days and can be delivered all at once or across months-long structured programmes (Rokstad et al. 2017). Internationally, these studies show that, regardless of topic or length, such training produces basic but positive impacts on staff-reported confidence, knowledge, and attitudes to dementia and person-centred care (Fukuda et al. 2018; Kaasalainen et al. 2019; Rokstad et al. 2017; Scerri and Scerri 2019). This may reflect that basic awareness of dementia remains low in the rapidly changing workforce of the care home sector across the world, and thus even short training is likely to improve staff outcomes at Kirkpatrick Level 2 (knowledge, attitudes, and confidence).

However, it is important not to overstate the assumption that improved staff outcomes at this level automatically equate to improved person-centred care and outcomes for residents through staff behaviour (Kirkpatrick Level 3) or wider impacts for staff in areas such as stress or burnout (Kirkpatrick Level 4). There are many factors external to staff that affect practice and thus focusing only on Level 2 outcomes, although simpler, provides only limited insight into the effectiveness of training.

A few training-only programmes evaluate the impact on residents and show positive effects. For example, training focused on end-of-life care for people living with dementia in 29 Italian nursing facilities resulted in a significant increase in comfort-hydration and palliative approaches to eating and drinking for residents (Di Giulio et al. 2019). Person-centred care training, tailored to feedback obtained from Dementia Care Mapping observations in a Japanese facility, resulted in an increase in well-being for all 40 residents (Yasuda and Sakakibara 2017). However, only one study using face-to-face training considered any impact beyond the immediate end of the training, demonstrating a maintenance of staff impact for a 24-month period following a person-centred training intervention (Rokstad et al. 2017). Considering the long-term impact of training is essential for the care home sector, especially given the high turnover of staff, and thus it is hard to draw significant insights from training-only programmes using face-to-face methods that have not explored their effectiveness over the longer-term.

Moreover, details of the delivery methods used in these training-only programmes are not always specified, meaning that there is no opportunity to further explore the effectiveness of particular strategies. However, one small study demonstrates the possibilities that could arise from rethinking the way that much face-to-face training is designed. McKay et al. (2021) compared a dementia training programme delivered using a 'skills-based' (SB) design (a traditional approach which relies on an individual learning new knowledge and applying it themselves in practice) with the impact of the same programme delivered using an 'occupational adaptation' (OA) approach. In OA, the delivery of training focuses on facilitating teams to better identify, analyse, and solve problems. Twenty-eight staff from a US retirement community undertook the same hours of training, with some receiving it as SB (via watching films and question-and-answer sessions) and others as OA (attending weekly facilitated sessions to find solutions to challenging cases). Those participating in OA showed significant improvement on measures of problem-solving and team development compared with SB. Observations and interviews also suggested that OA participants outperformed those who had received SB (by demonstrating increased questioning, team involvement, contributions to problem-solving, and resolving challenges). OA participants were much more likely to refer to teamwork and resolving challenges as core parts of their work than those who undertook the more traditional SB-style training (McKay et al. 2021). This highlights that the way that training is delivered (and the understanding of person-centred care that underlies it) has the potential to impact on outcomes, and that innovation is needed in both design and evaluation of formal training to be able to develop interventions that are impactful.

Simulation methods (including role-play)

A few training-only programmes use simulation methods as the primary method of education delivery. For example, a UK **advanced care planning** in dementia intervention was taught by successive rounds of role-play with actors and expert facilitators, resulting in increased confidence and understanding of the intervention for the 28 staff participants (Katwa et al. 2020). However, most often, when simulation is used it is alongside other training methods, making it impossible to identify the impact of simulation alone. In a worldwide review of training using simulation, Keane et al. (2020) highlight that role-play simulation (as opposed to technologically enhanced simulation methods such as manikin use) appears to be particularly favoured in dementia care programmes, especially with regards responding to distress behaviours. This is likely because of the value of body language in such interactions and the inappropriateness of using residents themselves to trial different approaches. However, reviewers noted the reliance on staff report and self-completed measures for determining results and the lack of research more generally in this area (Keane et al. 2020).

Case example: Using reflection, in-practice exercises, and role-play to develop empathy and appropriate caring attitudes in care home staff

A dementia care centre in Hong Kong that provides specialist dementia training has developed a reflective training programme to support staff working in care homes. The programme aims to develop an appropriate caring attitude and person-centred practice skills. The programme has the experiences of people living with dementia at its centre and develops a concept of 'DemenTitude®' (Man Chui and Lam 2019).

The programme contains six sessions delivered over 3 months, with each session lasting around an hour. It is suitable for all staff working in the organisation. The sessions are as follows:

Session 1 discusses the person-centred care approach and invites learners to share their perception of people living with dementia and their experiences of care in their workplace.

Session 2 focuses on the concept of personhood and on good communication skills. As part of the session learners will be asked to observe the experiences of and/or ask people living with dementia about their experiences of care and their environment.

Session 3 involves learners feeding back their collected information and the main messages about experiences of people living with dementia are shared and summarised by the facilitators. Learners are encouraged to reflect on any differences between their own perceptions shared in Session 1 and those gathered as part of Session 2.

Session 4 involves the facilitator undertaking role-play and scenario-building exercises to help learners feel how people living with dementia may experience difficulties in daily life. Videos related to 'dementia from the inside' are also used to facilitate reflection. The session also discusses dementia-inclusive language within the local context, and some key cultural questions about views of people living with dementia and dementia care provision are shared and discussed to help learners to develop an enhanced caring attitude.

Session 5 with the understanding of self-perception of people living with dementia gained during previous sessions, learners are encouraged in this session to consider how they can change their caring approach towards people living with dementia with alternative approaches based on person-centred care being presented and discussed. They are given an in-practice activity to complete after the session, which involves putting a new person-centred approach into practice, which they have to report their experiences of in the final session.

Session 6 the learners share their experiences of implementing the new approach and the differences they experienced in doing

> so. They are asked to commit to applying the person-centred care approach and a person-centred caring attitude in their future practice
>
> The training is currently being evaluated, with outcomes such as learners' appropriate caring attitude and their understanding of the person-centred care approach in dementia care being the focus.

Online methods

A number of studies, all from the USA, have established qualified success of online education for care workers and other care home staff addressing general person-centred care for dementia (Dobbs et al. 2018; Gleason et al. 2019; Inker et al. 2020) or specific topics such as use of music (Tompkins et al. 2020). However, all of these studies focus on relatively small groups and staff measures at Kirkpatrick Level 2 to judge effectiveness. Only one study was able to compare the results of online training with a comparable face-to-face version. The Changing Talk (CHAT) programme focused on use of communication to reduce resistiveness to care for residents living with dementia. The online version (CHATO) produced similar results of significant increases in knowledge and demonstrated ability to identify poor communication strategies in staff from seven nursing homes in the USA (Williams et al. 2017, 2020).

In contrast, a large **randomised controlled trial (RCT)** of online training to support management of distress behaviour in 63 UK care homes found no significant impact in relation to resident measures of neuropsychiatric symptoms or secondary measures related to quality of life, health, or medication. This led the authors to conclude that they may have miscalculated the accessibility and appropriateness of the online delivery (Keenan et al. 2020; Moniz-Cook et al. 2017). These opposing findings might suggest that, if online delivery is considered, it should be developed from an established and effective training programme and that learners' access and acceptance of the format needs to be addressed within development.

Overall, currently, whilst online approaches may have advantages for the care home sector in terms of reach and cost (and practicality during the COVID-19 pandemic), it is important that they are developed in awareness of the evidence and evaluated to examine both resident-focused and long-term outcomes. Otherwise, there is a real risk that research into online training will simply repeat the mistakes of the past by failing to understand the complexity of the care home sector and the only-partial role that training can play in changing practice. Across the last decade there has been a significant shift away from training-only interventions of all kinds, in favour of more complex interventions designed to deliver education *and* actively support implementation. This trend is in response to increasing recognition of the complexity involved in changing practice outcomes and the limited usefulness of research that overly simplifies training provision and impact.

Training-plus: Multi-component interventions to improve dementia care

Training-plus interventions recognise that training alone does not go far enough in supporting implementation of learning within a care home. Thus, they include elements that aim to enable and reinforce implementation during the course of the intervention period, with the aim that these will embed learning well enough to continue once the initial impetus has disappeared. Evaluated training-plus initiatives vary greatly, with some focusing on specific topics and others on comprehensive person-centred care programmes. This again demonstrates the range of specialisms care homes are expected to deliver within their dementia care. These interventions most often use resident outcomes as measures of success, committed as they are to examining the implementation of learning to practice.

Educational components within training-plus interventions

Successful training-plus interventions are more likely to demonstrate the features of impactful training design identified within Chapter 2 and Box 4.2, whether they deliver education about person-centred care overall or a specific topic within dementia care. The most commonly identifiable features are as follows:

- designed for the specific learners' job roles (Ballard and Corbett 2020; Brunkert et al. 2019; Gerritsen et al. 2021; Goossens et al. 2019; Jessop et al. 2017; Latham and Brooker 2017; Lichtwarck et al. 2019a; Oliveira and Sousa 2020; Reinhardt et al. 2020; Sævareid et al. 2018, 2019; Verreault et al. 2018);
- introduce structured tools for practical use (Ballard and Corbett 2020; Brunkert et al. 2019; Jessop et al. 2017; Latham and Brooker 2017; Lichtwarck et al. 2019a; Sævareid et al. 2019; Verreault et al. 2018);
- apply learning and tools to real-life cases and problem-solving from learners' own care homes (Ballard and Corbett 2020; Brunkert et al. 2019; Jessop et al. 2017; Latham and Brooker 2017; Lichtwarck et al. 2019a, 2019b; Oliveira and Sousa 2020);
- training for at least 8 hours in total, and individual sessions are of at least 2 hours' duration (Jessop et al. 2017; Latham and Brooker 2017; Oliveira and Sousa 2020; Reinhardt et al. 2020);
- use facilitators experienced in the setting, dementia care, and training (Ballard and Corbett 2020; Goossens et al. 2019; Jessop et al. 2017; Latham and Brooker 2017).

With regards to training delivery methods, a few successful training-plus interventions from Northern Europe utilise role-play as a significant component of the educational element (Goossens et al. 2019; Lichtwarck et al. 2019b; Sævareid et al. 2019). Notably, all three of these interventions apply highly structured role-play to a specific issue – advanced care planning (Goossens et al. 2019; Sævareid et al. 2019) and responses to agitation (Lichtwarck et al. 2019b) – suggesting that well-managed role-play may be especially useful to practise pre-formulated structured processes.

No recent training-plus interventions included the use of simulation methods beyond role-play and none used only e-learning approaches. Blended training was used to contrasting effect within two RCT studies. Kong et al. (2017) combined restraint reduction training with in-house expert consultations for Korean nursing homes and demonstrated statistically significant improvements, but on Kirkpatrick Level 2 staff outcomes only. However, in a German study combining pain management training with the introduction of pain-specialist roles in care homes, there was no effect on resident outcomes, with the authors identifying a lack of individualised interventions for pain as a factor in failure, suggesting the training content (rather than format) did not enable the right tools to be applied (Kutschar et al. 2020).

Additional components in training-plus interventions

It is important to consider the additional components included as part of these training-plus interventions to ensure that their effect is not subsumed within the training elements. These extra components are included with the specific aim of improving implementation, and usually in recognition of past failure of interventions to take hold or training to change practice. These extra components vary substantially between interventions (with many using several at once). Overall, they provide extra opportunities, support, and/or incentives to put learning into practice as part of the intervention itself, rather than solely relying on training to support intervention implementation. The most commonly used additional components within successful interventions are listed in Table 4.2.

These additional components are important because they potentially change the context within which the training is implemented, at least for the course of the researched intervention. It is possible that this change of context could be more significant in creating practice change than the training elements themselves. For example, it is not unreasonable to suggest that having an expert practitioner coaching staff or additional time available for specific staff to carry out certain tasks might facilitate change in practice irrespective of the training provided. This is not to suggest that training is not important, but that it may only be part of the picture contributing to success. Current research design and communication of findings does not generally consider the independent impacts of different elements within interventions. This is particularly significant when one considers the variation in impact seen across individual care homes within many studies, the challenges in implementing the intervention for many participating care homes, and the insight provided by unsuccessful interventions and studies exploring the experience of implementation.

Table 4.2 Common additional components used in addition to training in training-plus interventions

Intervention study	Components included in intervention (shaded area indicates component included in a particular intervention)				
	Use of 'champions' or similar within the care home. These are individuals receiving training and given responsibilities to implement the intervention and/or support the learning of other staff	**Provision of remote external support** for champions and/or all staff during the intervention either in person, by telephone or via e-mail, but not within the care home itself	**Facilitation of 'in-practice' assistance and coaching by external experts** within the care home itself as part of the intervention providing staff support but also tailored advice	**Introduction of specific assessments, tools, or documents** with reinforcement and auditing of their use in practice	**Organisational planning/change to support the intervention** such as action plans, separate leadership training, etc.
Jessop et al. (2017)	▓			▓	
Latham and Brooker (2017)	▓	▓			
Sævareid et al. (2018)	▓			▓	
Verreault et al. (2018)	▓	▓		▓	▓
Brunkert et al. (2019)	▓	▓			
Lichtwarck et al. (2019a)	▓	▓		▓	
Ballard et al. (2020)	▓	▓	▓		
Gerritsen et al. (2021)		▓		▓	▓
Goossens et al. (2019)			▓	▓	▓
Oliveira and Sousa (2020)			▓		
Reinhardt et al. (2020)					▓

Three interconnected issues provide food for thought for those concerned with training's role in improving person-centred care as a result:

Activating informal learning mechanisms

A significant way that the non-training components of these training-plus interventions could be affecting care home practice is through their influence on informal learning mechanisms. It is likely that measures introduced to aid the implementation of a particular approach could alter or activate these processes and thus have an impact above and beyond the training intervention itself. For example, introducing champions changes the members and interactions of the care home 'community of practice'; reinforcing the use of specific tools brings problem-solving and dilemmas that arise in the care home to conscious awareness; requiring focus on specific resident care issues changes the nature of relationships between staff and residents; and the use of expert coaching creates the space, time, and skills to facilitate reflective practice. These are not only factors that help put specific training into practice, they go beyond the features of impactful training design as identified in Chapter 2 and Box 4.3; they are also mechanisms that create opportunities for learning to occur at other times and in other ways. Essentially, what many of these additional components may be doing is formalising previously under-recognised and under-utilised (informal) learning processes occurring within the care home towards a specific outcome. Therefore, being able to explore and unpick the specifics of what is occurring creates the possibility of identifying, explaining, and replicating specific, effective informal mechanisms that influence practice regardless of the specific outcome desired.

However, this factor is rarely considered within evaluated training intervention studies at all, with any influence interpreted only within the frame of the training intervention itself. Only one intervention explicitly acknowledges the role of informal learning processes, describing the way in which a particular aspect of the 'TIME' intervention in Norwegian care homes (the use of regular case conferences led by trained nurse champions, to respond to resident agitation) resulted in a 'reflective learning process of learning how to learn at work' (Lichtwarck et al., 2019a, p.973) for those involved. It would be valuable for dementia care training and practice development generally to be able to distinguish the effective processes enabled by non-training components of these interventions from the specific intervention it is originally tied to. For example, would an appropriately resourced, structured case conference approach similar to that used in TIME be effective in improving other aspects of dementia care, such as increasing family engagement or meaningful activity? Moreover, this highlights that unpicking the 'how' of these processes may be particularly important when the uncertainty inherent to person-centred dementia care is acknowledged. Person-centred care needs to be adaptable and flexible, and so knowing *what* to do matters less than knowing *how* to work out what to do. Dealing with uncertainty has been identified as a need in scoping reviews addressing aspects of dementia care in care homes (Faraday et al. 2019).

Tailoring resources to educational outcomes

A second, significant way that the training-plus components change the context within which training is delivered for the care home is by enabling resources to be tailored specifically to the needs of the intervention; indeed, this is their explicit aim. Through allocating specific staff roles, protecting staff time, providing supervision, introducing new policies or processes, prompting assessments, initiating engagement of **multi-disciplinary** partners, encouraging managers to reinforce the use of particular paperwork, and so on, the care home's resources are organised to help achieve the desired outcomes. This is important for several reasons.

First, the marshalling of personnel, time, and other resources to affect care outcomes is the very essence of care home work and yet challenges with this are identified in every training intervention, whether as an explanation for the withdrawal of homes from an intervention, failure of homes to adequately implement the intervention, or as the cause of immediate or long-term failure or variable outcomes across participating homes (Aerts et al. 2019; Barbosa et al. 2017; Brunkert et al. 2019; Chenoweth et al. 2018; Fossey et al. 2019; Gerritsen et al. 2021; Goossens et al. 2019; Griffiths et al. 2019; Guzmán et al. 2017a; Keenan et al. 2020; Kutschar et al. 2020; Petyaeva et al. 2018; Surr et al. 2019b; Testad et al. 2016). This is regardless of country, type, or topic of training intervention, and despite the care homes actively opting into the expectations of the particular research project. This would suggest that achieving consistent and effective practice change for quality care may have more to do with adequate resourcing and appropriate management of those resources than it does to do with one particular input to those resources – education. Few studies, tied as they are to the exploration of education and training, have considered the consequences of these barriers outside of their effect on intervention implementation. The circumstances that result in poor adherence to an intervention are highly likely to affect the quality of care irrespective of training and on a long-term basis. Therefore, for care homes and those concerned with improving dementia care quality, establishing sufficient resources and strategies to support the effective use of existing resources should be the primary consideration when seeking to improve quality, rather than being addressed only after or through training.

Second, by enabling the tailoring of resources to intended outcomes, the training-plus intervention ensures scope for flexibility and adaptation of the intervention (or aspects of it) to individual care home circumstances. Dahl et al. (2018) explored this when tailoring a standardised training-only intervention designed to reduce restraint within a single Norwegian nursing home following a failed RCT of the programme (Testad et al. 2016). Successful impact was achieved by adding elements of bespoke training (based on needs identified by staff), facilitated discussions to improved staff interaction and confidence around restraint practice, day-to-day support with problem-solving, and reflection to apply learning from the training. Qualitative explorations suggested that these additional elements created the necessary conditions for positive impact because they ensured the intervention could fluctuate in response to three key factors: the staff's enthusiasm, their general workload, and the responses of the people living with dementia themselves to the intervention (because an intervention-learned solution could be successful one day but not the next). This suggests that both person-centred care and the care home are inevitably fluctuating situations and therefore any attempts to change practice and improve quality must enable a response to this fluctuation. The non-education components of training-plus interventions are what facilitate this responsiveness and thus increase the chance of successful outcomes.

Influencing (or not influencing) the culture of the care home

The final and perhaps most significant aspect of the care home context potentially altered by the additional elements of training-plus interventions is that of overall care home culture. This is discussed in depth in Chapter 9, but is important here because it is frequently highlighted as the 'x-factor' explanation for challenges in implementation, poor and variable outcomes to educational interventions, and reduction in long-term impacts (Aerts et al. 2019; Chenoweth et al. 2018; Fossey et al. 2019; Griffiths et al. 2019). Multi-component aspects of educational interventions may (perhaps unknowingly) address certain influencers of culture within the care home such as distribution of staff, boundaries of work roles, and leadership style in the name of facilitating implementation of learning into practice. However, this will result in very individualised outcomes for each participating care home depending on the acceptability of those influencers/ changes within its current culture, leading to failed temporary or long-term implementation depending on the care home's starting position.

For example, within care homes it has been identified that creating cultures towards positive care experiences requires addressing multiple elements at once rather than viewing change as a linear process (Brooker and Latham 2016; Killett et al. 2016). A multi-component education intervention may therefore tackle sufficient elements in some homes, but insufficient elements in another. This suggests that assessing the culture of the care home prior to an intervention is important, either to ascertain those care homes for which it will be most effective or to enable tailoring of the intervention towards specific care homes' needs. It also suggests that there may be prerequisites for care homes to truly benefit from training and that it cannot be seen as the single 'silver bullet' for correcting poor care cultures.

The findings from many of the training-plus interventions have enabled the initial identification of the building blocks for effectively using training in care homes by identifying common barriers and facilitators to effective implementation. These all point towards the need for an organisational approach to implementing such interventions.

Barriers and facilitators of successful training

Box 4.3 summarises the features of successful training-plus interventions, identifying not only the significant aspects of the intervention itself, but also the organisational and care home level features that enable success.

Box 4.3 The features of successful educational interventions

(in addition to training-specific factors outlined in Chapter 2)

The intervention itself

1 Includes multifaceted components in addition to education such as hands-on support, and auditing of practice.
2 Provides sufficient initial education and support to ensure key personnel (e.g. 'champions') feel confident and well-practised.
3 Is flexible enough to allow staff and facilitators to adapt the intervention to changing contexts in the home and with individual residents.
4 Includes availability of ongoing external support/advice for champions. In-house support is highly valued, particularly if it includes hands-on support with care.
5 Uses a model of having a 'champion' for the intervention within the staff group who has sufficient autonomy and authority.

Organisation and leadership of the intervention

1 There is an individual with dedicated responsibility for coordinating the intervention.
2 Alignment of priorities between organisational leadership and purpose of the intervention ensuring a top-down approach to change alongside the bottom-up approach instigated by the champions/specialists.
3 Organisational buy-in/no contradictory pressures (e.g. other changes).
4 Supportive ethos of organisation, e.g. active in supporting person-centred care and the aims of the intervention.

External relationships

1 Where intervention requires liaison with external actors (e.g. prescribers), support and authority to do this is provided within the intervention.
2 Alignment with local, regional, and national policy and guidance.

Care home factors

The *manager* of the care home is:

1 Present throughout the intervention.
2 Supports the aims of the intervention.
3 Able to see practical benefits of the intervention for the residents and care home.
4 Facilitates good communication throughout the team.
5 Active in support of person-centred care and the specific intervention (e.g. modifying work schedules, allocating time, enabling attendance at training, reinforcing care plan changes etc.)
6 Person-centred in their management behaviour (e.g. supportive of staff, accessible, proactive).

The *staff team* of the care home is:

7 Able to see practical benefits of the intervention for residents.
8 Sufficient for their daily work and stable (e.g. low turnover and sickness rates).
9 Able to work as a team and provide peer support in implementation.
10 Able and willing to take ownership of the approach.

Barriers to successful educational interventions obviously occur when sufficient facilitators are absent. However, it is worth noting that the following are by far the most frequently cited and most debilitating barriers experienced, leading to withdrawal from training, failure to implement, or limited success with implementation. These all point towards structural and resourcing issues within the care home sector as an important variable when considering the role for training in improving person-centred dementia care.

- Insufficient time for staff to complete their day-to-day tasks means that finding additional time to implement interventions and training is impossible for many. Often success results from staff using personal time and resources to complete implementation tasks, which is not a sustainable model (Barbosa et al. 2017; Fossey et al. 2019; Gerritsen et al. 2021; Griffiths et al. 2019; Kaasalainen et al. 2019; Latham and Brooker 2017; Surr et al. 2018a).

- Even when dedicated time/roles are supposed to be allocated for staff, separate from their day-to-day tasks, this does not occur because it is not facilitated and enforced by management and/or because daily workload and staffing levels do not allow it (Fossey et al. 2019; Griffiths et al. 2019; Kutschar et al. 2020; Latham and Brooker 2017; Surr et al. 2018a).

- Staff turnover in care homes is high, meaning that staffing levels are frequently problematic and that interventions relying on a few key individuals for implementation can easily be disrupted (Brunkert et al. 2019; Gerritsen et al. 2021; Goossens et al. 2019; Griffiths et al. 2019; Surr et al. 2018a).

- Lack of practical management support for the intervention means that organisational adjustment through communication, modifying work schedules, and empowering decision-makers does not occur. Implementation then fails not because of insufficient interventions but because management are not able to respond appropriately (Barbosa et al. 2017; Chenoweth et al. 2018; Griffiths et al. 2019; Guzmán et al. 2017a; Latham and Brooker 2017; Lichtwarck et al. 2019b; Petyaeva et al. 2018; Surr et al. 2018a).

- Organisational overload of a care home results in implementation being hindered by changes in, or conflicts with, other priorities (internal to and external to the organisation itself) and an increased workload on the care home and management to adapt to multiple changes at once. It also means statutory and regulatory requirements will always take priority (Abraham et al. 2019; Brunkert et al. 2019; Keenan et al. 2020).

Case example: Care homes using evidence-based training embedded within an organisational approach

A large care provider organisation with over 100 care homes in the UK has an organisation-wide dementia care strategy. In recent years, it has developed an accompanying training strategy that acknowledges both the need for evidence-based staff training, and an organisational focus to make that training effective in achieving and sustaining practice change.

Evidence-based training delivered by qualified professionals

In addition to a range of awareness-raising training available within the organisation, the organisation has committed to the evidence-based FITS into Practice programme (Brooker et al. 2015). This programme provides in-depth person-centred care training and ongoing support to designated champions within each care home. These staff are responsible for sharing their learning and implementing specific changes within their care homes. The provider is currently rolling out the programme to all its care homes. The champions are trained and supported by qualified dementia practice development coaches (DPDCs) employed by the care home provider organisation. These individuals, in addition to extensive experience in dementia care and training, have undertaken a master's level module focusing on the FITS into Practice approach.

These staff undertake the DPDC role alongside their existing role as 'Approach to Care' leads, which ensures they can tailor training to the needs of each care home. In addition, these roles have an existing remit to support person-centred practice in the homes by providing coaching support quality assurance, and by identifying and resolving barriers to implementation of person-centred care practice. This means the training is accompanied by the appropriate organisational focus and impact as well as focusing on staff.

As a result of this approach, additional training needs for managers have been identified. This training has been commissioned from the same university that delivers the FITS into Practice DPDC module so that coherence across programmes is maintained.

Thinking differently: The system of learning in care homes

As addressed in Chapter 3, informal learning opportunities within the workplace and daily work is a neglected area when considering the education of the dementia care workforce. In this chapter, we have highlighted that these informal processes may be significant (though often unacknowledged) within the success of training-plus interventions in care homes. In Chapter 3, we also shared the findings of one of the only studies examining how care workers in care homes learn to care for people living with dementia, presenting the 'system' of learning to care (Latham 2020). This illustrated: (1) the informal mechanisms of learning that influenced practice on a day-to-day basis; (2) how these interacted with formalised training in the care home; and (3) the way in which the system enables the 'culture' of the care home to play an influential role in learning and thus the outcomes of practice. Here we will share recommendations for how a care home might better influence their 'system' of learning towards person-centred dementia care.

For a discussion of the in-depth findings from this study, see Chapter 3. In summary, the system of learning to care in care homes identified three key elements for care workers that created a complex process through which practice was learned every day. Significantly, the same process could result in different practices being learned depending on the care home context. In this system, informal mechanisms of learning dominated the learning that occurred, interacting with each other, with formal attempts to influence learning (such as training) and with aspects of the care home culture to affect the outcomes of learning.

Recommendations for improving a care home's system of learning to care

The system of learning to care demonstrated in this small-scale study resonates strongly with the complexity revealed by training-plus interventions and the experiences of implementing them in practice. This would suggest that considering how to address the whole system of learning to care in a care home will be more effective in influencing person-centred outcomes than focusing on training alone. Moreover, recognising that much learning occurs continuously and often informally, highlights that effort should be directed towards what is already happening rather than introducing (and resourcing) something new. This enables the best use of resources in the care home and ensures that both formal efforts and informal dynamics are working together towards person-centred dementia care. There are two key areas to focus on so that a care home's system of learning to care will enhance person-centred care:

1 Creating a 'community of practice' in the care home that can maximise person-centred care.
2 Utilising informal learning mechanisms effectively towards person-centred care.

Boxes 4.4 and 4.5 contain recommendations for action to address these two areas in care homes.

Box 4.4 Recommendations for improving a care home's system of learning to care: Create the appropriate 'community of practice'

Consider culture
- Address definitions of 'success' in the care home overall: what is seen as a 'good result'? Does it relate to resident well-being or to achievement of certain tasks or expectations?

- Analyse how the organisation of work tasks and teams may impact what can be learned. Are opportunities to learn through performing work providing the broadest range of personnel and work types and promoting person-centred care?
- Enact the features of expansive learning environments (see Chapter 8) within the day-to-day functioning of the care home and wider organisation. How much does the day-to-day functioning of the care home facilitate discussion, reflection, consultation, etc.?

Organisation of staff

- Ensure that the organisation of staff's work and team enables them to work with a range of colleagues and experiences.
- Help staff to understand different roles and how they fit together to impact residents. Do care workers get to see the whole resident experience and understand how different roles contribute?
- Recognise the crucial role that senior instruction and shadowing can play in guiding person-centred care. Can more opportunities for feedback and reflection be created in day-to-day interactions?
- Improve the interpersonal skills of staff: communication, encouraging reflection, giving constructive feedback, etc. What characteristics are being rewarded with influence and promotion?

Role of residents

- Residents contribute to the learning environment. Assess the ways in which the organisation of work teams and tasks may affect the range of resident contact staff have. Do care workers get to experience residents in a variety of situations?
- Facilitate resident representation in feedback and reflective activities. How are outcomes for the residents articulated? How frequently are experiences of residents discussed and reviewed?
- Identify methods for observing and interpreting resident well-being and ill-being. Do staff have these skills for all residents? How and when are these interpretations used and discussed?
- Explicitly explore the challenges communal living poses for achieving person-centred care and support staff to negotiate them. When do staff encounter conflicts between different residents' needs and desires? How do they currently go about resolving them?

Box 4.5 Recommendations for improving a care home's system of learning to care: Utilise informal learning effectively

Connect formal and informal learning

- Push beyond minimum standards. How can you recognise and accredit the reflective, interpersonal, and dementia-specific skills you wish staff to develop?

- Ensure that training that determines when a person can officially 'be' a worker in the care home includes dementia-specific skills. What skills differentiate your care workers from others? Do these mirror person-centred care or only mandatory skills?
- Use the actions below to reinforce the desired message from formal training.

Reflection and feedback

- Maximise reflective opportunities in the home. Create in-work opportunities for reflection through time, space, routine events, and opportunities for feedback. What can be done every day to encourage reflection on tasks, problems, and resident experiences? What systems are in place to identify and respond to critical incidents?
- Skill certain individuals in the team with reflective, critical thinking and facilitation skills. Who in the home shows these abilities already? How can their influence be formalised in day-to-day interactions or after specific situations?
- Explicitly bring individual residents' experiences into discussion amongst staff. Is care work articulated according to completing tasks or resident outcomes?
- Assess how well resident interaction and behaviour are integrated into the way the home views and rewards success. How is 'success' talked about and rewarded day to day? How skilled are staff at interpreting resident well-being and ill-being?

Problem-solving and trial and error

- Identify the conflicting pressures negotiated by staff each day. Resolve those that are caused by structural factors such as organisation of work and work teams. When staff decide between different needs/pressures, are they able to choose a person-centred solution? If not, what needs to be in place to facilitate this?
- Encourage experimentation to improve outcomes for residents, where safe. How is negative knowledge (what not to do) from experimentation viewed and shared?

Language

- Address the language used to talk about care work in day-to-day interactions between staff. Address any shorthand that may transmit unintentional meanings rather than literally describe. If a new staff member hears staff-to-staff interactions, would they know what was communicated, or do they have to 'decode' the message?

Tacit knowledge

- Identify situations that occur where appropriate action is considered to be 'common sense' or is 'taken for granted'. Explore these further; what is meant by 'common sense'?
- When stand-out examples of good or poor practice occur, take time to reflect with individuals or teams as to why they occurred. What was their thought process? What opportunities exist to identify and draw out the tacit knowledge used by staff?

Summary

In this chapter, we have examined the needs of nurses, leaders, and paraprofessionals in care homes and addressed the wide range of evidence-based interventions that exist for care homes internationally. We have highlighted that whilst some lessons can be learned regarding the format of successful training, there is a need for more focus on outcomes for people living with dementia rather than the easier-to-assess staff measures. The biggest lesson points towards a need to think more broadly about learning and improving quality within the sector. The care home sector is primed to move this research and application forward, given the extent of training and training-plus interventions that already exist. Resourcing, effectively managing resources, and considering the impact of additional components of complex interventions on culture and informal learning, are areas that offer prospects to maximise the impact on person-centred care. In particular, there are several opportunities in which the role of people living with dementia themselves can be enhanced.

Implications for those delivering dementia training

Those leading and facilitating dementia training should:

- Seek to evaluate training effectiveness by focusing on higher-level outcomes related to resident well-being (Kirkpatrick Levels 3 and 4).
- Support commissioning organisations to review the whole learning system affecting care provision (e.g. resources, resource management, informal learning) rather than focus narrowly on training provision.
- Ensure that training is evidenced-based not only in terms of content and delivery methods but also additional components that enhance the effectiveness of implementation into practice (e.g. 'champion'-type roles, ongoing support, auditing of tools).

Implications for managers in dementia care settings and services

Managers in dementia care settings and services should:

- Guard against the view that training is a 'cure-all' for quality care issues. Training should be considered as part of an holistic review of the whole system affecting care provision.

- Be present and actively facilitative of the implementation of training within the workplace (e.g. protecting staff time, reorganising workloads, auditing use of tools, encouraging communication).
- Activate informal learning mechanisms within the care home environment such as recommended in Box 4.5.

Implications for staff providing care, services, or support to people with dementia

Staff working in dementia care should:

- Communicate the practical benefits for residents of training or other interventions to fellow staff in conversation and through demonstration.
- Contribute to good teamwork and provide support for peers who are implementing new interventions.
- Communicate to managers any factors in the care home which are preventing implementation of training or interventions such as environmental restrictions, contradictory guidance, or time pressures.
- Get to know residents' stories well and develop positive relationships with their family and friends so that their input is a key part of day-to-day practice and conversation with others.

Implications for those directly affected by dementia

To involve people directly affected by dementia everyone should:

- Ensure the purpose and benefits of training are articulated and measured in terms of impact on resident outcomes, not only staff outcomes.
- Increase the opportunities for resident and family/friend feedback to be integrated into the day-to-day informal learning of staff whether via direct means or indirect means such as observation.
- Enable staff to spend time with residents in a variety of different situations, times of day, and personal circumstances to encourage an holistic view of the person and how different parts of care home life affect them.
- Enable people living with dementia and their family/friends to share life stories and future goals as part of training and daily care.

5 | Learning and development in primary care

'Many of the services that have historically been specialist are in fact being provided in primary care. With enhanced opportunities for training in this setting there is hope that primary care staff can provide these services.'

Primary care is defined as first contact health care or continuing care provided for people in their communities by a range of professionals and paraprofessionals. For this reason, primary care is often seen as the 'front door' to health care services. Staff based in primary care have long been identified as being ideally positioned to respond to the needs of people living with dementia and those who support them as they are embedded in the community. A primary health care team in the UK will include people working in a range of roles, including doctors (or **general practitioners** (GPs)), nurses (including practice nurses, community/district nurses, nurse practitioners, palliative care and other specialist nurses), health care assistants, phlebotomists (who take blood), support staff (receptionists, secretaries, clerical staff), midwives, and health visitors. In the UK, primary care premises may also be used for secondary care services, including memory assessment services and allied health professional clinics such as physiotherapy, dietetics, podiatry, counselling, and so on. More recently, advanced care practitioners and physician associates (medical practitioners working with medical supervisors) have also been appointed to work in primary care in the UK. These roles are intended to provide more specialist care in multi-disciplinary teams under supervision.

The role of primary care for people living with dementia has often involved identifying and supporting people at points of crises or transition (into, for example, long-term care), as a point of referral to specialist services, or managing comorbid conditions. However, increasingly, primary care staff have also played a role in the assessment and diagnosis of people living with dementia (Wells and Smith 2017), despite this historically being a role associated with specialist services. In the UK, this work has been incentive driven, with financial incentives for primary care providers who complete an annual dementia review for people diagnosed with dementia, as mandated under the Quality and Outcomes Framework for practice (NHS England 2021). The annual dementia review requires that primary care staff provide data on advanced care planning and the future wishes of the patient.

Whatever the nature of the service provided, primary care staff are at the frontline in providing support for people directly affected by dementia, and this requires specialist skills and knowledge. For all primary care services, case-loads will include people living with dementia (or suspected dementia) and their informal caregivers. For example, in England, 43 people per 1,000 of the general population aged 65 years and over had a recorded diagnosis of dementia on their general practice primary care record in 2018 (Public Health England 2018). That being said, many people who are living with dementia do not have a formal diagnosis, so the number of people directly affected by dementia in contact with primary care staff is actually much higher. As an example, in the UK as of 31 February 2020 (prior to the COVID pandemic), only an estimated 67.6 per cent of people aged 65 or over who had dementia had a recorded diagnosis (NHS Digital 2021). In the US in 2018, it was estimated that 59 per cent of people with dementia either hadn't been diagnosed or were unaware of their diagnosis (Amjad et al. 2018).

Dementia-related services provided in primary care

Primary care staff can find themselves providing a wide range of services to people living with dementia or suspected dementia. Some of these services may be focused on the diagnosis and management of dementia, and some of these will be associated with the management of comorbid conditions. In both cases, staff are required to have the skills to communicate effectively with people living with dementia to involve them in decisions made about their care. Primary care services may include (but not be limited to):

- Screening or providing an assessment of cognitive impairment for onward referral or diagnosis.
- Conducting an annual dementia review of changes in cognition, changes in mood, or changes in level of need.
- Developing and contributing to care plans for people living with dementia.
- Ensuring that people are informed and aware of their future care options and rights.
- Providing advice about maintaining health and well-being to optimise outcomes for people living with dementia (e.g. diet, nutrition, exercise).
- Providing services to manage and treat comorbid conditions.
- Providing assessment and support for people to continue their everyday activities (e.g. occupational therapy or physiotherapy).
- Providing advice on continued activities such as driving.
- Offering support to people living with dementia in some long-term care facilities such as residential care homes.
- Providing palliative care and end-of-life care.

- Social prescribing for people living with dementia and their informal caregivers.
- Medication management, including prescribing and deprescribing.
- Providing advice, support, or treatment for managing non-cognitive changes in dementia (e.g. changes in behaviour and mood).

In fact, for a pathway of dementia care, such as the Well Pathway for Dementia described by NHS England and the National Collaborating Centre for Mental Health (NCCMH 2018), the phases of which are reproduced in Figure 5.1, primary care services are clearly relevant to the entire pathway – from diagnosis to end of life.

Furthermore, since primary care services are embedded in the community, this workforce is more likely than the wider dementia workforce to encounter people from minority communities, marginalised groups, and younger people living with dementia. The common misperception that people living with dementia are older and frail often leads to younger people living with dementia being overlooked, when in fact it is estimated that globally 119 per 100,000 people develop young-onset dementia. This equates to 3.9 million people worldwide (Hendriks et al. 2021). Younger people living with dementia are more likely to receive a delayed diagnosis, although will often present to frontline health care staff prior to receiving a diagnosis. In 2018 in England, the diagnosis rate (proportion of people living with dementia that have a diagnosis) for people over 65 was 67.8 per cent whilst for people under 65 it was 40.7 per cent. Therefore, although cases of young-onset dementia are rarer (which means it can be challenging to build up expertise), preparing the primary care workforce to identify signs of dementia in younger people and provide care and support for this group is nonetheless important.

Similarly, people with dementia from minority communities frequently experience a delayed diagnosis and are less likely to seek support for symptoms of dementia (APPG 2013). Therefore, primary care staff are ideally positioned to raise awareness of dementia and support people from these communities who may contact frontline services for other unrelated health care issues.

The dementia-related care provision provided by primary care is not limited to care of the person living with dementia. Often people supporting those living with dementia can experience a range of adverse physical and mental health outcomes. In the UK, it is recommended that people who are providing care for friends or relatives receive a caregiver assessment – a health check to identify any physical, mental health, or social impacts of their caring role (NICE 2018).

Figure 5.1 Phases of the Well Pathway for Dementia

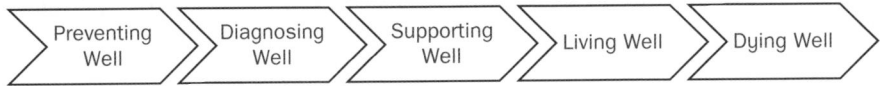

The landscape of dementia training for primary care staff

Education for those who will go on to work in primary care (including medical students and student nurses) will typically involve formal higher education in combination with short-term clinical placements throughout their training. Clinical placements also provide opportunities for informal learning, as reviewed in Chapter 3. This training is generally considered foundational rather than specialist. For example, Tullo and Gordon (2013) surveyed 23 of the 31 medical schools in the UK to establish the nature of dementia education being provided. Their findings showed that all the schools that responded provided some dementia-specific content, but this tended to focus more on knowledge and skills than behaviours and attitudes. In terms of assessment of learning, only 80 per cent of schools described formal assessment of dementia-specific learning outcomes. Overall, the authors concluded that the education provided failed to equip learners sufficiently to support people living with dementia.

Furthermore, placements in higher education programmes are frequently biased towards acute health care settings. Due to the short-term nature of the placements, they tend to equip learners to better understand acute illness rather than develop an understanding of the management of long-term health conditions. Overall, this model of learning has been criticised for overemphasising the importance of acute conditions treated in hospital settings whilst providing little opportunity to learn about dealing with and managing long-term conditions and providing community-based care (Banerjee 2015).

It has been proposed that health care education needs to adapt to meet the needs of people living with long-term conditions and comorbidities in the community (Cavendish 2013), which disproportionately burden health care systems (DHSC 2012). However, care for people with long-term conditions and comorbidities (e.g. dementia) requires a different set of skills and attitudes than care provided for acute conditions (Banerjee et al. 2017). Consequently, different models of education are needed that foster these skills and attitudes. One such approach has been the adoption of longer-term placements focused on the management of chronic conditions. Such placements provide opportunities to build relationships with patients, and their clinicians, over a sustained period whilst still providing the opportunity to demonstrate requisite clinical competencies across multiple disciplines during the placement (as is achieved through multiple short-term placements) (Norris et al. 2009). Some higher education providers have attempted to redress this through innovative approaches, as discussed later in this chapter.

Alternatively, higher education can be enhanced through engagement with continuing professional development (CPD) as careers progress. Where this is the case, attainment of dementia specialism (or arguably even sufficient knowledge) relies on the individual to take up further training for CPD. This chapter will focus on specialist and novel forms of training that have been developed to address the limitations of generic training, as well as the barriers and facilitators to training in this setting.

What dementia-specific knowledge and skills do primary care staff need?

As described above, the role of primary care staff is to support people directly affected by dementia across the whole dementia pathway – from the prevention of dementia to diagnosis and supporting people at the point of end-of-life care. This section addresses a few key phases in that pathway, and some of the knowledge and skills associated with these phases.

Knowledge and skills to support dementia identification, assessment, and diagnosis

One contentious issue in the field of primary care is the degree to which staff offer assessment and diagnostic services, due to conflicting views as to whether these services should only be provided as a specialist service. Historically, dementia diagnosis was considered the remit of specialist services located either in old age psychiatry or neurology. With the advocacy of more timely diagnoses in most National Dementia Strategies, specialist memory assessment services have become the norm (Brooker et al. 2014). While there is evidence that specialist memory services can be clinically and cost effective, diagnosis via this route can be affected by delays and waiting lists (Waldemar et al. 2007). In the US, primary care has picked up where specialist services cannot deliver. A recent study found that 85 per cent of people diagnosed with dementia in the US were diagnosed by a non-specialist (usually a primary care physician/GP) (Alzheimer's Association 2020). Five years after the non-specialist diagnosis in primary care, only 36 per cent of people had seen a specialist. Primary care therefore plays a significant role in the diagnostic journey for people living with dementia, although the degree to which primary care staff are active in the diagnostic process varies. In some cases, the involvement of primary care will be limited to screening, recognising the signs of dementia, and referring onwards to specialist services. In other cases, primary care services will take an active role in the assessment, diagnosis, and initiation of treatment where staff have been in receipt of specialist dementia training.

Primary care practices also often provide support for some people living in long-term care facilities in the community (such as residential care homes). Therefore, it will be the remit of staff who are caring for people living within these homes to identify cases of dementia and provide treatment where necessary. Often, referral to specialist secondary services for individuals in care homes for diagnosis is not practical, as well as potentially distressing for the individual. In England, tools have been developed to support this activity. For example, the DiADeM tool (Yorkshire and Humber Clinical Network 2018) is a diagnostic tool to support GPs in diagnosing dementia for people living with advanced dementia in a care home setting. The need for such tools further emphasises the need for primary care staff to be prepared to identify cases of dementia and provide the appropriate treatment for such.

A review of the role of primary care in diagnostic services noted that GPs can and do play an important role in diagnosing older and more frail people for whom progression through a more lengthy and complex assessment pathway may be inappropriate (Wells and Smith 2017). Furthermore, even partial involvement of primary care staff or services in the assessment and diagnosis of dementia has been shown to reduce pressure on specialist services and improve outcomes for patients. Nonetheless, primary care staff have reported a lack of confidence and skills in diagnosis and management of dementia (Ahmad et al. 2010; Thyrian and Hoffmann 2012). Limited basic dementia training and post-qualification training has been cited as driving their lack of knowledge and confidence (Ahmad et al. 2010).

Thus, primary care staff have a clear and important role to play in dementia diagnosis pathways. Having the right knowledge and skills associated with the identification, assessment, and diagnosis of dementia are essential for improving outcomes for people living with dementia or suspected dementia. Training initiatives have targeted these areas with positive effects. For example, a complex educational intervention that took place in the Netherlands (EASYcare) for dyads of GPs and primary care nurses indicated that training elicits positive benefits for adherence to diagnostic procedures as well as enhancing diagnostic accuracy (Perry 2011).

Knowledge and skills to provide post-diagnostic support and ongoing care

People living with dementia can frequently present to primary care with dementia-related health care issues as well as complex health care needs related to comorbidities where dementia adds complexity to its diagnosis and management, such as cancer or diabetes (Browne et al. 2017; Clague et al. 2017; Jones et al. 2020; Puts et al. 2010). Primary care staff are the most frequent providers and coordinators of ongoing care for people living with dementia and their informal caregivers from pre-diagnosis to end of life (Wells and Smith 2017).

There are a number of problems associated with providing ongoing primary care for people living with dementia outside of the diagnostic process, which necessitate specialist skills and knowledge. These include:

- People with cognitive impairment can have difficulties understanding, communicating, and retaining information, which brings additional challenges to the consultation and involving people in decisions about their care.
- Stigmatising views and perceptions of dementia can make people reluctant to engage with health care services until they reach a point of crisis.
- People living with dementia may not attend appointments alone, and there can be complex family dynamics to manage during consultations.

- People living with dementia and their families often seek the advice of primary care staff to address legal and ethical issues, such as whether to continue driving or not, or whether someone has capacity to make decisions.

There are also complications around approaching end-of-life conversations and advanced care planning. It can be difficult to identify the right time to have the conversation, meaning opportunities are missed and people living with dementia have their right to determine their end-of-life plans taken away. It can also be difficult to determine when someone is approaching the last year of life with dementia, and how to support patients, families, and friends to come to terms with this.

Primary care staff report feeling unprepared by their generic medical training to provide the types of services people directly affected by dementia typically need. A recent report published by the Alzheimer's Association (2020), relating specifically to the US, indicated that the responsibility of care for people living with dementia falls with primary care staff but that many feel inadequately trained to provide the level of care required. This finding is mirrored in other countries (see, for example, Foley et al. 2017).

Translation to training and education frameworks

There is no agreed consensus or unified framework regarding the dementia-related competencies required by primary care staff, and these will largely depend on the nature of the services that the primary care service provides. Despite this, there have been attempts to develop frameworks that can be helpful in informing the curriculum and content of dementia training for primary care staff, such as the Dementia Education and Training Standards Framework in England (Skills for Health 2018). This can be flexibly applied depending on the nature of care or service being provided (see Chapter 1). Applying this framework gives some indication of the breadth of curriculum content that would be required for those working in primary care (see Table 5.1).

Table 5.1 highlights that 13 of the 14 subjects proposed in this framework for England are likely to be relevant or essential for professionals working in primary care. The figure also provides some example learning outcomes from these subject areas. Primary care staff training needs to address a breadth of subjects because they are likely to come into contact with people at every stage of their dementia journey – from health promotion and risk reduction to end-of-life care. Furthermore, the Dementia Education and Training Standards Framework indicates that staff who have more frequent contact with people living with dementia need to cover a greater breadth of the curriculum. Higher levels of contact would be typical for those in frontline primary health care roles, as compared to those working in acute settings who are more likely to be faced with one-off episodes. This makes it even more important to consider the services that each primary care practice is providing and ensure that training is developed and delivered according to this need. See Chapter 1 for more information on conducting a training needs analysis.

Table 5.1 Dementia Education and Training Standards Framework in England applied to primary care

	Subject area	Is the Subject relevant to Primary Care workers?
	1. Dementia Awareness	Yes
Example	be able to communicate effectively and compassionately with individuals who have dementia	
	2. Dementia identification, assessment and diagnosis	Yes
Example	understand the different types of dementia, the stages or variants of these diseases and their primary symptoms	
	3. Dementia risk reduction and prevention	Yes
Example	be able to encourage behavioural change in individuals and organisations to promote health and well-being, reduce risk and potentially delay the onset and severity of certain types of dementia	
	4. Person-centred care	Yes
Example	understand the significance of a person's background, culture and experiences when providing their care	
	5. Communication, interaction and behaviour in dementia care	Yes
Example	understand common causes of distressed behaviour by people with dementia	
	6. Health and well-being in dementia care	Yes
Example	understand the complexity of ageing and co-morbidity in dementia	
	7. Pharmacological interventions in dementia care	Yes
Example	understand the range of cognitive enhancers, what they do, criteria for eligibility and sources of guidance	
	8. Living well with dementia and promoting independence	Yes
Example	understand the role of family and carers in enabling people with dementia to live well	
	9. Families and carers as partners in dementia care	Yes
Example	understand methods to assess a carer's psychological and practical needs and the relevant support available	
	10. Equality diversity and inclusion in dementia care	Yes
Example	be aware of the stigma, myths and stereotypes associated with dementia	
	11. Law, ethics and safeguarding in dementia care	Yes
Example	understand key legislation relevant to mental capacity, deprivation of liberty, equality and human rights.	
	12. End-of-life dementia care	Yes
Example	be able to contribute to the development of practices and services that meet the end-of-life needs of people with dementia	
	13. Research and evidence-based practice in dementia care	Yes
Example	understand how people affected by dementia may be involved in service evaluation and research.	
	14. Leadership in transforming dementia care	?
Example	be able to plan care to promote the use of appropriate, specific, evidence-based interventions	

Examples of training to enhance dementia knowledge and skills in primary care

Dementia training targeted to primary care staff comes in a variety of delivery modes and formats. The advantages and disadvantages of different methods and approaches to delivering training are addressed in Chapter 2. This section will focus on a few different approaches to developing dementia training for primary care staff as part of pre-registration courses and continuing professional development, and the evaluation of these approaches.

Dementia education and training for staff in primary care using online programmes

Online training has become increasingly common in health care education. The limitations of this approach are discussed in Chapter 2. However, online delivery is posited to have some advantages, particularly when delivering training at scale and to rural communities. An example of this type of at-scale specialist dementia training can be found in a recently evaluated Continuing Medical Education (CME) programme delivered in Australia (Casey et al. 2020). The CME programme offered the opportunity to enhance dementia-related awareness, practice, knowledge, and confidence of GPs in Australia.

This programme consisted of a minimum of 6 hours of thematically linked structured educational content, including at least two-thirds interactive or experiential content (such as case studies and discussion). It was based on Brodaty and colleagues' 'Dementia: 14 Essentials of assessment and care planning' (Brodaty et al. 2013a) and 'Dementia: 14 Essentials of management' (Brodaty et al. 2013b). The programme was offered in three formats: online modules, large group face-to-face workshops in major cities at the General Practice Conference and Exhibition, and small group face-to-face workshops. We focus here on the online format, which comprised six 60-minute modules; the findings speak to the accessibility and acceptability of this over the other two delivery formats that were available.

Over the course of the CME evaluation, 3,923 GPs participated, with 44 per cent enrolling for all modules in one of the delivery formats. Of these, 83 per cent completed all required activities (face-to-face, 647; online, 785). The online modules proved most popular, reportedly because learners were allowed to take their time and complete them at their own pace. Contrary to expectations, learners in city regions rather than rural regions preferred this format, with rural learners preferring face-to-face sessions. Whilst this was not fully explored, the authors assert that this may have been due to a lack of high-speed internet and poor phone signal for rural GPs.

Interestingly, in terms of scope and content of this programme, GPs requested more information on legal issues, assessing patient capacity, medication management, and community services in poorly resourced regional and remote areas. Online learners requested concise, practical information over theory-driven content and readings.

Similarly, Bentley and colleagues (2019) developed and delivered a 'Behaviour change in dementia care' online course in Australia. This comprised a 3-hour programme designed to assist primary care staff to develop a systematic framework to identify, diagnose, and manage patients with dementia within their practice. There were four modules: (1) Recognising Dementia in General Practice; (2) Diagnosing Dementia in General Practice; (3) How Does Dementia Progress; and (4) Managing Dementia in General Practice. Each module contained a video, assessment questions, and additional learning sources. The authors evaluated this programme using interviews and questionnaires. Learners' knowledge, confidence, and attitudes about dementia increased after completing the modules and they showed strong intentions to apply a systematic framework to identify and manage dementia. In the interviews, participants reported increased awareness, knowledge, and confidence in assessing and managing people with dementia. However, there was only limited evidence of behaviour change via the interviews, and no investigation of the impact on patients or sustained change in practice. This was a limitation of both studies and presents the challenge of evidencing the impact of training on sustained behaviour change and practice, particularly for interventions that are happening remotely.

Box 5.1 Key points to consider when developing online learning for primary care staff

- Those developing training should refer to national or international frameworks and standards.
- Training should be accessible to learners with consideration of the individuals who are undertaking the programme as well as equity of access (e.g. access to the internet or learning platform).
- Training providers should assess the services that the primary care practice offers in relation to the training needs of the staff.
- Training providers should consider learning outcomes related to attitudes and beliefs as well as skills and knowledge.
- The content should be practical rather than just theory-focused.
- Consideration should be given to the evaluation, especially with regards to impact of training on behaviour change.

Specialist postgraduate dementia programmes for primary care staff

A different CPD route is via accredited, dementia-specific undergraduate or postgraduate education programmes. A benefit of this approach is that it enables in-depth learning over an extended period incorporating assessment. However, this approach is extremely resource intensive in terms of cost and time for the learner (and the funder). An in-depth case study of one such accredited dementia programme for primary care was undertaken by two of the authors of this book as part of our research exploring effective approaches to dementia training (Sass et al. 2019). The case study was conducted in a single primary care organisation (a consortia of GP practices covering an area of more than 360,000 residents) providing a primary care-led Memory Assessment Service, with the aim of exploring:

- the models of dementia training being adopted;
- how staff perceived the training;
- the impact of the training on staff knowledge, attitudes, and practices;
- how people living with dementia and their informal caregivers experienced care in sites where staff had received training;
- the specific barriers and facilitators to effective training implementation.

Staff in the service had undertaken a Postgraduate Certificate in Dementia delivered via blended learning. Most of the teaching was online, with two face-to-face teaching days and compulsory practice-based learning within a Memory Assessment Service or similar (facilitated by a local practice mentor). The programme consisted of two 12-week, formally assessed, modules (Module 1 on assessment and diagnosis and Module 2 on post-diagnostic care).

Data was gathered from a wide range of sources and analysed using Kirkpatrick's evaluative model reaction, learning, behaviour change, impact on outcomes (see Chapter 10 for a more in-depth discussion of Kirkpatrick's model). Eight primary care staff took part in a focus group and completed questionnaires, an interview was conducted with the training lead, and people living with dementia and their informal caregivers were asked about their experience of the service.

Overall, learners appeared to have a positive reaction to the programme, which filtered through to self-reported changes in practice, such as improved communication. The learners and the mentors felt that the programme was successful at covering a broad range of content required for the role. It is recognised that accredited programmes are expensive and labour intensive, and for this reason are often designed to develop staff to be specialists in dementia within the service they are working, with the intention that they will go on to undertake a leadership role. Many GPs may already be undertaking this level of leadership inherently, whilst others plan to take up a specialist role. This was acknowledged by the learners who stated that they found the volume of work surprising, particularly after a break from studying. However, they also reported cascading information to colleagues within the service, meaning their own learning had an impact more widely.

Although it is difficult to evidence impact on the service (Kirkpatrick Level 4), the evaluation attempted to do this by gathering data from patients directly affected by dementia, who overall felt satisfied and cared for, although it is difficult to attribute this directly to the training.

Box 5.2 Key points to consider in relation to specialist postgraduate provision

- Does the programme identify and meet specific educational needs of primary care practitioners in relation to the leadership of care and support of people with dementia?
- Is learning provided in an accessible format, suitable for primary care practitioners?
- Are those attending adequately informed about and prepared for the workload involved in accredited postgraduate education?
- Does the programme involve a combination of theory and practice?
- Is there appropriate mentorship and support available for the practice-based components?

Training using practice-based workshops

An approach used to support education of primary care staff is practice-based workshops delivered in a small group face-to-face format. Evaluations of such programmes demonstrate variable outcomes.

In conjunction with an expert working group, Jennings et al. (2019) developed an interactive, interprofessional, 3-hour workshop for primary care teams, based around a case study approach. An evaluation of the pilot workshops with 54 participants from a range of primary care-based roles found over 80 per cent said it improved their knowledge, confidence, and understanding of dementia.

The multi-disciplinary peer learning aspect was particularly highlighted as beneficial by participants. Evaluation of a wider roll out of the programme (Foley et al. 2018) with 104 participants, where the 39 educational workshops were delivered by trained GP facilitators, again found that those attending the training reported improved dementia care knowledge and confidence. However, both studies relied on self-report of knowledge and confidence gains. A similar picture emerges from a programme delivered in Canada (Lee et al. 2011) whose aim was to develop primary care-based memory assessment services. This programme consists of a 2-day intensive, interactive, case-based workshop format, followed by a day of observation and training in a local memory service and 2 days of on-site mentorship while working in the primary care-based memory service. The authors again report very positive, self-reported learning outcomes from their pilot work. A formal evaluation of the programme (Lee et al. 2013) with 22 teams consisting of 124 health professionals, found significant increases in self-reported knowledge and confidence in assessing and managing dementia, with all but one team going on to form a memory service.

However, Wilcock et al. (2013) conducted a randomised controlled trial where 23 GP practices in England either continued providing usual care or attended tailored learning sessions for their health care and administrative staff (these comprised an average of three 1-hour sessions per practice delivered in-house). The primary object was to see if the training intervention increased the proportion of patients living with dementia who received at least two dementia reviews per year. The study found no differences between the training and care-as-usual on either the number of patients receiving two or more dementia reviews, or the number of cases of dementia detected over the trial period. The authors conclude that the intervention of a small number of workshops as a stand-alone approach may not be enough to change practice.

In summary, the benefits of this type of approach (an example of which is provided as a case study) are variable. A particular challenge is targeting the training at the right level when involving the staff with variable knowledge and abilities at the outset, as will be common in any primary care practice team. This is an issue explored further in the second part of this book, which considers factors that can support or impede implementation of training. Moreover, it is possible that practice-based workshops successfully increase the knowledge and confidence of primary care staff, but they do not necessarily provide the relevant learning to support translation into change of behaviour and practice-related outcomes (Kirkpatrick Levels 3 and 4). It may be that the in-practice components of the Canadian programme enabled staff to move from knowledge and confidence gains to effective implementation. Or, it may be that the setting conditions within these teams – who had committed to setting up a memory assessment service – may have provided the requisite context for implementation.

Case example: Creating dementia-friendly GP services

An initiative was developed with the aim of creating dementia-friendly primary care services in the UK. It began in one UK region and has been rolled out to hundreds of GP practices. The programme involves a number of key steps, which start with identifying and appointing a dementia champion or lead for the practice. This is followed by a programme of staff training that is specific to primary care. The programme requires promotion of partnership working with informal caregivers and linking to external agencies which can provide support for the person living with dementia and their informal support network. There is also a focus on assessment and early identification of dementia, development of person-centred care plans, and ensuring the environment is supportive for people living with dementia.

The training is interactive and discursive and includes the whole practice team (GPs, nurses, reception staff, and other allied health professionals).

Box 5.3 Key points to consider in relation to practice-based workshops for primary care practitioners

- Are the workshops delivered to the multi-disciplinary primary care team, including clinical and administrative and support staff?
- Are there opportunities for learners to apply learning in their own practice as part of the programme?
- Is input and support from dementia specialists provided where specific clinical skills are being taught and applied, e.g. dementia assessment and diagnosis?

Enhanced placements in dementia for health care staff

One of the criticisms of higher education for those who will go on to work in primary care is the unsuitability of the placements that form part of their pre-registration training. Short-term placements and placements that happen in hospital settings do not prepare learners to deal with the management of long-term conditions that will form a large part of their role when working in the community. One approach to address this has been to develop longer-term placements. The 'Time for Dementia' programme sought to implement this approach for nursing, paramedic, and medical students (Bentley et al. 2019). This approach was designed to enhance learners' knowledge of dementia, regardless of the setting in which the learners would go on to work in once registered. The programme aimed to provide learners with a longitudinal experience of how individuals and their families are affected by long-term conditions like dementia; improve attitudes, empathy, and knowledge of dementia; and ensure that the programme did not have an adverse effect on the people participating directly affected by dementia.

The programme involved recruiting people directly affected by dementia to work alongside pairs of learners for longitudinal placements (over 2 years with visits every 3 months). The visits were of 2 hours' duration and included having conversations with the person living with dementia and their family members, completing life story work, and completing a 'This is Me' document developed by the Alzheimer's Society (2021) that helps health care professionals to learn about the preferences and wishes of the person living with dementia.

The qualitative evaluation of the 'Time for Dementia' programme used interviews and focus groups with 77 learners. It indicated that there was a tangible benefit from this 'real-life' learning (Daley et al. 2020). The learners felt that work with real people in their homes made it easier and quicker to apply learning to their practice than it would have been from formal lectures. They also reported that they felt learning this way gave them enhanced insight and understanding about the condition and allowed them to see beyond stigmatising stereotypes about dementia.

Finally, learners reported an improvement in their communication skills, citing changes in behavioural practice such as explaining what they were communicating more clearly and checking understanding. Furthermore, they felt there was an improvement in their ability to support people living with dementia in practice, for example though the use of tools and approaches such as life story work.

Box 5.4 Key points to consider for implementing dementia-related placement opportunities

- Is there adequate central resource to sustainably develop and deliver the right number of placement opportunities and to provide appropriate preparation and ongoing support to participating families?
- Is it feasible to offer continuity in placements?
- How will this link to the curriculum?
- How will the placements be structured and students prepared in order to get the most out of the opportunity?
- How will students and families be supported to end relationships at the end of the placement period?
- Will students have appropriate supervisory support?

Barriers and facilitators to implementing training in primary care

In this chapter, we have covered a range of approaches to education and training that might be used to develop or enhance staff's ability to deliver high-quality care for people living with dementia in primary care. Whilst the different approaches can have distinct advantages and disadvantages, there are some commonalities in the barriers and facilitators to delivering education and training in this setting.

One of the areas of interest among this staff group has been their own attitudes and beliefs, which could act as a barrier to learning and motivation to change practice. Investigations of the attitudes of primary care staff have suggested that therapeutic nihilism (i.e. a lack of belief in their ability to improve patients' quality of life; Kaduszkiewicz et al. 2008) is a barrier to motivation to improve practice. Primary care staff have reported holding stigmatising views about dementia and finding it difficult to offer treatment for the condition due to poor envisaged patient outcomes (Gove et al. 2016; Kaduszkiewicz et al. 2008). Research has also shown that older GPs are less likely to feel that diagnosis is beneficial and more likely to perceive people living with dementia as a drain on resources than their younger counterparts (Ahmad et al. 2010). Addressing these views can be challenging and is why many of the training packages mentioned in this chapter specifically target attitudes and beliefs about dementia as part of the education provided. These interventions, as well as others, have shown success in addressing negative attitudes towards dementia as part of the training. Informal learning may also have a role to play in conferring positive attitudes and cultures of dementia care in the workplace, something that is explored in Chapter 3.

A further barrier to motivation for learning reported in the literature (and previously mentioned studies) is individuals' concerns about their competency and knowledge (Iliffe and Wilcock 2005). GPs report concerns that the management of dementia is a specialist role (Waldemar et al. 2007), although the reality is that many of the services that have historically been specialist are in fact being provided in primary care. With enhanced approaches to and opportunities for training in this setting, there is some hope and agreement that primary care staff can provide these services; and with additional training they will feel confident to do so (Leung et al. 2020).

There were several factors identified in the reviewed approaches that act as facilitators to delivering training with this group. Staff appeared to value the 'real-world' examples and applicability of their learning experience. Across the different learning formats this came in varying forms – from opportunities to share learning across different regions and services in the postgraduate certificate, to hearing about the experiences of patients over a long period in extended placements. This element of learning appeared to speed up learners' ability to apply these experiences to practice in their own settings. This is reflective of the wider dementia training literature, which identifies that learners benefit from opportunities to put theory into practice and hands-on learning (Surr et al. 2017a).

Summary

The take-home message from this chapter is that whilst there are many examples of quick and easy learning programmes (such as e-learning packages) designed to enhance awareness of issues facing primary care, realistically, training for this group must be tailored to the needs of staff and the broad remit they have in supporting the health and care needs of this population. A wide range of training approaches are available, and the chosen approach ought to be carefully considered based on evidence that the approach is best suited to that service and learners' needs at the time. For example, an online programme available nationally may enhance knowledge and awareness for many learners, but it can be difficult to translate this to change in practice (or provide evidence for practice change). Investment in an individual to undertake an in-depth accredited programme (such as the postgraduate practice certificate) may be more likely to instigate change in practice at a local level due to the individual becoming a leader and proponent of change. The limitation of this is the localised nature of the change and limited reach. Training designed to support the implementation of a particular practice initiative will look very different to that designed to enhance the knowledge and attitudes of a staff group, or to meet a predetermined benchmark standard.

A commonality in the approach to developing training for this group of staff is consideration of the breath of content that is needed. The evidence reviewed in this chapter suggests that this is often over and above what staff are prepared for via their basic pre-registration education, and that staff roles often involve tasks and services traditionally associated with specialist services. It is useful to use national or local guidance and frameworks to inform the content of training where possible. It may be worth looking to the published evidence for areas of consideration that may be overlooked, such as legal issues, assessing patient capacity, medication management, and community services. Across the board, the evidence suggests that to prepare these staff, as well as addressing knowledge and understanding of dementia, training should address individuals' attitudes and beliefs about dementia.

Finally, where new and innovative training initiatives exist, there needs to be more work done to understand the impact of the training on patients' experience of the primary care service. Presently, there is a lack of evidence to suggest that training in primary care services is having an impact on the behaviour of staff and thus the experience of people directly affected by dementia.

Implications for those delivering dementia training

Those leading and facilitating dementia training should:

- Develop the training with remit of the primary care service in mind, i.e. what is the nature of contact that the workforce has with people directly affected by dementia.

- Consider the different abilities and experiences of the learners where a whole-practice approach is taken.
- Undertake a training needs analysis and look to national or local benchmark standards to inform the content of the training where possible.
- Consider the mode of delivery that is most appropriate for the learners (e.g. online, group training, mentorship).
- Ensure training addresses attitudes as well as knowledge.

Implications for managers in dementia care settings and services

Managers in dementia care settings and services should:

- Provide all staff with the opportunity to participate in training.
- Consider how to measure the impact of training on users of the service.
- Provide support for learners undertaking CPD training (time and/or resources).
- Support placements for learners.
- Promote a person-centred dementia care environment.

Implications for staff providing care, services, or support to people living with dementia

Staff working in dementia care should:

- Reflect on their dementia-related knowledge and skills and seek to undertake training or CPD that is relevant to their practice.
- Provide leadership in promoting person-centred care to support other practice staff as appropriate.
- Challenge stigmatising views about dementia and promote a person-centred approach that engenders a positive attitude towards dementia training.

Implications for those affected by dementia

People affected by dementia should:

- Be visible and have a presence in placements offered to learners on health care courses who will be supporting people with long-term conditions.
- Have a presence in pre- and post-registration training to address attitudes to dementia and dementia diagnosis.
- Be offered opportunities to participate in training for primary care staff.

6 Learning and development in acute hospitals

'Staff working in acute hospitals need to access dementia-specific continuing professional development opportunities to enable them to develop the right knowledge, skills, and attitudes to deliver good care to people living with dementia, and to feel confident and competent to do so, no matter what a patient's presenting condition.'

Developing the health care workforce to be able to provide good quality person-centred acute or general hospital-based care to people living with dementia has been a relatively recent concern compared with settings more traditionally known to provide dementia care, such as care homes. There has been a corresponding growth in the development of dementia training for acute hospital staff and a similar increase in published research exploring the impact of dementia training in these settings. This chapter will explore the evidence on delivery of dementia training in hospital settings and provide guidance on best practice for those designing, delivering, and implementing dementia training for hospital-based staff.

Acute and general medical care in hospital settings for people living with dementia

In the UK, acute medical care is provided in acute or general hospitals. Hospital settings provide specialist services for a wide range of acute and chronic physical health conditions, typically through short-stay or outpatient care. They include emergency departments, cancer services, surgery, a full range of outpatient clinics, as well as access to a range of specialist health care professionals such as physiotherapists or speech and language therapists. This care, across a city or region, is usually managed by a single **National Health Service** (NHS) Trust, which may have several hospital sites. These may include smaller local or district hospitals through to larger regional centres providing a wider range of specialist services (e.g. specialist trauma, cancer, and surgery). Around 25 per cent of inpatient beds in acute hospitals in the UK are occupied by people living with dementia (Alzheimer's Society 2009). Given the increase in numbers of older people that will be living in the UK in the coming decades, both the absolute numbers of people living with dementia requiring hospital care and the proportion of beds occupied by people living with dementia are likely to increase.

In the UK, mental health services are usually provided by specialist mental health or community NHS Trusts in separate hospital sites and within the community. It is these services that largely provide dementia diagnosis and post-diagnostic support (although this is also provided via primary care in some areas – see Chapter 5). Mental health services also provide care and support for people living with dementia with complex needs or behaviours associated with their dementia, for example via inpatient assessment wards and community-based mental health teams. Therefore, these specialist mental health services are typically not co-located with physical health care. In some hospitals, multi-disciplinary liaison psychiatry teams (Royal College of Psychiatrists 2019b) may work to support staff to meet patients' mental health needs. However, access to such services is not widespread (Naylor et al. 2016). Therefore, NHS services that provide support for physical health-related conditions often have inadequate provision for also meeting patients' mental health needs, including dementia.

Internationally the way in which physical and mental health services are structured varies and as in the UK the two are often poorly integrated (Triliva et al. 2020). In some countries, mental and physical health care may be provided on a single site, but on separate wards with separate teams of staff. Therefore, the input of staff with specialist mental health and/or dementia care expertise, to support the care of people living with dementia who are in hospital for a different medical condition, may be variable and limited to the most complex cases or where additional problems such as delirium are present. Thus, internationally there is a need to improve the ability of acute hospital services and staff working in these settings to deliver care that considers the needs associated with a comorbid dementia.

In the UK at least, most dementia care delivered by specialist mental health practitioners is provided in Memory Assessment Services, by community-based mental health teams, or through liaison psychiatry teams working in acute settings. Where there are a limited number of inpatient wards for people with dementia, these provide specialist assessment and care for those who have the most complex needs. Despite the assumption that staff working in mental health services have more in-depth expertise in care of people living with dementia, there is limited literature examining when and how such skills are acquired or concerning their ongoing professional development needs in relation to delivery of dementia care. Where published studies have focused on mental health specialist teams working with older adults, evaluations have examined training staff on specific interventions such as recovery models (Daley et al. 2019) and cognitive stimulation therapy (Streater et al. 2017). Where relevant, examples and evidence related to specialist mental health staff working in the community are discussed in Chapter 7. This chapter focuses predominantly on dementia training for acute hospital staff.

Dementia adds significant complexity to the management of chronic and acute physical and mental health conditions. People living with dementia often have poorer outcomes as a result of a stay in hospital than older adults without dementia, including more frequent and longer hospital stays and a greater chance of being readmitted following discharge as well as being discharged to a different place of residence such as a care home (Fogg et al. 2017; Reynish et al. 2017). Being acutely unwell, alongside a change of routine and an unfamiliar physical environment that is not designed to meet the needs of people living with dementia, can lead to an increased risk of a person becoming more confused and agitated.

People living with dementia are also at high risk of developing delirium, an acute severe neurological syndrome often seen in older people who are in hospital, and which can cause increased confusion and agitation. Dementia is one of the main risk factors for developing delirium, with people with both dementia and delirium making up around 65 per cent of all cases of people with delirium in acute hospitals (Jackson et al. 2017). People living with dementia and delirium have the worst outcomes of people in acute hospitals.

It is therefore unsurprising that acute hospital staff consistently report struggling to meet the complex needs of this patient group and highlight how their education prior to and since entering the profession has not adequately prepared them for this role (Brooke and Ojo 2018; Gwernan-Jones et al. 2020b). Physical and chemical restraint are commonly used approaches, across many countries, for what is often called the 'management' of people living with dementia who are confused, distressed, or agitated. Physical restraints include the use of bedrails, belts, recliner chairs, or positioning tables to prevent people from getting out of their chair (Abraham et al. 2020). Chemical restraints include the use of **antipsychotic** and other sedating medications. Restraints are used despite no clear evidence of effectiveness and a range of potential risks for harm, often because staff feel there are no other alternatives.

In the UK, a number of guidelines and initiatives have encouraged and promoted the provision and uptake of training on dementia in acute hospital settings over recent years, including: the National Institute for Health and Care Excellence (NICE) Dementia Guideline (NICE 2018), which underpins all health and care delivery to people living with dementia; the Alzheimer's Society 'Fix Dementia Care: Hospitals' campaign (Alzheimer's Society 2016), which called for increased dementia training including annual reporting of awareness and higher tier training figures; the Dementia-Friendly Hospital Charter (National Dementia Action Alliance 2020), which provides a framework of dementia-friendly principles against which hospitals can self-assess; and John's Campaign (John's Campaign n.d.), which campaigns for families to be welcome in hospitals and for the right for informal caregivers to stay with (for 24 hours if needed and desired) and support their family member living with dementia during a hospital stay; and a programme of work encouraging the creation of supportive physical hospital environments for people living with dementia in hospitals (Waller et al. 2013). The context, then, is one that is supportive of dementia training as an important foundation of good dementia care.

It is clear then that staff working in acute hospitals need to access dementia-specific continuing professional development (CPD) opportunities. This will enable them to develop the right knowledge, skills, and attitudes to deliver good care to people living with dementia, and to feel confident and competent to do so, no matter what a patient's presenting condition. A broad range of staff work in acute hospital settings, and this chapter will consider dementia training for individuals working across all these roles. These include, but are not limited to: nurses, doctors, allied health professionals, associate practitioners, health care support workers/assistants, pharmacists, managers, clerks, reception and telephony staff, porters, catering, domestic and house-keeping, and estates staff. In the UK, it is a requirement that all NHS staff complete dementia awareness training and an expectation that relevant staff groups will undertake more in-depth training appropriate to their role (Department of Health 2013, 2014, 2015). Whether staff have received an appropriate level of training and the priority that is given to this amongst other mandatory training is variable across different hospitals. The National Audit of Dementia Care in hospitals in England has reported a steady increase in dementia training, with an average of 89 per cent of staff asked reporting they had received some training. However, 47 per cent of hospitals were unable to provide hospital-level training numbers (Royal College of Psychiatrists 2019a). Hospitals therefore need to improve their recording of staff trained in dementia care.

There is a growing body of research evidence examining the implementation and impact of dementia-specific formal training for acute hospital staff. In this chapter, we summarise the key features of this before outlining in more detail the implications of this for those tasked with dementia workforce development in hospital settings. It is important to acknowledge that many dementia training programmes are not formally evaluated or published (Schneider et al. 2019), and so what is included in the research literature is not necessarily reflective of the full range of dementia training available internationally. Research carried out in the UK by the authors of this book (Smith et al. 2019) has indicated that there are a wide range of different dementia training programmes available nationally for staff working in acute hospital settings. While some are locally or nationally available free or commercial programmes, the majority are developed and delivered in-house. Those tasked with training and workforce development in acute settings are often faced with developing their own materials, deciding whether to use freely available materials that can be found online, and whether to commission external commercial providers to meet some training needs. These decisions are often made with little or no available guidance. The Dementia Training Design and delivery Audit Tool (DeTDAT) (Surr et al. 2017b), developed by the authors of this book, based on the research evidence on effective dementia training, can provide a useful resource to help inform such decisions. There has also been very limited research exploring informal learning within acute hospital settings, particularly in relation to dementia care and so the mechanisms and influences of this on learning and care practice remain poorly understood.

What is the impact of dementia training on acute hospital staff?

The majority of published studies on dementia training in acute hospitals are from the UK, with others emanating from the US, Australia, Canada, and

Malta (Gkioka et al. 2020; Surr and Gates 2017). Most research studies include mixed staff groups in the training programmes they aim to evaluate. However, despite this, the majority of staff actually attending evaluated training programmes are nurses (Gkioka et al. 2020; Scerri et al. 2017), reflecting the composition of the patient-facing workforce, of which the majority work in nursing roles (Rolewicz and Palmer 2020). A handful of studies have, however, focused only on single groups (e.g. nursing assistants in the USA; Pfeifer et al. 2018). No research we have identified has evaluated training for those working in patient-facing, non-clinical roles such as porters, reception and administrative, estates, catering, or housekeeping staff.

The research evidence that is available provides a consistent picture that providing formal dementia training programmes to acute hospital staff significantly increases staff knowledge, improves their attitudes towards people living with dementia, and increases their confidence and sense of competence in caring for this group (Brooke and Ojo 2018; Gkioka et al. 2020). Training also leads to changes in individual staff behaviours, improved performance, and can positively influence wider practices in the hospital, including the use of positive communication techniques, delivery of more person-centred care, improved clinical skills, implementation of action plans, a decrease in use of **antipsychotic medications**, changes to the physical hospital environment, and modification of policies (Gkioka et al. 2020). Another benefit of providing dementia training programmes is an improvement in staff job satisfaction (Murray et al. 2019). One limitation of most studies, however, is their failure to evaluate how sustained these benefits are, with most having only short follow-up periods of 1–3 months after the end of a training programme (Scerri et al. 2017). There is evidence to suggest that refresher training needs to be provided at regular intervals in order to maintain benefits. In addition, as will be discussed further in Chapter 10, measuring impact of dementia training can be challenging and in many of these studies changes were evaluated using staff self-report rather than via more objective measures of change. Therefore, some caution is needed when interpreting the findings. A further limitation is that no studies have involved the direct engagement of people directly affected by dementia in the training delivered. Some studies have used indirect methods such as videos. Therefore, little is known about the possibilities and potential benefits of involvement of those directly affected by dementia in hospital-based dementia training.

What do acute hospital staff need to know about dementia?

Acute hospitals have a large workforce who work in a range of patient-facing and non-patient-facing roles. In England, the expectation is that all staff working in the NHS, in any role (patient- or non-patient-facing) should have undertaken dementia awareness level training (Skills for Health 2018). Staff who have regular contact with people living with dementia are expected to have more in-depth training relevant to their role. Across patient-facing roles, there is also significant diversity in prior education and dementia training among staff groups and individual staff members. For example, registered health professionals such as doctors, nurses, and allied health professionals in the UK will have completed university level education as part of qualifying for their role, although the dementia content covered within this will have been variable (Alushi et al. 2015; Tullo and Gordon 2013). Staff in other roles, such as health care assistants, porters, and domestic services will have received induction and ongoing development opportunities once in post but may have had variable exposure to and experiences of prior education and formal learning.

Therefore, as was discussed in Chapter 1, conducting a dementia training needs analysis to determine the knowledge and skills needed by different staff is required. This should be in the context of any national standards for dementia training but should also consider local priorities and needs. For individual staff, a learning needs assessment should consider prior exposure to dementia training alongside their priorities and preferences for what they feel will best support them to work effectively, recognising the time they have allocated to training and development within their role.

The design and delivery of continuing professional development dementia training for staff working in acute hospital settings

While the principles of good dementia training design and delivery discussed in Chapter 2 apply to training for acute hospital staff, there are also some setting-specific issues and evidence that should be considered.

Face-to-face training including experiential learning and simulation

Most training programmes for staff working in acute hospital settings that have been evaluated and published have adopted a wholly or partial face-to-face delivery. Our own experience suggests this is generally the most widely adopted approach in acute hospital settings. We recognise that it can be logistically challenging to deliver face-to-face training to an entire acute hospital workforce, due to the limited group sizes that can be accommodated, shift-working patterns, and difficulties giving staff time away from their duties to attend (Brooke and Ojo 2018; Surr et al. 2018c). However, evidence consistently indicates that face-to-face delivery is most impactful in terms of staff experiences of training, and improvements in learning and behaviour change (Gwernan-Jones et al. 2020b; Surr and Gates 2017), compared with e-learning or other methods.

In general, face-to-face training programmes that use a range of methods are most likely to be impactful because they meet a variety of preferred learning styles and offer opportunities to cover similar content in different ways to reinforce learning and support its application in practice. For example, combining lectures to provide theoretical and knowledge-based content with simulation (for example, with trained actors taking on the role of patients), real-life video clips, small group discussions, and work-shop-style activities has been shown to be effective in increasing staff knowledge about good communication, leading to behaviour change in practice and this being sustained over at least a one-month period (Harwood et al. 2018).

One particularly successful resource for dementia education in acute hospitals in the UK has been the ethno-drama film *Barbara, the Whole Story* (Guy's and St. Thomas' NHS Foundation Trust 2014). The film depicts the experiences of Barbara, an older lady living with undiagnosed early dementia, as she attends hospital for appointments and investigations for a health problem (Baillie et al. 2016). It was developed by a large NHS Trust in England. An initial 12-minute film was delivered to staff in multi-disciplinary sessions, with facilitated discussion after viewing the film. The training was made mandatory for all staff whether working in clinical or non-clinical roles. A second phase of the project developed a further series of short films following Barbara through a deterioration of her health and her care in hospital and community settings. Evaluations indicated the film-based training raised awareness of dementia across the organisation, helping staff to develop empathy for people living with dementia and to see the experience of hospital care through their eyes (Baillie et al. 2016). Staff reported thinking more about how they interacted with patients living with dementia they supported and modifying their practice in response to the film (Baillie and Sills 2015). A key factor identified for the success of the training was its mandatory status for all staff, meaning there was a shared experience, and all staff gained the same knowledge and understanding, creating a shared culture. Strong leadership for the project from senior staff in the organisation was also identified as vital to this success (Baillie et al. 2016).

Face-to-face delivery methods such as experiential learning and simulation support development of empathy. Small group discussion facilitates peer-to-peer learning, and interactive exercises support structured and informal reflection as well as underpinning the application of theory into practice. Development of staff empathy towards people living with dementia has been identified as important in enabling the delivery of person-centred care in acute hospital environments, alongside knowledge and understanding to recognise when and why care practices may need to change as well as practical, dementia-specific skills that can be readily applied in practice (Handley et al. 2019). This can be achieved, for example, through direct involvement of people living with dementia in the delivery of training, the use of audio and video materials of people with dementia discussing their experiences, and through more creative, experiential activities.

Case example: Using reflective practice in training about pain assessment and management in people living with dementia

A health care provider delivering care over multiple hospital sites developed a specific pain training course. Pain assessment and management training had always been a part of the wider dementia study day; however, the organisation felt that full engagement with dementia-specific pain assessment in practice had never been achieved. To address this, they introduced a two-part Pain in Dementia course, accompanied by a workbook.

The first session (Pain 1) is aimed at updating the learner on pain theory in relation to dementia, assessment, and management. Having completed this, the learners are asked to read the workbook and complete four reflective exercises before returning to undertake Pain 2. The second session begins with an informal discussion about the learners' reflections and is followed by information about non-pharmacological interventions, touch, and a practical session on how to deliver a simple hand massage.

The training has been very successful; the learners state that they have felt that the gap with reflection has helped to embed the learning more effectively. The process of returning and having the opportunity to discuss thoughts and concerns has consolidated the learning as well.

E-learning

The potential uses and limitations of e-learning were discussed in some detail in Chapter 2. These limitations are replicated in programmes where e-learning is a major component of delivery for acute hospital staff. In particular, completion rates of e-learning are often poor as a result of a lack of dedicated time to complete the training, a lack of access to an appropriate device in the workplace through which to complete training (Scerri et al. 2017; Surr and Gates 2017), and low staff motivation, given e-learning is regarded by many staff to be insufficient to meet their learning needs (Gwernan-Jones et al. 2020b). The National Audit of Dementia conducted in hospitals in England found that staff receiving only e-learning felt least well prepared to care for people with dementia (Royal College of Psychiatrists 2019a). Where e-learning programmes have had some success in being acceptable and useful to learners, their design has included interactive content. For example, a US e-learning intervention included video interviews, video scenarios using footage of real interactions between staff and people living with dementia as an indirect method of involvement, interactive text entry, and 'what would you do?' case scenarios (Hobday et al. 2010).

There is strong evidence, then, that e-learning as the sole approach to dementia training is inappropriate for acute hospital settings, despite the appeal of potentially reaching a large workforce in a resource-effective and time-efficient way. The limited effects of e-learning on the knowledge, attitudes, and confidence of learners completing it suggest this may represent a false economy, meaning training becomes a 'tick-box exercise' of achieving volume with little consideration for effectiveness. However, if an organisation makes a decision that some dementia training content must be delivered via e-learning, then this should always be as part of a blended approach that also uses face-to-face (or similar alternative online methods) and practice-based delivery approaches (DeSouza et al. 2020).

Mentor-supported and in-practice learning

To address challenges with enabling staff to leave the ward environment during working hours to attend training, some training programmes have attempted to adopt other methods that might build formal learning opportunities into day-to-day practice. For example, in one UK study, Smythe et al. (2013) developed a programme of mentor-supported in-practice training and compared this with their standard classroom-based training offer. The training aimed in particular to give staff the opportunity to work directly with people living with dementia and to learn from this through observation and feedback with a more experienced clinician. On a range of standard measures related to knowledge, attitudes, self-efficacy, and burnout, there were no significant differences between this method of delivery and the standard face-to-face training usually offered in the hospital. The authors also interviewed staff from both groups and found that staff found it equally challenging to engage in mentor-based training while on-duty due to the busy ward environment. It was also unable to be delivered in the planned small group format due to shift patterns and many patients living with dementia being situated in individual rooms, meaning having more than two staff members present was not feasible. Some staff reported feeling self-conscious about being observed during in-practice learning while others preferred the practical approach. Overall, the approach did not prove to be more impactful than, or a more practical solution than, face-to-face training. However, it might provide a useful blended approach alongside shorter face-to-face learning sessions.

Multi-disciplinary or single-role learning?

The majority of studies that have reported on evaluation of dementia training in acute hospital settings have involved staff working across multiple wards and roles, including medics, nurses, allied health professionals, nursing assistants, and occasionally ancillary staff (Scerri et al. 2017). While there may be challenges in ensuring training programmes can meet the needs of a diverse group of staff working in acute settings, the evidence suggests that, overall, multi-disciplinary learning is valued by those attending training (Harwood et al. 2018), in particular for the peer-to-peer learning that takes place. If taking this approach, it will be important to consider carefully which training programmes are suitable for true multi-disciplinary learning (e.g. including staff from patient-facing and non-patient-facing roles and all roles within these). However, it may be that some training is better delivered with a more limited range of staff roles involved, or to single professional groups in order that training can be best tailored to individual learner needs and job roles.

Case example: Accessible dementia training for all

A large health care provider in a regional city is one of the largest employers of its community, representative of a diverse and multi-cultural society. As part of its whole-hospital dementia programme, one of its objectives was to design a dementia awareness and training programme for all staff. In line with the national tiered dementia training standards of the country the health care provider is located in (see Chapter 1), it was agreed that all staff should receive Tier 1 (awareness) and Tier 2 (specialist) training. Tier 3 (leadership) training was offered to volunteer dementia champions and more senior health care professionals. To achieve this, the team responsible for the design and delivery of its dementia awareness and educational programmes took into consideration the educational needs of all staff, providing a variety of training sessions that staff could choose to attend. The content and delivery methods reflected the different skillsets and roles of staff, recognising that not all staff had the same prior educational experiences or confidence in learning.

As an example, the health care provider had undertaken a programme of award-winning work in creating dementia-friendly environments through its aesthetics, buildings, and infrastructure. To provide staff with the knowledge to use the environment to help people living with dementia orientate and feel relaxed during their hospital visit, training sessions were developed. Hospital porters play an important role in moving people around the hospital environment. The hospital facilitators identified that it would not be appropriate to deliver their training using approaches such as PowerPoint slides and theoretical content that might be used with other staff groups. Porters were instead provided with a shorter, bespoke, interactive session facilitated through discussion and simulation, with no written resources. Content focused on transportation of patients, discussing how to utilise the hospital's environment to engage patients (e.g. through prompting conversation, orientation, and providing a stimulating or relaxing environment), how to recognise a patient in need, and knowing when to report or escalate concerns. The training aimed to empower and validate the important role porters play in patients' overall hospital experience.

Developing dementia training and practice leadership

The development of staff within acute services to act in a role to lead change is a common and successful approach adopted across several existing training programmes within acute hospital settings. Dementia leaders, in some cases called dementia champions, are staff with a greater level of knowledge about dementia who are there to support implementation of dementia training into practice. They may also be involved in the delivery of dementia training to the hospital's workforce. There is evidence that having staff acting in this role can help to support embedding and sustainability of dementia training into practice (Brooke and Ojo 2018; Gkioka et al. 2020; Surr and Gates 2017). They also aim to foster a person-centred approach to dementia care within wards, developing an organisational culture that positions the psychological as well as physical health of people living with dementia as important (Gwernan-Jones et al. 2020b).

Jack-Waugh et al. (2018) developed a Dementia Champions programme for staff working in acute hospital settings across Scotland. Their role is to demonstrate leadership through modelling good person-centred practice, work in partnership with relatives of people living with dementia, disseminate learning through educational activities, and lead the implementation of practice development plans within their teams. The programme is delivered through a range of learning methods such as face-to-face content, which includes sessions delivered by people living with dementia, mentoring by personal tutors, peer discussion, participation in a community activity with people living with dementia, and reflective activities. It is delivered over an 8-month period and includes distance learning study, five face-to-face learning days, and a half-day in a community setting. It is assessed via three written assignments. Over 500 individuals registered for the programme between 2014 and 2017, with 430 completing, the large majority of whom were health care staff. The programme demonstrated significant improvements in knowledge and a large effect on the post-training self-efficacy scores compared with those recorded before learners commenced the programme. This shows this type of in-depth champion training provides people with the increased confidence and self-belief to work with people living with dementia, which is necessary to both role-model and lead practice change. Many of the champions have gone on to lead effective and sustained care and practice improvement in their organisation. Therefore, a robust approach to development of dementia champions, alongside a defined leadership role on training completion, seems to be an effective and sustainable way to implement a programme of dementia training and practice development.

The practicalities of training delivery and implementation in hospital settings

Who delivers training?

Acute hospital settings employ large numbers of staff. Therefore, it is important to consider how programmes of dementia training might realistically be implemented across a workforce. One approach to this is the use of train-the-trainer programmes (upskilling a group of existing staff to deliver a specific dementia training programme to other staff), whilst another is to rely on a smaller staff team whose roles are primarily focused on training delivery or who have specific contracted time dedicated to this.

Train-the-trainer programmes have the benefit of creating a large enough pool of staff who are able to deliver a programme of training in a cost-effective way (Pearce et al. 2012). This can be beneficial in terms of an organisation having a pool of staff who are able to offer a specific programme of training, both flexibly and sustainably. However, there are challenges with this. The more staff who are involved in the delivery of dementia training, the greater risk the core messages or learning becomes diluted. In addition, as was discussed in Chapter 2, skilled facilitation of formal dementia training is important. Training facilitators need to be both experienced clinicians, with an in-depth knowledge of dementia care theory and practice who role-model good practice, as well as competent, confident, enthusiastic teachers who are able to work flexibly. Train-the-trainer programmes often focus on upskilling individuals on delivery of the content of the training but may focus less on ensuring they have the necessary skills needed to facilitate learning and understand teaching techniques. They may also overlook important skills such as best practice in involvement and engagement of people living with dementia in training.

Research by two of the authors of this book explored the implementation of acute hospital-wide dementia training programmes in England (Surr et al. 2018c). We selected sites to take part in the case studies based on indicators of good practice regarding their training content and delivery methods, based on responses to a survey. Of the three case study sites that took part, Sites 1 and 2 employed a full-time lead nurse for dementia who coordinated training and was supported by a small group of clinical staff with expertise in dementia and training facilitation. Site 3 employed a small private training company to deliver its dementia training, supported for some sessions by Trust dementia champions who were clinically but not training facilitation experienced. In this site, the dementia training lead was one of the external training facilitators who was allocated one day a week to this role. The training delivered was evaluated well by staff in all sites, although sessions in Site 3 delivered by the dementia champions were noted to be less engaging for staff. In Sites 1 and 2, staff were able to describe how the training had impacted their staff knowledge, confidence, and practice behaviours. In Site 3, attendance at training was problematic and staff were less able to identify its impact on them or their practice. Overall training was patchy in Site 3 and this seemed to be related to the lack of a full-time dementia lead and allocation of responsibility to external staff who were less able to influence the organisational commitment to dementia care, or its culture towards training and its implementation.

Selection and development of facilitators therefore warrants careful consideration, alongside leadership for dementia care and associated training (which is discussed in more detail later in the chapter and in Chapter 9). A fine balance may be needed between ensuring an adequate pool of staff who are willing to deliver dementia training, alongside ensuring they have the required depth of experience and knowledge (both in terms of training facilitation and dementia care) to deliver it to a high standard. There is also a risk when developing staff as facilitators (who will be expected to deliver training as part of their existing clinical role) that they will be unable to make time to deliver sessions and thus training programmes may not be sustainable. This may also impact their ability to continually review and update training, or potentially to develop new and innovative approaches to training delivery. Limited time and resources can also mean opportunities to involve people directly affected by dementia in training may not be utilised, due to the additional time and financial resources this incurs. In addition, use of in-house facilitators may reduce the possibility of training programmes effectively challenging current ways of working, due to individuals being embedded within existing organisational cultures, the impact of which is discussed in more detail in Chapter 9.

However, despite these challenges, having internal staff to deliver training and support its implementation in practice, is likely to be the most cost-efficient, impactful, and sustainable approach for most health care organisations. Studies from the UK that have adopted a train-the-trainer model in **acute care** indicate that it can be as effective as training delivered by specialists, with regard to impact on learners' dementia knowledge and feelings of competence (Elvish et al. 2014; Heward et al. 2021b; Sampson et al. 2017), and it has the benefit of training being able to be delivered to a large number of staff. All these successful programmes ensured careful selection of staff to develop as facilitators and thorough preparation of them for their role via train-the-trainer programmes.

Features of impactful training in acute hospital settings

Surr and Gates (2017) conducted a review of the literature on dementia education and training in acute hospitals. They identified several features of training that were most likely to have a positive impact on staff reactions to the training, their knowledge and attitudes, and to support change in their practice behaviours and to lead to impacts on outcomes. These are presented in Box 6.1.

Box 6.1 The features of impactful education and training for acute hospital staff based on Surr and Gates (2017)

Training should:

- Be relevant and tailored to the staff role and workplace (e.g. use case studies relevant to those working across a range of roles or to the care scenarios staff commonly face).
- Include approaches, tools, or strategies that staff can apply directly to their own practice, such as pain assessment tools or communication strategies.
- Consider feasibility of placements in other settings that provide dementia care.

- Be facilitated by someone who is knowledgeable, able to role-model good practice, and who can engage and motivate staff.
- Carefully consider the use of e-learning. Avoid it as the sole method for dementia training and ensure that, where it is used, it is used alongside face-to-face learning activities that can ensure consolidation of learning.
- Ensure that time to attend training or engage in learning activities is scheduled for learners and is conducted in paid time.
- Include face-to-face, group-based discussion, exercises, and activities. These may be part of a blended approach, alongside other learning methods.
- Ensure the time allocated to learning is enough to provide adequate depth of learning (at least one full day is optimal with individual, face-to-face formal learning sessions of at least one hour's duration).
- Develop a number of staff as experts, facilitators, or 'champions' who can provide ongoing support to other staff and facilitate implementation of training into practice.
- Be led by a dedicated dementia lead whose role involves promoting good dementia care within the hospital, alongside organising the programme of dementia training, leading the team of training facilitators, and supporting implementation of training and delivery of person-centred care in practice.

Supporting implementation of learning into practice

The challenges of how to transfer learning from a training programme into practice are well documented across all settings, and Part 2 of this book is dedicated to considering these issues in more detail. Here we will briefly explore some of the factors that relate specifically to acute hospital settings.

It is well established that training alone is not enough to change care practice in acute hospital settings (Abley et al. 2019; Hung et al. 2019), and that a range of barriers and enablers exist that must be considered. Acute hospital settings are unique in the sense that people living with dementia have particularly complex needs due to the combination of being acutely, physically unwell alongside having dementia, which is usually not the reason for their hospital admission. The physical and emotional challenges of delivering person-centred care to people living with dementia with complex needs, within a context of high physical/medical care workload are widely acknowledged, and this may be accompanied by a perceived lack of support to meet these needs (Brooke and Ojo 2018). In some cases, the dementia diagnosis and subsequent impact dementia symptoms have on a person's behaviours and actions, can overshadow other physical care needs and symptoms. This can lead to misdiagnosis and unmet needs. A lack of support can be felt in various ways by staff, including disempowering policies, procedures, and practices focused on safety, legal issues, and liability (Brooke and Ojo 2018). However, evidence shows these can be mitigated by developing an organisational culture that gives staff the authority to act to address or adapt care practices, with a focus on person-centred care (Handley et al. 2019). This should include ongoing support to implement training through adopting a multi-disciplinary collaborative approach that supports the building of a common understanding and shared values base across staff teams. This can support development of team resilience, which can help with sustainability of implementation and practice change. As an example, in a Canadian study where general medical and mental health services were provided in one hospital site, mental health specialist nurses facilitated regular 'team huddles' during which practice related to care of people with dementia could be discussed (Hung et al. 2019). This provided an ongoing informal learning mechanism that helped to build on and sustain the formal training that staff had accessed.

Time is one of the major challenges identified in acute hospital settings, including that needed to attend training or engage in work-based learning opportunities (Smythe et al. 2013; Surr and Gates 2017). In some NHS Trusts, for example, dementia training is considered mandatory and therefore a strong case for dedicated time to attend training is able to be made for every staff member (Surr et al. 2018c). To achieve high levels of training completion and implementation, support for this needs to be clearly demonstrated throughout the organisation, including from the Hospital Board/Executives/Directors. There also needs to be widespread management buy-in and provision of clear clinical leadership to oversee and support implementation (Handley et al. 2019; Hung et al. 2019).

Summary

This chapter has outlined acute hospital care and the challenges staff working in these settings face in delivering person-centred care to people living with dementia. It has highlighted how the majority of training delivered in hospital settings is provided in-house, with nurses as the main learner group. The chapter identified how undertaking dementia training has been consistently found to provide benefits for staff knowledge, attitudes towards and confidence in caring for people living with dementia, alongside increased job satisfaction. Given the diversity of staff roles within acute hospital settings, ensuring training is tailored to the staff and their learning needs and role is important. Multi-disciplinary learning opportunities are valued by learners.

Implications for those delivering dementia training

Those delivering dementia training should:

- Tailor the training to the learners' individual needs and role, including dementia awareness for all staff and more in-depth training for those with regular contact with people living with dementia.
- Develop dementia leaders who can help to role-model good practice, mentor staff, champion dementia training and good dementia care, and support implementation of training into practice.
- Consider opportunities for multi-disciplinary learning.
- Ensure e-learning is not the sole method of training for any staff. When used, there should also be opportunities for face-to-face learning and small group discussion.
- Combine learning methods to provide the greatest impact and potential to put learning into practice (e.g. theory and knowledge-based content alongside experiential learning or simulation).
- Ensure training programmes include content that supports the development of empathy for people living with dementia.
- Ensure the voice of people directly affected by dementia is central to the training delivered, through use of direct and indirect methods of engagement, which are consistently and sustainably implemented.
- Consider ways to evaluate the impact of training (see Chapter 11), including long-term follow-up, impact on patient outcomes, and the potential need for refresher training.

Implications for managers in dementia care settings and services

Leaders and managers in hospital settings should:

- Make dementia training mandatory for all staff, facilitate attendance, and maintain an accurate organisational record of training completion.
- Create a culture that recognises the importance of person-centred care and the provision of good psychological as well as physical care to people living with dementia.
- Identify staff who can take on the role of dementia leaders to champion dementia training and care, and support implementation of training into practice.
- Identify and implement approaches to support the application of training into practice.
- Provide time and supplementary opportunities for staff to implement learning.
- Ensure those tasked with the delivery of dementia training are skilled clinicians and skilled training facilitators.
- Ensure there are enough skilled facilitators to be able to sustainably deliver dementia training to all staff who need it across the hospital.
- Ensure the hospital has at least one person whose primary role is to support the delivery of good dementia care across the service, which includes responsibility for dementia training and its implementation.

Implications for staff providing care, services, or support to people with dementia

Staff working in hospital settings should:

- Recognise the importance of delivering person-centred dementia care and the value of dementia training in enabling this.
- Identify ways that learning from dementia training can be implemented into practice and commit to making changes in how day-to-day care for people living with dementia is delivered.
- Seek support from dementia leaders (e.g. dementia champions) around delivery of person-centred dementia care and implementation of training into practice.
- Create opportunities to reflect on practice and use this as an opportunity for learning.

Implications for those directly affected by dementia

- There is very little research on hospital-based dementia training that has adopted direct or indirect methods of engaging with or ensuring the voice of those directly affected by dementia are heard.
- The time and resource limitations experienced in hospital settings may present a barrier to direct involvement in training by people living with dementia.
- There are many possibilities for engagement that remain unexplored and there may be innovative examples of engagement in practice that have not been more widely shared. Those working in the field should commit to broadening the scope of research and practice knowledge in this area.

7 Learning and development in community settings

> 'Care in the community sector is less homogeneous than statutory care provision and is subject to less dedicated research and development of training. This is despite most people with dementia living in the community.'

The majority of people living with dementia, with and without a diagnosis, will spend most of their time living in their communities: in their own or family home, or supported accommodation. In the UK, two-thirds of people living with dementia are living in the community in their own homes, with one-third living alone (Prince et al. 2014). In lower-income countries, almost all (96 per cent) of people living with dementia live at home (ADI 2021). This is significant because by 2050, 71 per cent of people living with dementia will be in low- and middle-income countries (Wimo et al. 2018). Access to statutory dementia services (social care and medical care) is often limited in low- and middle-income countries, meaning informal caregivers – or the third sector – are critical to providing support.

Whilst most of the support in the community is provided by family or friends (informal care), formal support can be delivered by a wide range of health and social care staff or volunteers. This workforce needs to be as well equipped as any other to provide person-centred care. This is particularly so because community services meeting people early in their journey of dementia have an opportunity to set expectations for person-centred care that will improve the trajectory of a person's experiences as their dementia progresses. Community services most often provide support alongside the unpaid, informal support of families and friends and thus, when done well, offers fortification to this vital component of living well with dementia.

Community care and support is complex and entails a range of services: government funded, private, third sector, and volunteer led. A range of health and social care services are provided in the community, including care provided in people's homes (homecare), housing, **housing with care** options, day services, and community-led support initiatives such as dementia cafes, advocacy services, support groups, meeting centres, and befriending services.

The range of professionals and paraprofessionals involved in the delivery of these services makes it challenging to systematically review and make generalisable recommendations for training and education for the sector. Furthermore, given that many of these services are delivered by non-health care staff, the application of training standard frameworks, such as those described in Chapter 1, can be more challenging, at least without substantial adaptation to fit different service types. The purpose of this chapter is to select some of the services, professionals, and paraprofessionals involved in providing support for people in the community and review the evidence base for best-practice training in these services as well as some novel initiatives associated with these areas, so that targeted recommendations for people providing training or support for these areas can be made.

It is important to state at the outset that many of the initiatives aimed at enhancing dementia care by volunteers, community groups, and/or informal caregivers focus on raising awareness of dementia by highlighting the things that people can do to help people living with dementia to live well and safely in their communities. We refer to this level of training as 'dementia awareness training' (i.e. basic information about dementia that everybody should know). One example of this type of dementia awareness raising is the Dementia Friends initiative delivered by the Alzheimer's Society in the UK. This type of training is useful as a route to enhance dementia knowledge for the general public, to improve 'dementia-friendly' communities, or for volunteers working in generic settings. Nonetheless, as stated by the Alzheimer's Society, dementia awareness is not formal training, and is positioned as an awareness-raising initiative only. If this dementia awareness training were to be equated to a training level outlined in the Dementia Training Education Standards Framework in England described in Chapter 1, it would be equivalent to Tier 0. This is not to detract from the value of such initiatives, but rather to illustrate that they are distinct from training of interest to learning and development practitioners and the intended readership of this book.

Care provided in people's homes (homecare)

More than half of people (60 per cent) who receive formal care and support at home (as distinct from informal care from family and friends) in the UK are living with dementia (Carter 2016). Similarly, across Europe more people living with dementia are cared for via homecare services than in institutional settings (Hallberg et al. 2016). Homecare, also known as domiciliary care, can range from ensuring that people are safe, preparing meals, and administering medication, to providing support with personal hygiene and activities of daily living. Supporting people to stay at home where possible is important, as the longer people can be supported to live independently at home the better outcomes people experience in terms of well-being.

Homecare is most often provided by homecare workers, known internationally as support workers, healthcare assistants, or home health aides. Although the systems within which they operate vary, these workers are often paraprofessionals. In a study of eight European countries, it was established that frontline care was most often provided by those with little or no formal training for the role, and rarely by anyone with dementia specialist education (Hallberg et al. 2016), although some countries do integrate professional nursing services with paraprofessional support. Historically in the UK, this workforce has been overlooked, falling through the gap with regards to regulation, recommendations, and training provision. In 2016, a large-scale survey conducted by the Alzheimer's Society and the trade union UNISON established that 38 per cent of homecare workers had not received any dementia training, and 71 per cent had not received any accredited training. Moreover, only 2 per cent of respondents directly affected by dementia felt that homecare workers received enough dementia training (Carter 2016). Several recommendations were made following this report, including linking homecare services to The Care Certificate, training frameworks and regulations affecting care home and hospital paraprofessionals outlined in Chapter 1 and elsewhere in this book. However, as highlighted in Chapter 1, these are not unproblematic, not least because they are not dementia specific.

Despite more people living in community settings than in long-term care settings, there is significantly less research evidence concerning dementia training for the homecare workforce, suggesting a need for researchers and practitioners to focus on homecare for people living with dementia. This chapter will review the international evidence for innovative approaches to delivering training and education to the homecare workforce. In the first instance, there are a small selection of studies that seek to identify the training needs of this group across various countries.

Training needs in the homecare sector

In Australia, an evaluation of the experience of homecare recipients (Polacsek et al. 2020) revealed that there are gaps in homecare workers' knowledge about dementia. The evaluation indicated that an understanding of the lived experience of dementia, effective communication and rapport, and continuity of care, all contributed positively to their experience of receiving care, suggesting that training for this workforce should focus on these areas. These findings are particularly pertinent because researchers more commonly conduct studies in which educational needs are determined by workers themselves or chosen from selections provided by academics. For example, a number of topics were identified by homecare workers in rural Canada as a priority for continuing education, including recognising different dementia sub-types, providing palliative care, managing behaviour, and discussing changes with patients and families (Morgan et al. 2016). In addition, a review of literature on homecare workers' experiences of aggression in dementia care identified that specific training in communication skills and responding to behaviour could be helpful for homecare workers (Schnelli et al. 2020).

These studies are not directly comparable because they were conducted in different countries and in different ways. However, they do suggest that, whilst there may be some overlap between worker-identified and recipient-derived training needs, there may also be differences that are worthy of further exploration. Therefore, a way forward in this under-explored area should include investigating the implications of these differences in terms of how person-centred homecare is understood by those living at home and needing care and those delivering it.

Training interventions in the homecare sector

There are fewer evaluated training interventions in the homecare sector than in other sectors. This suggests this an area that requires more focus within research, but also hints at some of the challenges to accessing this sector for the purposes of both training and research. As in other sectors, training interventions generally show an impact on staff outcomes at Kirkpatrick Levels 2 and 3. For example, in Japan a 2-day programme (one day training and one day follow-up/debrief) focused on supporting people experiencing behavioural changes in dementia which resulted in significant improvements in homecare staff attitudes to dementia with no associated increase in burden of care (Nakanishi et al. 2018).

As indicated in Chapters 4 and 10, attempting to assess the impact of training on people directly affected by dementia is also important. However, because so many other factors can affect the translation of staff knowledge, attitudes, and confidence into changed behaviour and improved outcomes, it is also very challenging.

There is plenty of opportunity for future development and research of training interventions in this sector to take this into account and demonstrate a more sophisticated understanding of what is important for achieving real-world impact. For example, two rural homecare organisations in Canada explored the role of 'knowledge brokers' to identify and design 'knowledge translation strategies' (bespoke education solutions to regular problems faced by workers). Evaluation via interviews established that these bespoke solutions not only enhanced knowledge but also enhanced client and family well-being and enabled more tailored solutions for clients.

It could be argued that online training may be well suited to workers who are mobile, work varied hours, and often lack a central 'hub' for their work. It is perhaps surprising, therefore, that there has not been greater exploration of online education delivery with this group. One study using a unique online, 12-week person-centred dementia care training intervention that combined mobile e-learning and social networking was subjected to a randomised controlled trial in Taiwan. When compared with conventional day-long lectures, the intervention significantly improved the knowledge, attitudes, and sense of competency of homecare workers, retaining this impact 12 weeks after the end of the programme (Su et al. 2021). This is promising. However, a study of rural homecare workers in Canada established that there was low interest in computer-based, online delivery for continuing education and high interest in locally delivered courses (Kosteniuk et al. 2016). The authors suggested that homecare workers' professional isolation is likely to contribute to this preference and thus this is important to consider when planning provision.

Whilst the lack of homecare-specific training interventions is marked, this does not mean that learning from other sectors is not transferable. It is important that the homecare sector does not 'reinvent the wheel' when it comes to developing person-centred educational interventions but is instead mindful to adapt existing evidence-rich solutions to differing circumstances. For example, a Norwegian study explored the implementation of the VIPS practice model, a training-plus intervention successfully introduced within care home settings (Rokstad et al., 2013; Røsvik et al., 2011) that uses 2-day training and weekly 'consensus' meetings built around the VIPS framework. It identified that similar facilitators existed across care homes, day care and homecare services. These included a supportive management ethos, stable staff team, dedicated time for both training and for consensus meetings, and leadership of the intervention within the service (Røsvik and Mjørud 2021).

Training has also been explored as a route to reducing job strain within the homecare sector. In the UK and elsewhere, the pressures on homecare staff have been extensively reported, regarding pay, status, and restrictions on time given for visits, travel between visits, and pay to attend training (Carter 2016). High levels of job strain and stress have been reported in homecare workers worldwide (Hanson et al. 2015). A targeted education intervention in Sweden was designed to address job strain. The intervention involved enhancing knowledge and skills concerning evidence-based care and person-centred care, thus improving staff's ability to deliver high-quality care, as a means of reducing job strain. Training was delivered by researchers in small groups over 12 months (meeting ten times), involving a range of learning activities and exercises, including working through challenging experiences from learners' own practice. Overall job strain was shown to be reduced by the training, although the efficacy of person-centred care in practice was not assessed (Fallahpour et al. 2020).

Finally, mention of informal learning within the homecare sector is rare, perhaps simply reflecting the lack of focus overall on this sector. However, it is important to note that the isolation of homecare workers, lack of daily oversight, and the variability of their work environments (every individual home presents a new challenge compared with more standardised environments such as hospitals) will lend themselves to certain types of informal and self-directed learning, such as problem-solving and reflection. These present some interesting possibilities for approaches to support informal learning towards person-centred care that may be particularly important given the relative lack of daily interaction with colleagues experienced by homecare workers. For example, a small innovative study exploring the impact of reflective diary writing for 11 homecare workers suggests that the process (which included short training in reflective diary writing, but not in dementia care) enabled workers to better make sense of their work and stress and improve their caregiving because it prompted reflection and self-directed learning about clients, self, and situations (Travers et al. 2020).

Dementia training within the housing sector

In the UK, supported, sheltered, extra care or housing with care services – in which a person owns or rents a self-contained property within a housing complex that also offers the option of additional facilities, social and/or personal care support – has been suggested as an option to maintain independence and quality of life for people living with dementia, and to reduce the need for long-term care in care homes (Department of Health 2009). Internationally, the term 'assisted living' is also used for these types of services, although there is an overlap between the level of care provided within assisted living and that provided by care homes. For example, assisted living is the primary provider of non-nursing 24-hour care for people living with dementia in the US, with an estimated two-thirds of residents having dementia (Zimmerman et al. 2014). This is a demographic more akin to residential care homes in the UK.

Internationally and domestically, such housing services can vary substantially in their organisation and the services they provide, and they have changed over time to cater for the increasing needs of tenants. Typically, an extra care type service would include on-site management with optional care services provided either by an on-site team of staff or by an external homecare provider. Services with higher levels of support (in particular, newer-style services) often include optional facilities such as restaurant dining, activities, and support with housekeeping. Whilst there will be similarity in training needs and lessons to be transferred between the care home and extra-care housing sector, it is also true that unique issues and needs arise in this sector (Hyde et al. 2007). For example, studies have identified that staff in extra care housing faced very specific issues in implementing person-centred care that could have implications for their training, such as navigating independence, environmental barriers and social stigma on behalf of tenants (Evans et al. 2020), and responding to walking with purpose (Barrett et al. 2020).

One of the few examples of focused research into housing-specific training is the randomised controlled trial of the Enriched Opportunities Programme (Brooker and Woolley 2007). This is a training-plus intervention in which four components (a specialist expert role; individual assessment and case work; activity and occupation programme; and leadership) occur alongside comprehensive training for staff. This approach demonstrated positive outcomes for residents living with dementia in terms of increased quality of life, reduced depressive symptoms, and reduced admittance to a care home or hospital across an 18-month period (Brooker et al. 2007). The design of this training matches those features shown to be impactful: occurring across multiple days, including reflection, experiential exercises, and application of tools to practice (Surr et al. 2017a). This would suggest that specialist training is important to improving person-centred care but only in the context of a comprehensive intervention that addresses the setting holistically. In Chapter 4, the implications of this were discussed in depth with reference to care homes, most notably that it could be the other non-training components of comprehensive interventions that are most significant in changing practice. As Dutton (2010) highlights, specialist and well-trained staff are only one organisational attribute that helps to enhance quality of life for people living with dementia in extra care housing.

The lack of a specific focus in research and training on the housing sector is more stark when looking to more generic forms of housing. As an example, the UK has a large and diverse non-specialist social housing sector. Whilst often overlooked by dementia researchers and practitioners (due to a lack of targeted funding) in favour of specialist housing services, or other health and social care provision (Lipman and Manthorpe 2017), this type of generic landlord provision is important to promote person-centred outcomes for people living with dementia because increasing numbers of older people will be living in social rather than private accommodation (Bligh 2016). Moreover, social housing providers often contribute additional services such as property maintenance, welfare advice and signposting, and have a significant presence in underprivileged communities (Bligh 2016) and communities with high cultural and ethnic diversity (Lipman and Manthorpe 2017). This suggests that staff in these settings could be a significant route of influence towards positive experiences for those living with dementia across society.

Staff training has been identified as an essential component of enabling non-specialist generic housing to become (Hucker 2013) with those in customer-facing roles such as maintenance operatives identified as being of significant importance (Bligh 2016). People living with dementia themselves identified training as a key component of the dementia-friendly housing charter (Miles and Pritchard-Wilkes 2018). However, evidence-based approaches to training this workforce are lacking. Training for this workforce was identified as a key issue in the UK in a 2021 government report on housing for people living with dementia, specifically stating that there are gaps in the knowledge and skills in the workforce, and that there was an educational need for families (APPG 2021). The report goes on to state that the housing workforce should be trained in line with the Dementia Training Standards Framework (outlined in Chapter 1). In summary, the development and implementation of evidence-based training for people working in the housing sector remains a pressing international issue.

Dementia training in day care and respite services

Even more varied than the housing sector is the provision of day care programmes, centres and day respite services for people living with dementia. Not only are there a variety of different names given to this type of service both nationally and internationally, their organisation and management is disparate. They may be run via statutory services or third sector organisations, or attached to other facilities such as care homes. There can also be a significant overlap between such services and those for the general community; some may develop specifically for those people living with dementia, whereas others may spring up within community settings such as libraries, community centres, and leisure facilities or as offshoots of generic community provision. More-over, staffing of these services also reflects this variation, with a combination of health and social care workers (commonly paraprofessionals) and volunteers operating these services in the UK and internationally.

Specific research evidence of specialist dementia training programmes in this sector is notable by its absence. However, there are studies that identify training as an important component in improving stakeholder experiences and uptake of respite services (O'Shea et al. 2017) and transforming the organisational culture of services towards person-centred care (Kirkley et al. 2011). As with other community sectors, there may be some overlap between the para-professional workforce within day care settings and those of housing, home-care, care homes, and hospitals. However, there are also likely to be differences and as such, additional research could be useful. The most significant difference within day care services is likely to be the interface between paid professional/paraprofessional staff and volunteers, particularly when a service is primarily focused on social support and occupation for people living with dementia. The following case example illustrates how evidence-based training programmes developed for care home settings have been successfully adapted for use in community settings. In this particular case, the location of the service is also important. We have previously identified that community care for people directly affected by dementia is vastly more relied upon in low- and middle-income countries than in higher-income countries, and will be a growing issue.

Case example: Adapting a UK training programme combining formal training and in-practice coaching with use in community care in Southern Africa

According to Alzheimer's Disease International (2019), Sub-Saharan Africa is expected to experience the greatest proportionate increase in the numbers of people living with dementia by 2050, thus making it the key focus for awareness and policy development. An evidence-based training programme from the UK adapted for use with community-based practitioners in Zimbabwe, is already proving to be invaluable in equipping staff in the region with skills and knowledge to tackle local dementia-related challenges.

Whilst initially designed for implementation in care homes, the training programme uses a training and coaching model to support the ongoing development of individual dementia care champions, who progress person-centred care within their own services. A dementia practice development coach (DPDC) trained in the evidence-based training approach has adapted the programme to the community context in Zimbabwe. In this Southern African version, the 10 days of interactive training content includes additional country-specific knowledge and enhanced teaching on basic person-centred care, alongside the standard learning outcomes intended to develop comprehensive understanding of topics including:

- dementia, the brain, and the principles of person-centred care;
- behaviour as communication;
- tools for using person-centred interventions to provide care instead of restrictive practices and inappropriate prescribing of antipsychotics;
- the role of life history, supporting families, the environment, and meaningful occupation in providing good dementia care;
- delivering training to support others.

In addition, the six, monthly, group-coaching sessions facilitated by the DPDC focus on the practicalities and real-life experience of trainees as they apply that learning in their day-to-day work and support people living with dementia in their own homes.

The first cohort of ten dementia champions working under the supervision and guidance of the DPDC have completed their training and are putting their skills to use in Zimbabwe. Alongside this, a day care centre for older people founded on person-centred principles, is providing a service to the community in one locality in Zimbabwe. The day centre, which operates as a private voluntary organisation, adopts close and collaborative working together with two care homes within the city and the director has been invited to share its principles and success in neighbouring countries. It has helped to equip trainees of the evidence-based programme with invaluable experience and opportunities for coaching and reflection-in-practice at the centre.

Dementia training for the third sector and volunteers

Dementia care is frequently provided by people working or volunteering in third sector organisations and community groups. The nature of services provided by this sector is vast and again involves paid professionals (such as nurses) and volunteers. For example, a leading dementia charity in the UK (Alzheimer's Society) provides services that range from dementia cafes, run by paid staff and volunteers, to conferences showcasing dementia research, to online support services.

It is often the case that these services expand or provide more support when there are reduced statutory services for people living with dementia, for example in low- and middle-income countries. In the context of dementia care in the UK, where health and social care services are available, the third sector still plays a pivotal role in reducing pressure on health and social care services by providing support and care for people living with dementia (Bull et al. 2014) as well as filling gaps. Furthermore, third sector organisations can often better reach marginalised and minority communities, where individuals may be reluctant to engage with statutory services. In the UK context, this opportunity was identified in the All Party Parliamentary Group on Dementia report 'Dementia Does Not Discriminate' (APPG 2013). The report provides two examples of specialist ethnic minority dementia services that have successfully met the needs of the local population, a day centre service and a befriending service. The report identifies a large ethic minority voluntary third sector providing health and welfare support in a culturally sensitive manner, where statutory dementia services fail to meet these needs.

There is limited research evidence concerning training provided for this sector. Given the importance and scale of this sector, particularly for low- and middle-income countries, research is needed to establish a consensus in best practice. Furthermore, funding for training in this sector can present a significant issue. Despite the third sector often relying on people giving freely of their time, there are staffing costs associated with training volunteers in order that they can deliver safe person-centred care (Hansen 2014). Some volunteers are encouraged to sign up to national programmes that are freely available online, such as those available via the UK Social Care Institute for Excellence websites. A limitation of this is that it relies on the individual and there is no follow-up as to the efficacy of training outcomes. On the other hand, a feature of this sector is that many volunteers will be coming to their volunteer role with experience or an interest in dementia, which means that their level of pre-existing knowledge may be higher than that in the general population.

Training needs for third sector organisations and volunteers

The disparate nature of staff and volunteers working for the third sector means that it is hard to suggest a one-size-fits-all approach for identifying training needs. In this section, we provide an example of an approach taken which provides a suggested way to tackle this issue. The Alzheimer's Association is a leading US-based international dementia charity. Their mission is related both to supporting research to end Alzheimer's and to provide support and advocacy for people living with dementia. Therefore, ensuring that their workforce is aligned to their beliefs and philosophy is important. If a workforce is not prepared to deliver care in line with the core philosophies and values of the organisation, this represents a risk (Hansen 2014).

Training which addresses stigmatising views about dementia and addresses beliefs and values about living with dementia is central to many of the dementia training standards frameworks presented in Chapter 1. In a small-scale study (Herrmann et al. 2019), training that addressed dementia-related stigma was delivered to non-health care professional Alzheimer's Association staff. The training intervention was delivered in group sessions over 2½ hours, and involved communication experts, example scenarios, and opportunities for interactive discussions. The study found that the training which aimed to improve awareness of stigma had positive effects on knowledge and plans to change behaviours. Most Alzheimer's Association staff felt the training helped them to better identify stigma surrounding Alzheimer's, made them more comfortable about talking about these issues, and said it would change the way they interacted with people and families impacted by Alzheimer's-type dementia.

This study highlights the importance of providing targeted training to third sector and voluntary staff. The training did elicit benefits in intended behaviour as well as knowledge. However, the duration of the training was short, and this is a limitation of the study. If we are to take the standard of 8 hours of training (to elicit positive effects) outlined in Chapter 2, the duration is short by comparison.

Training interventions for the third sector

As well as limited studies of dementia-specific training in the third sector, it can be challenging to draw comparisons between training provided by third sector organisations and that provided by statutory services due to the nature of the staff and organisational differences. One difference is that third sector organisations are often not subject to the same benchmarks or standards, although aligning to benchmarks or standards can be a useful reference point for developing and evaluating training outcomes. The following provides an example of this approach being adopted. Wilesmith and Major (2020) describe a course provided by a third sector organisation for volunteers providing a 'sitting' service for people living with dementia. The training course involved attending six, weekly, 3-hour sessions, delivered by a mental health nurse. The course was developed to align with the Dementia Training Standards Framework in England (Skills for Health 2018), and was underpinned by a person-centred approach. The course, attended by 13 volunteers, involved open discussions, case study work, and role-play. There were opportunities for practical advice throughout, which enabled discussions for the translation of theory to practice, which was also facilitated by the role-play. The varied nature of delivery methods was specifically designed to engage people with different learning styles (see Chapter 8). The course was evaluated by a pre-post questionnaire designed to capture knowledge of dementia, confidence, and awareness of safeguarding in their role, which showed positive effects because of the training.

This small-scale training intervention adheres to many of the best-practice recommendations for developing training described elsewhere in this book, such as aligning to an established training standards framework, meeting the minimum duration of training, having a face-to-face component, enabling opportunities to translate theory into practice, and being responsive to the learning styles of different learners. A further feature of this training was that it involved simulation via role-play. The use of role-play in dementia training has been a contentious issue. From an experiential learning perspective, this kind of approach can have positive effects as it engenders empathy and can help practise managing scenarios which can be challenging, such as when people experience behavioural changes. However, it can also overgeneralise the experience of living with dementia and perpetuate myths and stigmatising views about living with dementia. As such, it is an approach that should be incorporated into training with caution and care. In this study, the learners reported that they valued the opportunity to understand how to manage the behaviours that people find challenging through the opportunities to engage in role-play, although three of the ten volunteers declined the role-play opportunity as they did not feel confident enough to take part.

Case example: Developing a nursing academy incorporating an in-house competency model

A charitable organisation set up to provide specialist dementia nurses who support the needs of families of people living with dementia has developed a nursing academy with its own in-house competency framework. The academy facilitates continuing practice and professional development for the nurses, where possible providing the opportunity for peer-to-peer support. The charity is currently supporting around 350 specialist nurses based in a variety of different settings, including the community, hospitals, care homes, and hospices.

All the specialist nurses are qualified to the standards identified in professional registration frameworks – however, these standards are not tailored to prepare the nurses for undertaking their more specialist dementia-specific role.

To address this, the charity worked in partnership with a higher education institution to develop their own competency framework. Developing a personalised competency framework is a means of ensuring that education and development is fit for purpose and tailored to the needs of learners. The competency framework was first developed in 2003 and subsequently updated in 2012 and 2016. The framework is currently being reviewed to ensure that it aligns with the Specialist Practitioner Qualification standards that the Nursing and Midwifery Council will release in 2022.

The charity engaged in a period of consultation in 2019 to assess the best ways of delivering the educational resources that support the implementation of the competency framework. Educational resources had initially been made available to the specialist nurses online and as printed documents. However, the evaluation indicated there was limited engagement with these resources, with nurses citing issues with lack of support and having to work through things by themselves as barriers to engagement.

To address these barriers, educators at a university worked with the charity to deliver the competency framework and associated resources using more interactive approaches. Workshop-based activities were provided to groups of nurses to promote understanding and critical reflection. The workshops were divided into three exercises: one focused on sharing perspectives, the second on critically reflective conversations, and the third on the competency framework and sharing examples from practice.

The COVID-19 pandemic meant the charity had to adapt the means of providing practice and professional development for the nurses. The charity adopted a virtual model with a dedicated online space for supporting the nurse academy and which facilitates learning and development. The online space provides independent learning opportunities and facilitated modules, with time built in for shared learning and peer support. The academy also includes webinars, special interest groups, communities of practice, and leadership programmes. Throughout their learning, the nurses are expected to reflect on and identify which elements of the competency framework they are demonstrating and the implications this has for their practice.

This case speaks to the importance of two facilitatory factors for education and development of professional staff working in dementia specialist roles within a range of settings:

1 The benefits of developing tailored competency frameworks to ensure the preparedness of staff to meet their role.
2 Ensuring that the delivery of resources is supported in practice using a wide variety of interactive methods and opportunities for reflective dialogue with peers. Competency frameworks in themselves are not sufficient; it is important to enable the opportunity to apply critical reflection to one's own practice.

Summary

In this chapter, we have discussed a range of evaluated education and training relevant to the homecare, housing, and day care sector, including approaches to volunteers and the third sector. Care in the community sector is less homogeneous than statutory care provision and is subject to less dedicated research and development of training. This is despite most people with dementia living in the community. Community-based services make a significant difference to the personal experiences of people affected by dementia, so it is vital to grow the evidence base concerning approaches to learning that are feasible and effective to ensure that the paid and volunteer workforce is equipped to promote person-centred care for people living with dementia.

Implications for those delivering dementia training

Those leading and facilitating dementia training should:

- Refer to benchmarks or standards where available for the sector or explore the development of such.
- Evaluate the real-world impact of training interventions.
- Consider the impact of sector-specific issues on ability to engage with training, mode of delivery, and willingness to engage – for example, home-care workforce is often mobile, volunteers may have limited capacity to engage with training.
- Use methods of training that are appropriate for the staff or volunteers' experience and learning style.

Implications for managers in dementia care settings and services

Managers in community service settings should:

- Understand the training priorities identified by staff, volunteers, and recipients of support.
- Assess the extent to which the values of the workforce align to the organisation.
- Consider the ways in which people directly affected by dementia can be better integrated into training provided to staff and volunteers.

- Pay particular attention to the needs of marginalised and minority communities who may have contact with the service and ensure training addresses their needs.

Implications for staff or volunteers providing care, services, or support to people living with dementia

Staff and volunteers working in dementia care should:

- Reflect on their values and learning needs.
- Recognise that basic 'awareness' level knowledge of dementia is not sufficient when working closely with people directly affected by dementia – further training will be required.

Implications for those directly affected by dementia

- Consider ways to better integrate direct experiences of people affected by dementia in training provision, as outlined in Chapter 2.
- Pay particular attention to the diversity of people living with dementia: reach out to organisations working with hard-to-reach and minority groups to ensure their perspectives are heard and represented in training.
- Establish and integrate what people directly affected by dementia want and need from their community services into the design and delivery of training.
- Involve people affected by dementia in the evaluation of training interventions when assessing the impact on changes in the behaviour of staff or volunteers.

Part **2**

Theory and evidence underpinning the implementation of effective education and training for the dementia care workforce

8 The person at the centre of the learning experience

'It is important that facilitators create a learning environment in which learners feel welcome and supported, and which recognises not everyone arrives with confidence, excitement, and openness to learning. Flexibility is paramount.'

This chapter will explore the individual needs of learners that are important for supportive and successful learning to take place. It will include factors such as learning styles, prior educational experiences, neurodiversity, learning difficulties, physical and sensory disabilities, literacy, and culture. It is not meant to provide a comprehensive guide on how to provide training that is inclusive, supportive, and accessible to all, but instead to highlight specific issues that need to be considered when designing dementia training. This chapter will also consider the opportunities and issues surrounding use of training explicitly as a mechanism for improving poor individual job performance.

Learning styles

Learning styles are commonly discussed in relation to tailoring the way training is delivered to the specific ways individual learners prefer to learn (Riener and Willingham 2010). An individual's learning style might be established through completing a questionnaire or learning styles test such as those listed in Table 8.1.

Before the start of the millennium, learning styles were commonly accepted as being based in evidence. However, recent research indicates there is little evidence to support the existence of learning styles, or that tailoring training to learning style improves learning (Cuevas 2015; Pashler et al. 2008; Riener and Willingham 2010; Rohrer and Pashler 2012). It may be that learners feel they have a preferred mode of learning, but evidence suggests they can learn equally as well when using other modes. Whilst there remains little evidence or evaluation of some learning styles models and further research is needed in this area (Riener and Willingham 2010), the current evidence base provides no support for using learning styles models to underpin how individual learners are taught.

Rather, it is suggested that those designing and delivering training should consider the most appropriate method for delivering a particular component of learning, based on learning theories (see Chapter 2). Providing variety in the

Table 8.1 Common learning styles models

Authors	Components/styles
Kolb (1985)	Individuals prefer to learn in one of four quadrants across the dimensions of Do vs. Watch and Feel vs. Think. • Accommodators: prefer to actively do and feel an experience. • Convergers: prefer to actively do and think about an experience. • Divergers: prefer to watch and feel and experience. • Assimilators: prefer to watch and think about an experience.
Honey and Mumford (1986)	Builds on Kolb's learning styles. • Activists: enjoy having and immersing themselves in an experience. • Pragmatists: like to try out new ideas and experiment. • Reflectors: like to stand back and observe and think about experiences from different perspectives. • Theorists: like to analyse and bring together information and observations and draw logical conclusions.
Butler and Gregorc (1988)	People have natural preferences that position them in one of four combinations of: • Concrete (dealing with the here and now information via the senses) vs. Abstract (visualise and conceive beyond what can be seen) *combined with* • Sequential (preference for linear or step-by-step ways of organising information) vs. Random (information organised in chunks but without a particular order) e.g. concrete sequential learning style.
Dunn and Dunn (1992, 1993)	Learning style is an individual's reaction or preference to elements across five strands of processing: • Environmental: learning environment including sound levels, lighting, temperature, and seating type/layout. • Emotional: motivation, feelings of responsibility for learning, imposed structure vs. personal choice. • Sociological: learning alone vs. with peers, with an instructor, in a routine/pattern or ad hoc. • Physiological: perceptual preferences (*auditory*, e.g. listening; *visual*, e.g. texts, pictures; *tactile*, e.g. hands-on via experiments or making models; *kinaesthetic*, e.g. experiential learning/total involvement), time of day, movement/static. • Psychological: global vs. analytic (preference for global content/concept followed by details and facts vs. details and facts building up to global content/concept), reflective vs. impulsive (preferring a thorough process to reach a conclusion vs. concluding quickly with little fear of failure). Perceptual preferences are seen as the most important aspect.

way content and materials are presented is one way to support effective learning that would accommodate a range of approaches different learners may feel more comfortable with and thus feel more inclusive. This chapter will outline a variety of dimensions on which learners will differ, which can impact on how they learn, and which those designing and delivering dementia training must consider.

Prior educational experiences

Staff working in dementia care have diverse backgrounds and experiences regarding prior educational attainment, experiences of education and training, and in the subsequent impact this may have had on their learning self-efficacy, confidence, and motivation (Hussein and Manthorpe 2012). Social cognitive theory (Bandura 1986) puts forward a three-way framework to explain this (see Figure 8.1). It states that learners who have high self-efficacy or confidence in learning (personal processes) are more likely to engage in learning activities and to make efforts to learn (behaviours). A learner's feelings of self-efficacy are influenced by their prior experiences of education – whether they have been told they are 'bright', 'intelligent', 'academic', or, as may be the case with many learners working as paraprofessionals in non-academic sectors such as care, they are 'stupid', 'not a natural student', or 'lazy'. For those with this latter experience, their confidence in learning and thus feelings about attending training programmes are naturally impacted. This can lead to them feeling anxious, worried, and disengaged from learning or to even avoid attending training, for fear of being belittled or made to feel stupid, as they did when they received these negative messages during prior educational experiences.

It is important that facilitators create a learning environment in which learners feel welcome and supported, and which recognises not everyone arrives with confidence, excitement, and openness to learning. Flexibility is paramount. Understanding learners' existing knowledge of a topic and what they hope to gain from attending a training programme can be an important starting

Figure 8.1 Social cognitive theory's triadic reciprocal framework (based on Bandura 1986)

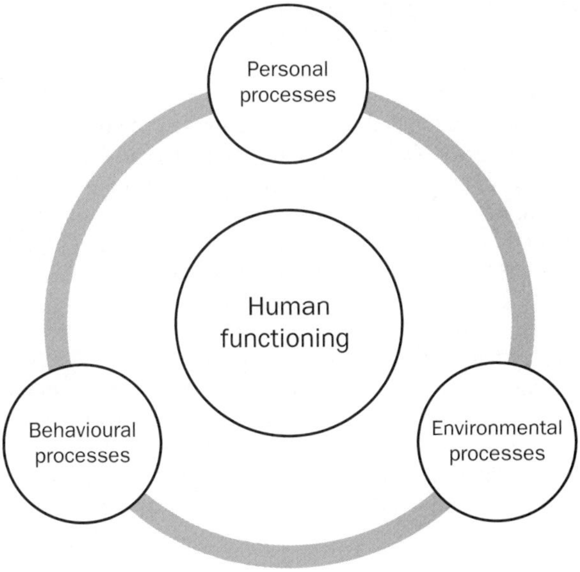

point from which to build delivery of content in a way that is tailored to both groups of learners and specific individuals. This may mean, for example, ensuring training is pitched at the right level for those attending to build confidence, and including exercises and activities that can help to assess learners' understanding, so training can progress at the right pace. Facilitators may also need to spend time building confidence, encouraging engagement, recognising and praising achievements, and undoing the damage caused by negative prior educational experiences, which may have been present since childhood for some learners. It can also be helpful to provide learners with full information about the training programme and what it will entail in advance. Box 8.1 includes examples of approaches training facilitators can adopt that may help to build learner confidence. These are things which are easier to implement in face-to-face training situations and may be more challenging to achieve where delivery is online.

Box 8.1 Approaches that can help to build learner confidence

- Help learners to feel prepared. Give learners enough information about what the training will involve so they are not unsure about or fearful of what to expect.
- Know your learner group and pitch the training at their level. This will mean advance preparation to gather the required information and may mean being flexible and able to adapt what you are doing.
- Do not put people on the spot, or force people to answer questions or speak out in front of the group as this can raise fear and anxiety levels.
- If people do speak out or share answers to questions, then encourage this and welcome their response and insights. Even if you feel the answer is incorrect, sharing is an important part of learning and feeling safe.
- If you feel an answer is incorrect, then use careful questioning and ideas from others in the group to explore alternative views. For example, you might say 'That is a really interesting answer. Can you explain more about why you think that?' Or, 'I can see exactly where you are coming from there. Situations like this are very complex and there are often different perspectives. Can you think of any alternative ways of seeing this/ approaching this situation that you also think might be helpful?' Or, 'Does anyone else in the group have a suggestion about this?'
- Ensure there is time to provide support within the session, during breaks, or at the end for anyone who seems to be struggling. For example, you might spend time with individuals when the group is completing learning activities. Having two facilitators can be helpful in such circumstances.
- Offer different approaches to learning the same content, so that confidence and skills can be built slowly. For example, talking through information in a short lecture, followed by a video and then a case study-based exercise can help to build learning step by step through different methods.

- Offer praise – tell the group they are doing well, that they have given some excellent answers to the exercises, etc.
- Draw and build on their existing knowledge and expertise – think about what they already know and use that as building blocks for learning.
- Build learning activities in small steps, with tangible outcomes so both you and the learners can see their progress. Don't move on if the group is not understanding the content; find another way to go over it again.

In Chapter 2, the potential benefits of multi-disciplinary learning were discussed. One of the potential challenges of true multi-disciplinary learning (which includes management, professionally registered, non-registered clinical/care, and ancillary staff) is ensuring training content and pace are able to meet the potentially diverse needs of such cohorts – a diversity which may include prior educational experiences. Recognising that each learner brings with them unique skills and knowledge and can make a valuable contribution and then building exercises and activities within the training to draw these out is one approach. For example, case study activities may ask for different perspectives on a care scenario and can be used to explore what those in different roles within the setting contribute to the care of a person living with dementia.

Neurodiversity and learning differences

Neurodiversity means recognising we are all different in the way we think and learn. Some people's ways of thinking and learning are labelled as neurotypical, whereas others think and learn in neurologically diverse ways. All of these are natural human differences and should not be pathologised (Rentenbach et al. 2017). Barriers to learning can occur if those providing training consider only neurotypical ways of learning and do not consider or design for neurodiversity. People who identify as neurodiverse or as having a learning difference may include autistic people, those with dyslexia, dyspraxia, dyscalculia, or attention deficit (hyperactive) disorder (AD(H)D) (Pollak 2009). People living with dementia as learners, or indeed as co-educators, should also be considered as having a learning difference. The concept of adapting to neurodiversity aligns with that of person-centred care and recognising, valuing, and working with the uniqueness of individuals.

Box 8.2 provides some strategies and approaches that can be helpful in providing a learning environment supportive of neurodiversity. The UK Department for Education (DfE n.d.) has developed a useful guide to teaching for neurodiversity, which provides more information about learning differences and some of the difficulties these may present for learning and considerations for those facilitating learning.

Box 8.2 Practical approaches for educators to design and deliver training that is inclusive of neurodiverse learners

- Where possible, request information on any learning needs from learners ahead of time so you can plan for these.
- Ensure regular opportunities to check in with learners individually during the training so you can see how they are getting on and can identify any additional individual needs or required support.
- Provide information in different formats, such as handouts, presentations, and discussion.
- Read out the content of any case studies or other materials that form part of exercises and summarise what you want learners to do. Never ask a particular learner to read out content to others.
- Limit the amount of text you have on any PowerPoint slides or other materials.
- Ensure any training materials and handouts are written in plain English.
- Make sure training programmes offer enough time and are not rushed or packed with too much information and content. This should include time for reflection and breaks.
- Break a training session down into chunks or shorter sections and allow time to consolidate this learning before moving on.
- Offer learner choice of how they participate in exercises or activities – working alone, in pairs, or with people they know.
- Offer quiet space outside of the training room for people to sit when taking part in exercises and activities so there is less background noise or distraction.
- Never ask a learner to answer a question in front of the group or other learners during training. Ask for volunteers to give responses and notify groups in advance if you want feedback from them so they can nominate someone who is happy to take on this role.
- Think of alternative ways learners can ask questions or respond to exercises and activities – for example, you could create an online space where they can post anonymously using apps such as Mentimeter or Padlet.

It is worth noting that some learners may have undertaken a formal assessment for learning difference needs related to autism, dyslexia, dyspraxia, or ADHD and may have clear and specific information about their learning and support needs, for example from school or university. Facilitators should provide an opportunity for people to contact them ahead of delivering a training programme, to share this so any required reasonable adjustments can be made ahead of time. However, other learners may not have had a formal assessment of their learning needs because they have remained unidentified, due to lack of availability or costs of assessment services. Therefore, it is important training programmes are designed in ways that are supportive to all and which allow flexibility in delivery.

Physical and sensory disabilities

Learning facilitators need to ensure that training is accessible for those with physical or sensory disabilities, remembering that not all disabilities are immediately visible. This might mean paying special attention to the training location, room layout, lighting, space and positioning of tables and chairs, formats of training materials, and the types of and ways exercises and activities are run. Again, it is helpful if facilitators are aware of any needs in advance so they can ensure the training room is accessible and materials are available in appropriate formats. Ideally, training sessions should always take place in venues and rooms that are accessible to wheelchair users, and are close to other facilities such as restrooms/toilets and refreshments. If a learner has a visual impairment, they may find it helpful to have materials sent to them in advance in a particular format, such as pdf, so they can familiarise themselves with the content in advance or access them on an electronic device during the session. If someone has a hearing impairment, facilitators will need to consider if there is equipment to support hearing aids (such as a hearing loop) and ensure the learner can see the presenter clearly throughout the training if they lip read. In some cases, they may need to consider using sign language interpreters.

Literacy skills and confidence

In England, approximately 17 per cent or 7.1 million people have very poor literacy skills (National Literacy Trust 2012). In the US, 19 per cent of the population has very low literacy skills and there are significant literacy gaps between adults who are White and those who are Black or Hispanic, the latter having significantly lower literacy levels (National Center for Education Statistics 2017). Globally, literacy skills vary significantly, with countries such as Japan, Finland, and the Netherlands having fewer people with low literacy proficiency and countries such as Indonesia, Turkey, and Chile having larger percentages of the population with low literacy proficiency (OECD 2016). Literacy skills and confidence will also differ by job role. Staff working in roles requiring professional training and qualifications may have higher literacy skills or confidence in reading and writing than those working in settings or roles where qualifications are not required, such as ancillary staff (cleaning, transport, or catering) or paraprofessionals. Some of the practical approaches to designing training that are inclusive of neurodiversity, such as writing in plain English or using minimal words on PowerPoint slides, can also be helpful to those who have lower literacy skills or confidence in reading. Likewise, the approaches to supporting people with different prior educational experiences are also applicable in considering training that is inclusive of those with different levels of literacy.

Culture

The dementia care workforce in many high-income countries is culturally diverse. In 2021 in England, 21 per cent of the health and social care workforce were from minority ethnic groups, compared with only 14 per cent of the population as a whole (GOV.UK 2021; Skills for Care 2021), although this varies by region of the country and staff role. Additionally, non-British workers (including those from the European Union) make up 14.6 per cent of the NHS (Baker 2021) and around 16 per cent of the social care workforce (Skills for Care 2021). In the US, there is a similar picture with the health care workforce being more ethnically diverse than the general population (29 per cent from Black, Asian, Hispanic, and other non-White ethnic groups vs. 25 per cent of the general population) (Snyder et al. 2015). Again, there are disparities by occupation, with White non-Hispanics making up a higher proportion of professionally qualified roles (Salsberg et al. 2021) and care aide roles being occupied by a more ethnically diverse workforce (Snyder et al. 2015). In Australia, foreign-born workers are estimated to comprise around one-third of the nursing and midwifery workforce, over half (53 per cent) of medical practitioners (Negin et al. 2013), and up to 37 per cent of the aged care workforce (Eastman et al. 2019; Mavromaras et al. 2017).

This cultural diversity of the workforce must be considered for several reasons. In English-speaking countries, the points raised above about prior educational experiences and literacy in English apply, particularly for those for whom English is a second or additional language. It is also important that dementia training acknowledges and is respectful of the diversity of experiences and values of this workforce. For example, stigma and understanding or beliefs about the causes of dementia can differ greatly between countries (Gauthier et al. 2021) and cultures, meaning people attending training may not share a common understanding about dementia that is aligned with that adopted in many Western high-income countries (Johnston et al. 2020). They may not share the same perceptions of the value of help-seeking (Mukadam et al. 2015), institutional care, or understand the need to deliver person-centred dementia care. They may also have personal experiences of barriers in health and care services for support for dementia or other conditions (Sagbakken et al. 2018) alongside experiences of wider societal discrimination.

Additionally, training materials such as pictures, case studies, exercises, activities, and video content used should reflect both the diverse workforce and the diversity of people affected by dementia. This should not only include cultural but other forms of diversity, including sexual orientation, disability, religion, biological sex, and gender identity. One challenge the field needs to address is ensuring that those directly affected by dementia who are involved in dementia training, either directly or indirectly, reflect the diversity of people affected by dementia who access services. In high-income Western countries such as the UK, there is currently a predominance of White, middle-class people who contribute in these ways. Whilst their engagement within dementia training is invaluable, we need to work harder to make this a more diverse, and thus more representative, voice.

Summary

This chapter has outlined several individual learner factors that are important to consider when designing and delivering dementia training. It has discussed the concept of learning styles and argued that there is little evidence that tailoring methods to an individual's specific learning style is effective at producing improved learning, although use of a variety of learning approaches is likely to be beneficial for all. It has described various individual factors that may affect learners and their confidence and ability to learn, and suggested ways training facilitators can meet their needs.

Implications for those delivering dementia training

Those delivering dementia training should:

- Ensure they consider individual factors when designing and delivering dementia training.
- Recognise the diversity of individual confidence and prior learning experiences and the impact these may have on willingness and ability to learn.
- Ensure neurodiversity and learning differences are considered and the methods used in training are inclusive for all.
- Ensure training venues, environments, and content are accessible for people with physical and sensory disabilities.
- Ensure that training content and materials are tailored to learners' literacy levels, recognising people may have low literacy or may speak English as a second or additional language.
- Recognise and be respectful of culture and diversity, understanding that this may impact understandings of dementia. Training materials should also reflect the diversity of people affected by dementia and in the workforce.
- Provide opportunities before or during training for learners to share individual learning needs and then respond to these.
- Consider the most appropriate method(s) for delivering specific knowledge or skills and adopt a variety of methods to achieve this.

Implications for managers in dementia care settings and services

Leaders and managers in hospital settings should:

- Where possible, identify or ask learners to identify any individual learning needs and provide this information, with permission, to training facilitators.
- Identify if additional support may be needed for some staff to attend training – for example, in preparation to attend or afterwards in consolidating learning and considering how they might apply it.

Implications for staff providing care, services, or support to people living with dementia

Staff working in health and social care settings should:

- Speak to their manager if they are concerned or worried about attending training, so that appropriate support can be provided.
- If they feel comfortable to do so, let their manager or the training facilitator know of any learning needs they have so the facilitator can ensure these are met.
- Let the facilitator know if training is too fast, difficult to understand, or they are struggling or feeling left behind.

Implications for those directly affected by dementia

- People living with dementia as learners or co-educators will have similar needs to those with learning differences. Educators need to understand these and what the person living with dementia may need to support them to fully participate.
- People living with dementia who are involved in dementia training, whether directly or indirectly, should reflect the diversity of the people affected by dementia who access health and social care services.

9 Training implementation and driving practice and culture change

'Far from being a remedy for non-person-centred organisational culture, training and its implementation is often at the mercy of that culture itself.'

In this chapter, we will outline some commonly used implementation and behaviour change theories and discuss how these can be applied to planning the delivery and implementation of dementia training programmes and to sustainably drive forward practice change. In planning programmes of dementia training, it is important to consider readiness for change and approaches to achieving implementation and behaviour change at organisational and individual levels. Implementation science is the study of methods and strategies to support the implementation or uptake of evidence-based practice or research into regular use within health and social systems (Bauer et al. 2015). This includes the implementation of training programmes and associated interventions. We will also explore organisational culture as a key component of readiness for change and how the deployment of organisational resources can act as a barrier or facilitator for practice change.

Organisational readiness for training implementation and practice change

Organisational readiness is essential to consider ahead of embarking on any change process driven by a programme of dementia training. Organisational readiness is multifaceted, and there are several useful frameworks from implementation science that can help those responsible for developing, delivering, and implementing training. We explore three models in this chapter. While each has a slightly different focus, any can be chosen to underpin a programme of workforce development and it may be helpful to adopt components of each depending on the context. For example, the first two models, i-PARIHS and the Theoretical Domains Framework, focus more on the broader organisational picture. The Behaviour Change Wheel and COM-B model, in contrast, includes greater detail on individual factors impacting behaviour change.

The i-PARIHS (Integrated Promoting Action on Research Implementation in Health Sciences) Framework

The i-PARIHS Framework (Harvey and Kitson 2016) presents the key components required for successful implementation of interventions (including training) into practice within health and care settings through four core constructs: innovation, recipients, context, and facilitation (see Figure 9.1).

Innovation relates to evidence and new knowledge in its broadest sense. It recognises that individuals rarely take evidence in its purest form, for example from a published clinical guideline or review, but will incorporate them into practice through adaptive and inductive methods blending the explicit knowledge gained from the source with their own tacit or practice-based knowledge. In this way, external evidence is aligned with local priorities and practices, supporting compatibility and facilitating implementation. However, if this new knowledge does not fit well with existing practice, it faces a disadvantage compared with evidence-based approaches that are more compatible with usual ways of working.

In the context of dementia training, the external evidence is the theory and knowledge-based content presented in the training programme. Learning facilitators have the advantage that they can also provide activities within a training session, which can help learners start the process of alignment and

Figure 9.1 The i-PARHIS Framework (based on Harvey and Kitson 2016)

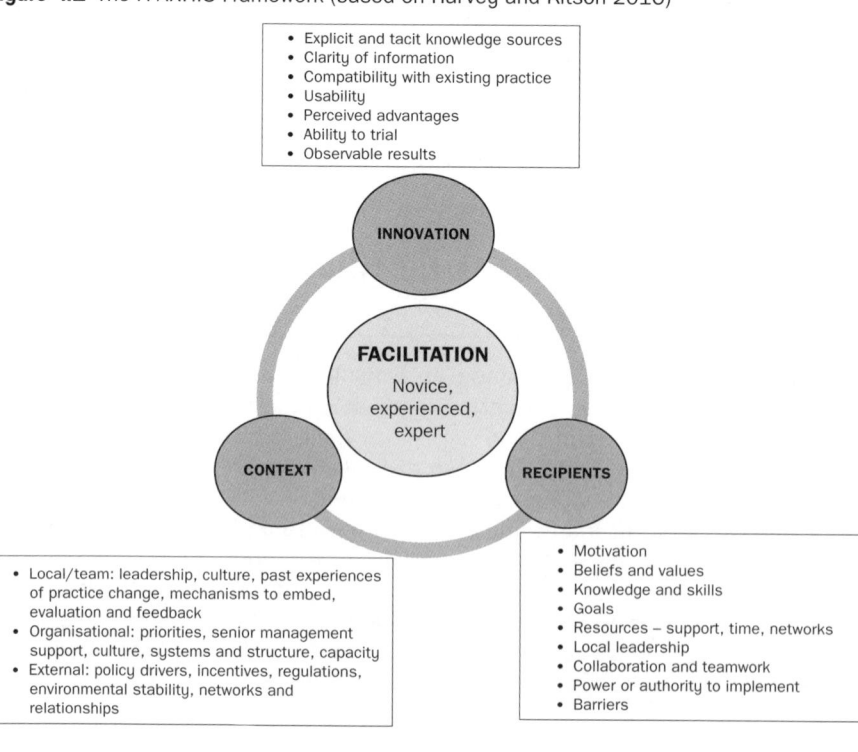

• Explicit and tacit knowledge sources
• Clarity of information
• Compatibility with existing practice
• Usability
• Perceived advantages
• Ability to trial
• Observable results

INNOVATION

FACILITATION
Novice, experienced, expert

CONTEXT

RECIPIENTS

• Local/team: leadership, culture, past experiences of practice change, mechanisms to embed, evaluation and feedback
• Organisational: priorities, senior management support, culture, systems and structure, capacity
• External: policy drivers, incentives, regulations, environmental stability, networks and relationships

• Motivation
• Beliefs and values
• Knowledge and skills
• Goals
• Resources – support, time, networks
• Local leadership
• Collaboration and teamwork
• Power or authority to implement
• Barriers

embedding into practice. However, as has been discussed in Chapter 3, outside of formal training, informal learning and tacit knowledge can either serve to support or undermine this process. Therefore, organisational culture, openness to change, and informal methods of influencing what good practice looks like must be considered and addressed if they may potentially present barriers to implementing new ways of working.

Recipients are the individuals who are involved in implementing the intervention, including individuals and teams who are affected by or influence implementation (through supporting or resisting it). Individual or collective views, beliefs, and established ways of practice, and organisational culture all have a significant effect on how easy or challenging practice change, underpinned by formal programmes of dementia training, is. Recipients may be staff, managers, and people directly affected by dementia. Figure 9.1 outlines some of the key attributes of recipients that may serve as motivators or barriers to change. The role of the facilitator is to consider how recipient barriers to change can be addressed, whilst building on motivating drivers.

When considering the implementation of dementia training into practice, there are opportunities to design training programmes to be delivered in ways that will best build on supportive factors and address potential resistance (see Chapters 2 and 3). For example, face-to-face learning including experiential and simulation exercises alongside reflective practice can build empathy in individual staff, which is a strong driver for recognising a need to change. Alongside this, delivering content that provides practical approaches to addressing practices that need to change, and opportunities to apply these in the training room and in practice, can assist in breaking down perceptions of change being too difficult or demanding. This can be supported by ongoing role-modelling and mentorship, for example by experienced dementia champions, which can assist in providing informal learning opportunities that support rather than undermine learning from formal training. All of this must be underpinned by strong, local leadership that is supportive of dementia training and the implementation process. This process may also require effective engagement and consultation with people directly affected by dementia, so they too are on board with and able to inform planned changes.

Individual change is examined later in this chapter when we discuss the Behaviour Change Wheel and COM-B model.

Context operates at three levels: (1) micro or local/team, (2) meso or organisational, and (3) macro or external, including the wider health and social care system. Factors at each of these levels can serve to facilitate or constrain implementation and change.

Therefore, before embarking on a programme of training, those leading this should take time to consider the context at each of these levels. Is there likely to be a supportive context for what they hope to achieve? If so, how can they use this to their advantage and build on it? If not, what are the likely barriers and what could they do to address these? It may be that supportive factors at one level can help to address potentially undermining factors at another. For example, at the macro level, English government policy that has mandated dementia training for all NHS and social care staff has led to this being prioritised over recent years. Publication of practice guidelines (e.g. NICE dementia guideline in England and Wales; NICE/SCIE 2011), incentivising practices through monetary rewards (e.g. the Quality Outcomes Framework in England; Sutcliffe et al. 2012), and inspection and regulation standards can all provide strong influencing factors that can potentially help to address barriers that may be in place at the meso and micro levels. When leading the implementation of dementia training, an individual will need to consider what macro-level factors might support what they are trying to achieve and use these as leverage.

Likewise, meso-level factors need to be considered, both where they may facilitate implementation of training or where they may act as barriers that will need to be addressed. This may include organisational culture and available resources, which are discussed later in this chapter. Micro-level factors can also provide a strong driver for change. For example, areas for change identified by staff can provide support for attendance at training, where staff and managers feel it will be beneficial to addressing day-to-day practice challenges. This must come alongside empowerment of staff to apply problem-solving using knowledge from training to initiate bottom-up led change.

Facilitation is the active component of the framework. Any change process must be led by one or more Change Facilitators, who develop and employ a set of strategies and actions designed to enable implementation. A Change Facilitator within this framework takes on a wider role than a training facilitator but may well include training as part of their strategies. The strategies and actions employed are based on an assessment of the innovation itself and its characteristics (what needs to be done), alongside those of the recipients (will individuals and teams be open to and supportive of this?) within the context (what local and wider issues are likely to support or undermine what we want to implement?). The role of the Change Facilitator is to enable recipients to implement the change, by supporting adoption or adaptation of the innovation so that it can work within the particular context. This may mean tailoring different approaches on a ward or unit level if the local context is different. Without someone driving forward and leading change, delivering a programme of dementia training will not lead to improvements in care for people with dementia.

It is clear, then, that this individual (or preferably individuals) must be empowered to lead and make change and have the right knowledge, skills, and qualities for the role, and so need to be selected carefully. They will also need ongoing mentoring and support to be able to lead change sustainably. Being an expert practitioner or training facilitator does not automatically mean an individual will also possess the full range of qualities and skills to lead these ongoing programmes of practice change (Griffiths et al. 2021). However, this clinical and training expertise will be essential to understanding the training programme as an intervention and being able to adapt the knowledge from this to each local context. Therefore, it is important to also consider how Change Facilitators will be prepared for this role and supported on an ongoing basis. Without doing so, they may be set up to fail. Leadership as a resource to support training implementation and drive practice change is discussed in more detail later in this chapter.

Harvey and Kitson (2016) identify three levels of Change Facilitator (novice, experienced, and expert) and highlight how all three are required for an effective facilitation process. As such, they must be empowered and supported by the organisation to lead change and support training implementation. Expert Facilitators take on an overall coordinating role and work at a macro level supervising and guiding other facilitators, working across a range of networks and evaluating success. Experienced Facilitators work at the meso or organisational level with a particular focus on the system-wide context, activities, and actions. They may, for example, develop an organisational action plan and engage in work on organisational culture and leadership. Novice Facilitators work at a local level by understanding teams and individuals and what motivates them to change and how they can be supported to work effectively together. They might, for example, be a local dementia champion or clinical leader. Change Facilitators may therefore comprise a range of staff working in and external to an organisation.

The Theoretical Domains Framework

The Theoretical Domains Framework (TDF; Cane et al. 2012; Michie et al. 2005) is a model comprised of 14 domains that determine behaviour (see Table 9.1) as it relates to the implementation of evidence-based practice or quality improvement. It has been used to explore barriers and facilitators to the implementation of interventions, to support intervention design, and to inform behaviour change techniques and intervention implementation strategies (Atkins et al. 2017). It is equally applicable to considering implementation of programmes of dementia training.

One way the TDF can be applied is by asking staff to complete a questionnaire based on the behavioural domains to identify perceived barriers and facilitators to the implementation of training in practice (see, for example, the Determinants of Implementation Behaviour Questionnaire (Huijg et al. 2014) and the Influences on Patient Safety Behaviours Questionnaire (Taylor et al. 2013). This can help with planning implementation and support for staff, through building on facilitators and developing approaches to address barriers. One challenge identified with use of the TDF is the need for facilitators to develop familiarity with the framework and the terminology it uses, to be able to interpret and apply the domains appropriately (Phillips et al. 2015). This can feel challenging for those who do not have a background in psychology. However, it is not necessary to apply the TDF in an in-depth or systematic way when designing and implementing training; using it in an informal manner may give useful insights. For example, this could include thinking about the different domains and whether they might pose barriers to implementation, or talking to staff before, during, and after training about potential barriers and facilitators in the context of the TDF domains.

Table 9.1 The Theoretical Domains Framework (Cane et al. 2012) and its application to dementia training programmes

Domain name	Constructs	Examples of application to dementia training programme design, delivery, and implementation
Knowledge	Knowledge Technical/ scientific Procedural Environmental	• Training content (delivered via formal and informal methods) should be aligned to outcomes to be achieved. • Ensure a blend of theoretical, technical, and skills-based content. • Tailoring of training content to staff roles and individual needs.
Skills	Skills development Competence Ability Interpersonal skills Practice Skills assessment	• Use of practical methods for training delivery (see Chapters 2 and 3) through which skills aligned to theoretical knowledge can be developed. • Use of appropriate formal and informal methods to support self and external assessment of skills and competence, e.g. reflection, mentorship, feedback.
Social/ professional role and identity	Professional identity Professional role Social identity Professional boundaries Professional confidence Group identity Leadership Organisational commitment	• Training content is tailored to the specific professional role of learners. Where learning is multi-disciplinary, exercises should include opportunities for learners to consider how this relates to their own professional role, but also their contribution to a wider collective approach to delivery of person-centred care. • Programmes of training need to be delivered with appropriate engagement, buy-in, and support from managers at all levels. • Training delivery and implementation needs dedicated, skilled leadership.
Beliefs about capabilities	Perceived competence Self-efficacy Perceived behavioural control Beliefs Self-esteem Empowerment Professional confidence	• Conduct individual learning needs assessments and plan tailored programmes of training to develop knowledge, skills, and confidence in identified areas of need. • Offer routes and support for ongoing self-assessment in the context of training delivery and implementation in practice, e.g. reflection, supervision. • Create an organisational culture supportive of learning, professional development, risk-taking, and individual ability to suggest and make practice changes
Optimism	Optimism Pessimism Unrealistic optimism	• Training facilitators and those supporting implementation in practice must create an environment where implementing learning into practice is seen to be possible and desirable. • Encourage development of realistic individual implementation plans with ongoing support, e.g. via supervision, mentorship, etc.

(continued)

Table 9.1 (*continued*)

Domain name	Constructs	Examples of application to dementia training programme design, delivery, and implementation
Beliefs about consequences	Beliefs Outcome expectancies Anticipated regret	• Use training methods that encourage the development of empathy (e.g. experiential learning, simulation, reflection) to encourage a perspective that practice change is necessary and to do nothing is not an option. • Use practical training methods (e.g. in-service learning, role modelling, simulation, practical exercises, in-practice projects) to illustrate possible positive outcomes of implementing training in practice.
Reinforcement	Rewards Incentives Punishment Consequences Sanctions	• Rewards for training attendance might include certificates, badges, and the opportunity to take on additional duties. • Dementia education and training should provide a route to career progression. • It may be helpful to make dementia training mandatory as this can give greater legitimacy to supporting staff to attend.
Intentions	Stability of intentions Stages of change model	• Create a context where learners see a need to change their current behaviours/practices. • This needs to be sustained over the long term through an organisational context and culture that maintains and supports this intention.
Goals	Goals (personal/external) Target setting and prioritising Goals (autonomy/control over) Action planning	• Ensure dementia training is embedded within a process of individual and organisational learning needs assessment and personal and professional learning and developmental goal setting.
Memory, attention, and decision processes	Memory Attention Decision-making Cognitive overload/tiredness	• Individual factors influence the ability and willingness to learn (see Chapter 8). These may relate to prior educational experiences, impairments, learning differences or health problems, and levels of stress and burnout. Training needs to support equity of access for all and to be able to be delivered flexibly to meet individual needs.
Environmental context and resources	Environmental stressors Available resources Organisational culture Events/critical incidents Barriers and facilitators	• The cultural, social, and physical context and available resources to support training delivery and implementation, must be considered as part of its design. • Barriers and facilitators to implementation should be mapped and mechanisms to address barriers identified. This needs to be an ongoing process.

(*continued*)

Table 9.1 *(continued)*

Domain name	Constructs	Examples of application to dementia training programme design, delivery, and implementation
Social influences	Social pressure/ norms Group conformity/ norms Social support Power Conflict Group identity and alienation Modelling	• The ways in which organisational culture play out in day-to-day practices and group norms in which training is facilitated and implemented are crucial (see later in this chapter), and must be considered when designing and implementing training. • Informal learning mechanisms include opportunities for social pressures, norms, and conformity to regulate whether what is taught in formal training can, and will, be implemented into day-to-day practice (see Chapter 3). How informal and formal learning experiences can be aligned must be considered when implementing any programme of training.
Emotion	Fear Anxiety Stress Depression Positive/negative feelings Burnout	• Staff readiness or willingness to engage with learning must be understood. Trying to implement programmes of training at times of high stress and burnout is unlikely to be welcomed or produce the desired outcomes. • Staff well-being needs to be supported in order to ensure they have the energy and physical and mental capacity to engage with training and subsequent practice change.
Behavioural regulation	Self-monitoring Breaking habit Action planning	• Training should include opportunities for reflection and planning and practising implementation, for example through having in-practice exercises to complete between training sessions.

The Behaviour Change Wheel and COM-B system

The Behaviour Change Wheel (BCW; Michie et al. 2011) is a framework or 'behaviour system' that aims to provide a link between the determinants of behaviour and techniques for behaviour change. It provides a representation of the relationship between policies (actions by organisations to enable or support interventions), interventions (approaches or activities that aim to change individual behaviour), and individual behaviour change in a series of layers (see Figure 9.2). The BCW supports exploration of the question, 'What conditions internal to individuals and in their social and physical environment need to be in place for a specified behavioural target to be achieved?' (Michie et al. 2011).

Education and training are two intervention functions that might be used to change behaviour within the BCW. Modelling might operate, for example, via both formal (such as mentoring and development of dementia champions) and the informal learning processes we identified in Chapter 3 as important to learning. The BCW advocates for selecting the most appropriate intervention function or functions to support behaviour change, dependent on the desired

Figure 9.2 The Behaviour Change Wheel (adapted from Michie et al. 2011)

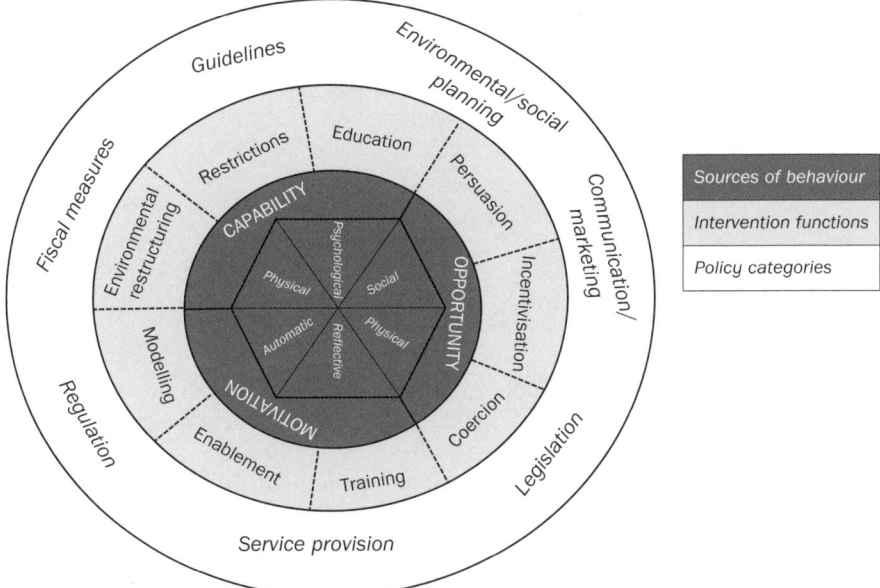

outcome. Therefore, education, training, or modelling may be the only method, one of a selection of methods, or deemed an inappropriate method for supporting practice and behaviour change, depending on the outcome(s) to be achieved. It is, therefore, important to consider if and how training is appropriate to achieving delivery of person-centred dementia care and whether additional intervention functions or approaches also need to be employed.

Sitting outside the intervention functions are the policy or contextual categories. These are potential policies, approaches, or actions by organisations or authorities that can serve to enable or restrict interventions and their implementation. For example, in England the NICE Clinical Guideline on Dementia (NICE 2018) sets out expectations for good practice for health and social care, founded on the principles of person-centred care. Regulatory bodies such as the Care Quality Commission set inspection standards that are underpinned by person-centred care (CQC 2017). Legislation such as the Mental Capacity Act (Department of Health 2005) and Liberty Protection Safeguards (Anon. 2022) serve to protect the rights of people with dementia, particularly when capacity to consent and make decisions is diminished. While these aim to help ensure the delivery of person-centred care and can be used successfully to do so, they can also be used as mechanisms to support poor practice if misunderstood or applied in an unchallenged way. For example, within a poorly resourced, risk-averse culture, they may be used to justify restrictive practices such as preventing a person spending time outside on ill-defined grounds of 'safety', when a more person-centred approach would recognise the benefits to well-being and use policies to enable safe risk-taking.

Figure 9.3 The COM-B system (adapted from Michie et al. 2011)

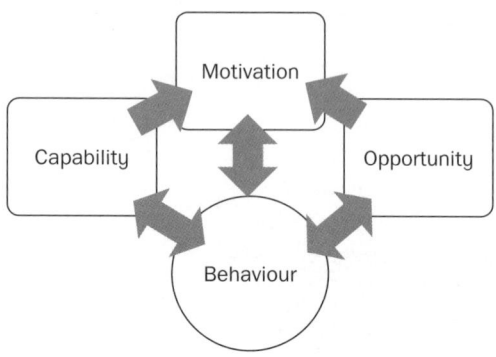

At the centre of the BCW, individual behaviour is understood as part of a behaviour system comprised of Capability, Motivation, and Opportunity known as the COM-B system (Michie et al. 2011) (see Figure 9.3). Capability is comprised of two components (physical and psychological) and relates to an individual's capacity to engage in the intervention and behaviour change activity. Motivation (including automatic and reflective) reflects the cognitive processes that direct and influence behaviour, including goals, decision-making, habits, emotions, and analysis. Opportunity is the external factors that facilitate or prompt a behaviour. The arrows in Figure 9.3 reflect how each component can influence the other.

Capability may relate to aspects such as individual factors discussed in Chapter 8, as well as a learner's health and well-being. If a learner is feeling stressed and burnt out, for example, then attending training and placing expectations on them to implement this in day-to-day practice may feel unachievable and add to their burden. Individual factors that can impact learner motivation include prior educational experiences, and the fact that staff do not see the need to change practice or consider alternative approaches. If this is the case, then it may be necessary to include activities before or during training that will increase motivation and desire to learn. Chapter 2 explored learning theory that considers methods to increase empathy and motivation to learn and change. Opportunity factors include those identified in Chapter 3 in the context of informal learning, as well as in the form of the broader organisational culture discussed later in this chapter.

The Behaviour Change Wheel and COM-B model emphasise the complexity of the context into which dementia training is delivered and highlight the inadequacy of seeing training alone as an intervention to improve care practice. For training to have any possibility of having a sustained impact on staff knowledge, skills, and practices, and subsequently on outcomes for people directly affected by dementia, approaches to ensure the right conditions for training to be implemented are necessary. Without this, training is unlikely to have the desired effects and is unlikely to result in a good return on investment of time and resources. Chapter 10 will explore approaches to evaluating training impact.

Organisational culture and its role in implementation of training to drive practice change

Organisational culture was recognised as important in the delivery of person-centred care by Kitwood (1997) and was introduced in this context in Chapter 1. It is also a key consideration of the implementation science models that underpin practice or behaviour change. In this section, we will explore organisational culture in more detail, presenting models for how it can be understood and research evidence about its influence on care practices and ability to implement interventions such as training.

Models and frameworks for understanding organisational culture

There are many different theoretical models and frameworks of organisational culture. Schein's (2017) work underpins a great deal of existing research. He described components of organisational culture at three levels: *artefacts* (what can be observed about an organisation); *norms and attitudes* (how people describe their thoughts and feelings about an organisation); and *assumptions* (what influences people's behaviour in an organisation). These levels are inter-related, but assumptions are particularly influential because they are used by people in daily problem-solving and are reinforced when they are shown to be successful in helping solve the day-to-day dilemmas and situations they face in their work. New members of staff are then taught these assumptions as expected practice (Brooker and Latham 2016; Schein 2017). As well as being particularly influential, assumptions are often much harder to identify, as they are hidden in habits, unquestioned actions, and what goes on when people are doing very routine aspects of their work, often 'behind closed doors'. This mirrors Kitwood's understanding of how and why non-person-centred practice, such as malignant social psychology, could spread so easily. Within this view of culture, the effectiveness of any training initiative therefore depends upon its success in recognising and influencing all levels of culture simultaneously. If it only focuses on promoting a particular vision of care (an 'artefact' of the culture) without also addressing day-to-day realities and problem-solving, then efforts will be undermined by the norms and assumptions of the culture itself.

Another useful model, the Competing Values Framework (CVF; Cameron and Freeman 1991; Cameron and Quinn 2011; Quinn and Rohrbaugh 1981), often applied within health and social care organisations, describes the way that structures and values can influence an organisation's effectiveness in different circumstances. Based in substantial research, it describes two axes of organisational operation that matter: whether the organisation is oriented towards what is going on *internally* or *externally*, and whether the organisation is structured for *stability* or *flexibility*. Depending on where the organisation sits on these axes will determine the culture type it exhibits: clan, adhocracy, hierarchy, or market. Figure 9.4 depicts this framework and the four culture types.

Figure 9.4 The Competing Values Framework (based on Cameron and Freeman 1991; Cameron and Quinn 2011)

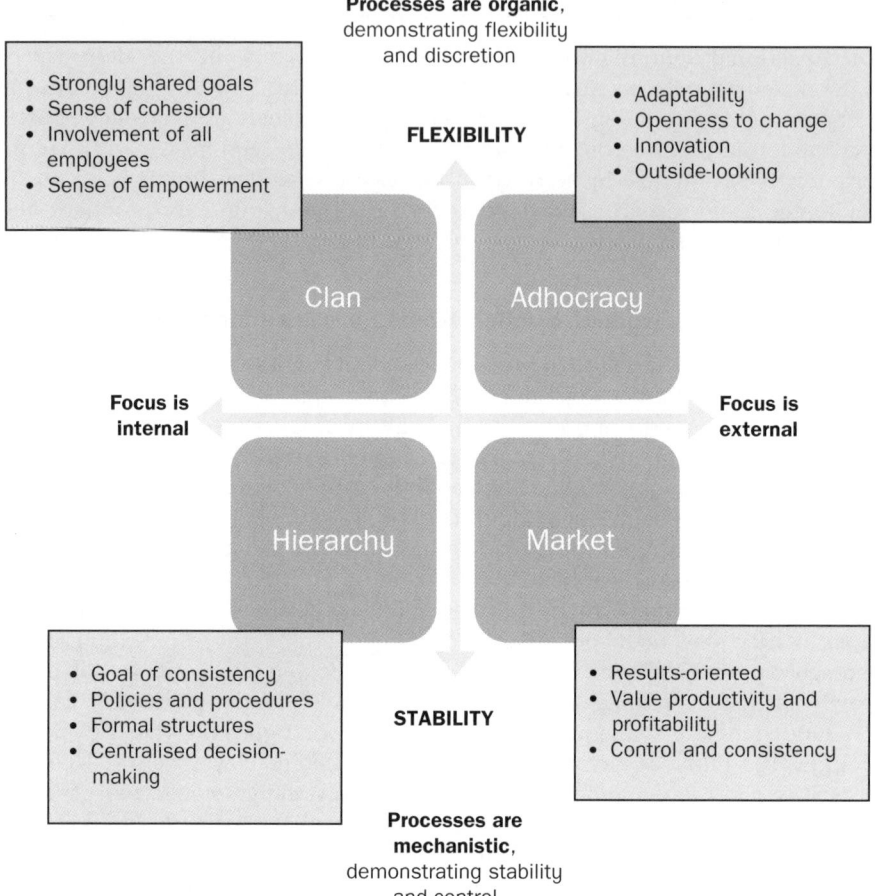

Processes are organic, demonstrating flexibility and discretion

- Strongly shared goals
- Sense of cohesion
- Involvement of all employees
- Sense of empowerment

FLEXIBILITY

- Adaptability
- Openness to change
- Innovation
- Outside-looking

Clan

Adhocracy

Focus is internal

Focus is external

Hierarchy

Market

- Goal of consistency
- Policies and procedures
- Formal structures
- Centralised decision-making

STABILITY

- Results-oriented
- Value productivity and profitability
- Control and consistency

Processes are mechanistic, demonstrating stability and control

It is not that there is a 'best' or ideal type of culture; both ends of the two CVF axes are necessary at different times, in different situations, and for different purposes. What makes an organisation effective is when its activities and values are aligned (Cameron and Quinn 2011). For example, if an organisation needs to be able to conduct its 'process' (day-to-day work) in a flexible way and be responsive to changes internally, it will do that effectively if it operates a clan- or adhocracy-type culture. However, if it adopts a market-type culture, it will struggle to be flexible and responsive to daily challenges because the culture is set up to promote an external focus and to utilise static processes.

Using a framework such as the CVF *before* planning training can be useful for considering how an organisation currently functions or where problems may be rooted. This means training can be designed and focused on what needs to change to produce certain outcomes, rather than relying on assumptions about where the problem may lie. For example, as person-centred care requires flexibility in response to people living with dementia, in many situations a clan or adhocracy culture will be most effective. However, training staff in this flexibility is only part of the picture; cultural practices need to shift as well, such as enhanced empowerment of staff, less reliance on policies, or reduced focus on external results and consistency. Each of these factors will require its own development (which may or may not include training) to align with the intentions of increasing flexibility in response to the needs of people living with dementia. If not addressed as well, training will likely be undermined, particularly in the longer term. The Organisational Culture Assessment Instrument (OCAI) has been robustly developed to assess against the CVF. It is widely used and is accessible online (Cameron and Quinn 2011).

Organisational culture's interaction with training and learning

It is important to consider the relationship between training, learning and organisational culture and the role that both can contribute towards the process of culture change. Moreover, and perhaps more importantly, it also necessary to address the ways in which organisations can and should marshal their other resources, alongside training, to facilitate ongoing change and create cultures that are supportive of person-centred care. The relationship between organisational culture and training is complex, since without a supportive organisational culture, training programmes and wider practice change initiatives are unlikely to be successful. However, where a supportive culture does not already exist, some form of intervention – which is likely to include formal training and informal learning – will need to be implemented to enable person-centred care.

Formal training as a means of influencing organisational change

Thinking about organisational culture demands that those concerned recognise that achieving person-centred outcomes for people living with dementia is a much more complicated process than simply imparting knowledge by delivering training to staff. Indeed, far from being a remedy for a non-person-centred organisational culture, training and its implementation is often at the mercy of culture itself. For example, more flexible organisation types (e.g. clan/adhocracy) have been shown to demonstrate much more successful learning transfer from training than stable market/hierarchy culture types (Chatterjee et al. 2018).

The superior influence of culture over training is something that has in recent years begun to be acknowledged within research and practice development, as interventions to improve outcomes have become more complex and organisationally focused rather than relying on training-only approaches to initiating change. In Chapter 4, this was discussed with reference to care home interventions. We argued that the development of educational programmes that contain additional components (training-plus interventions, including elements such as the use of in-house champions, ongoing coaching support, and organisational action planning alongside staff training) achieve successful outcomes because the additional components help to accomplish organisational outcomes that support implementation. These outcomes include activating informal learning mechanisms, helping to tailor resources towards specific outcomes, and influencing the overall organisational culture. This suggests that there is a role for training to play in facilitating culture change towards person-centred care, but that it must be recognised as just one component of a much more comprehensive effort, rather than viewed as the primary route to success. It is important, but it is not sufficient.

Embedding training within a cycle aligned to culture change

There is research evidence to suggest approaches that are effective in utilising training can be used to successfully achieve culture change. One such approach is action research, by delivering training on the cycle of planning, action, observation, and reflection that underpins action research alongside support to learn from application in practice. Cultural shifts in communication, teamwork, and staff empowerment were evident after participation in one such programme applied in Australian care homes, which is now available as a stand-alone toolkit (Etherton-Beer et al. 2021; Venturato et al. 2020).

Outside of care homes, in a primary care facility in South Africa, Mash et al. (2016) achieved a significant change in culture and leadership style through an 18-month action research project. In addition, a community-based project in Australia reported significantly improved relational care for people living with dementia in its services because of a long-term participatory action research project, which helped to foster common experiences, trust, and appreciative relationships (de Witt and Fortune 2019; Dupuis et al. 2016; McKeown et al. 2016).

Although not widespread, the success of these programmes appears to suggest an avenue where training could play an effective role in supporting culture change, which may then provide an environment in which practice change interventions with training components may be successfully implemented. Action research processes may help services and individuals to learn about the processes of achieving change: learning the *how* in addition to the *what* of change. This is not as simple as imparting knowledge, but includes using training to create supportive learning environments.

Informal learning as a means of influencing organisational change

In Chapter 3, we highlighted the importance of recognising the role of informal learning in influencing practice towards person-centred outcomes for people living with dementia. We highlighted that it is currently an under-utilised resource within all settings, especially when compared with the attention paid to formal training. The significance of organisational culture to achieving person-centred care and for influencing the impacts from training, emphasises the importance of understanding what goes on within the workplace. Organisational culture is so important precisely because it informs the environment in which highly influential and ongoing informal learning takes place. It is an arena within which all learning is tested out in the real world to see if it provides 'workable solutions to everyday problems' (Schein 2017).

Latham (2020) illustrated the significance of this when describing the system of learning to care, as described in detail in Chapter 3. Dementia care workers draw on three sources of knowledge and skills to apply in their day-to-day learning mechanism of finding out 'what works is what matters', the most significant of which is care home cultural knowledge gained via interactions with colleagues. This creates a self-reinforcing cycle between organisational cultural knowledge and informal learning because workers draw on that knowledge to apply in day-to-day learning and the results of that learning are then passed on to others through interactions with colleagues, thus becoming part of the 'new' organisational cultural knowledge. This cycle explains why culture's influence can be so pervasive and hard to change. It highlights that, when seeking to influence culture, it is vitally important to address informal as well as formal sources of learning.

Creating the right organisational culture means ensuring that it offers ongoing opportunities for person-centred practice to be modelled, reinforced, and thus learned. This not only means paying attention to the components of person-centred care cultures and using available resources to achieve them (as we will discuss in the next section), it also means addressing the overall attitude and approach to learning and development within an organisation. Organisations can adopt practices that create either expansive or restrictive learning environments, with the former more likely to make the most of informal learning opportunities and influence them towards particular outcomes as well as being better able to develop personnel (Evans et al. 2006; Fuller et al. 2005). Expansive environments also better facilitate learning from the responses and experiences of service users (Bridges and Fuller 2015). The key features of restrictive and expansive learning environments are summarised in Table 9.2.

A concept such as expansive-restrictive learning environments helps to highlight that routine practices and mundane, day-to-day decision-making such as rotas, teamwork, and work allocation can be very significant contributors to organisational culture, because they shape what and how work is learned by determining how empowering, safe, and encouraging of learning a workplace feels for those who work within it. Achieving these organisational-level factors mean a workplace is also more likely to be able to also address the individual learning needs of each worker, as discussed in Chapter 8.

We will now move on to discuss the resources available within organisations that can be used to create person-centred and expansive learning cultures that provide a positive informal learning context and setting for implementation of formal learning into practice.

Table 9.2 The features of restrictive and expansive learning environments (based on Evans et al. 2006; Fuller et al. 2005)

Restrictive	Expansive
• Restrict participation to single/few communities of practice	• Allows participation in multiple communities of practice
• Restrict range of learning opportunities to within specific boundaries (specific area, role, etc.)	• Breadth of learning experiences fostered by opportunities across organisation and boundaries (work type, role, etc.)
• Restrict communication and teamwork to within role boundaries	• Encourage cross-boundary communication and teamwork
• All learning is on-the-job, no planned time off	• Planned time off-the-job for training and reflection
• Managers are controllers of access to development	• Managers are facilitators of access to development
• Skills and knowledge of only key workers are developed and valued	• Skills and knowledge of whole workforce are developed and valued
• Specialist skills are restricted to only parts of the organisation	• Specialist skills are distributed widely throughout the organisation
• Top-down view of expertise and innovation	• Wide-ranging view of expertise and innovation
• The vision of workplace learning is static and for the job role only	• The vision of workplace learning is about development and progression for individual
• Workforce development is used to restrict individual development to what the organisation needs	• Workforce development is aimed at aligning individual development and organisational capability

Organisational facilitators for the successful implementation of training

Thus far we have discussed the overall concept of organisational culture and the role training can play in shaping it to achieve person-centred care for people living with dementia. We have also highlighted organisational culture as a barrier or facilitator to the implementation of training. There is no one simple solution for creating the right kind of culture, rather what is needed is ongoing attention to the many different components of culture. Training and fostering expansive learning environments can help with this ongoing process. However, any service setting also needs to know how best to use the other resources available to create the best environment for person-centred care training to be successful and thus help foster the right culture. The specifics of these resources can vary between settings and circumstances and are often subject to change, but in broad terms any organisation regardless of size, ownership, or purpose will have the following resources to consider: leadership, staff, people directly affected by dementia, and physical resources.

Leadership

The importance of leaders has already been highlighted when discussing models for the implementation of training to drive practice change and organisational culture, not least because of the influence and authority leaders have to institute the necessary changes to the environment, care approaches, staff roles, and so on that may be required to support implementation of learning from training. It is highly unlikely that substantial changes will be successful, especially in the long term, without the support of key decision-makers, who usually occupy management roles. Strong and committed leadership is identified as an important and early step in most culture change programmes – usually developed initially through training – and cited as a reason for failure of many person-centred interventions (Doll et al. 2017; Eliopoulos 2013; Karrer et al. 2020; Schick 2017). These are also applicable to considering implementation of learning from training to support delivery of person-centred care.

There are a number of features of leadership that are particularly significant to facilitating person-centred care. First, the adoption of non-hierarchical approaches in which leadership is diffuse within a setting and staff are empowered to make decisions and take action on behalf of those they are supporting enhances person-centred cultures and thus potential outcomes for people living with dementia (Brossard Saxell et al. 2021; Cornelison 2016; Doll et al. 2017; Duan et al. 2021; Grant et al. 2014; Hamiduzzaman et al. 2020; Killett et al. 2016; Lima et al. 2020). Rokstad et al. (2015) compared three different leadership approaches to changing cultures following the use of Dementia Care Mapping in Norwegian nursing homes. The most successful approach entailed collaboration and widely distributed points of authority and influence because this helped to share the new vision, help staff feel valued and appreciated, and motivated different groups of staff to join forces in reflecting and implementing changes.

A second influential feature of leadership for implementing training and creating person-centred cultures is leaders and managers that are present and involved in the day-to-day functioning of the organisation and its delivery of support to people living with dementia (Killett et al. 2016). This creates trust between managers and staff and ensures that the practicality of any intervention is understood and well considered before implementation; both are identified as barriers to sustaining complex person-centred care interventions (Colón-Emeric et al. 2016). Moreover, being present and involved enables a leader to role-model and problem-solve using person-centred solutions and provide back-up for champions or interventions amongst the staff team. These are facilitators of person-centred informal learning (Latham 2020) and of successful implementation of training interventions (Chenoweth et al. 2018; Kelley et al. 2020; Rokstad et al. 2015).

Third, culture change requires leadership that recognises that achieving person-centred outcomes creates ongoing challenges and therefore requires flexible solutions (Killett et al. 2016). Corazzini et al. (2015) described this as 'adaptive' leadership because leaders identified that they needed to engage in adaptive work (rather than seeking technical, permanent solutions) to respond to the many ongoing challenges of implementing person-centred care, such as maintaining quality in staff–resident relationships, managing multiple expectations, and respecting individual personhood. Adaptive leadership involves behaviours that enable finding new and changing solutions rather than simply generating new rules and procedures. For example, an adaptive (and person-centred) solution to implementing new approaches to occupational activity following training is to consult with residents and staff to find possible solutions. In contrast, a technical or procedural solution would be to create a new activity schedule and allocate staff to set times when they should engage residents in activities. The flexible, adaptive style of leadership makes particular sense in light of the understanding that the most successful person-centred training interventions are those which have in-built flexibility to enable adaptation to the particular circumstances of a setting or situation (Dahl et al. 2018; Eliopoulos 2013).

Finally, as highlighted when discussing both informal learning and the concept of enabling/restrictive learning environments, leaders need to adopt approaches that are thoughtful about the learning process itself. By being aware of learning opportunities that are available (both formally and informally) and how they can be influenced towards creating person-centred cultures, a leader can maximise (or limit) their input. In a study of managers in the elderly care sector in Sweden, leaders who approached learning and development as an administrative task produced constraining learning environments, whereas those leaders who approached it with a 'development-orientation' saw it as a chance for growth and a central part of their work (Ellström and Ellström 2018; Ellström et al. 2008; Fuller et al. 2005). A leadership programme using action-learning sets for hospital ward nursing teams developed leadership practices to foster expansive learning environments resulting in 'expansive outcomes'. These outcomes included high-quality interactions between team members and service users, positive care experiences, and high levels of empathy. These leadership practices involved good relational practices between managers and staff, including dialogue, reflective learning, mutual support, and peer observation of practice (Bridges and Fuller 2015).

Furthermore, it is particularly valuable for leaders to have an awareness of the dynamics of informal learning, and the way that structural decisions about work tasks, organisation of teams, time and space, and boundaries of work roles can influence who and what staff can learn. With this awareness they can use previously mundane day-to-day decisions to ensure breadth of opportunity through interactions, communication and interpersonal relationships, create opportunities for reflective practice and feedback, and influence occasions of problem-solving and application of tacit knowledge (Latham 2020).

Staff

Staff and leadership are of course interdependent, and many ways of how best to utilise staff resource require action from organisational leadership. There are several staff issues that appear to be particularly significant to promoting person-centred cultures and outcomes for people living with dementia, driven through formal and informal learning opportunities. However, before addressing these, there is an obvious but important issue to address. Sufficient staffing – that is, adequate in number, satisfactory in experience and skill, and appropriately stable – is pivotal to the success of any change initiative driven or supported by a programme of training and this has been demonstrated repeatedly in research and practice (Brossard Saxell et al. 2021; Colón-Emeric et al. 2016; Fossey et al. 2019; Gerritsen et al. 2021; Griffiths et al. 2019; Gwernan-Jones et al. 2020a, 2020b; Kutschar et al. 2020; Lawrence et al. 2016; O'Shea et al. 2017). It is therefore also essential to achieving appropriate cultures for person-centred care. Sufficient staffing requires appropriate financing and governance at organisational, local, and national level and there is no substitute for it. Whilst different organisational cultures may be able to make more, or less, effective use of their available resource, no model or programme can compensate for sustained, structural underfunding of dementia care and its workforce. There is a significant and two-fold danger in focusing solely on initiatives to train and 'change culture' whilst ignoring this wider issue. First, it contributes to a prevailing public perception that the issue is one of individual behaviour and organisational management rather than public policy. Second, it means the pressure for compensating for structural underfunding is placed on individuals who make up the dementia care workforce, which is unsustainable and, in the long term, reduces resilience. We only have to look at the crisis in staffing following the COVID-19 pandemic to recognise the consequences of an exhausted and devalued workforce.

Notwithstanding this issue, there are four areas where staff resources can be supported towards achieving more person-centred outcomes. First, and interacting with leadership, staff empowerment is a key component of person-centred cultures (Berridge et al. 2018; Cornelison 2016; Doll et al. 2017; Duan et al. 2021; Killett et al. 2016; Lepore et al. 2020) and a facilitator of successful training implementation (Ballard et al. 2020; Chenoweth et al. 2018; Grant et al. 2014; Venturato et al. 2020). Therefore, it is important to recognise that cultural and personal change need to be addressed simultaneously rather than viewing one as the route to the other. Practices which enable staff to develop their skills and knowledge, take responsibility, and make decisions within their roles alongside appropriate support are likely to improve person-centred outcomes, with opposite activities likely to reduce person-centred experiences. For example, high inappropriate usage of psychotropic medications in nursing homes has been found to be associated with hierarchical leadership structures (Peri et al. 2015) and staff perceptions of helplessness in influencing experiences (Sawan et al. 2018).

Second, practices that show staff that they are valued and support their well-being will also help to create person-centred cultures and outcomes. Indeed, emphasising the clear connection between staff well-being and the well-being of those they care for is a central tenet of culture change movements (Hermer et al. 2017; Nolan et al. 2006; Power 2010; Thomas 2004). Staff need to be cared for in order to be able to care for others. Keady and Elvish (2019) highlight the significance of well-being and mental health on staff performance in caring professions. Kadri et al. (2018) identify that care workers' own personhood can be forgotten by employing organisations. It feels like common sense, but it is surprising how frequently dementia care staff are expected to demonstrate person-centred behaviours towards people living with dementia, without experiencing such behaviours from their colleagues, managers, and organisations. This was something Kitwood (1997) highlighted in *Dementia Reconsidered* in his discussion of the 'caring organisation', and that has been further developed within relationship-centred care philosophies (Nolan et al. 2004).

Applying the same principles of person-centred approaches to interactions with staff can be a good starting point for creating supportive workplaces: valuing people in words and actions, honouring people's individuality and life history, respecting their personal perspectives, and providing supportive social environments (Brooker and Latham 2016). Kitwood (1997) noted that at an organisational level these may be provided through pay and conditions of service, good induction, the creation of a team, ongoing quality assurance, as well as opportunities for ongoing personal development and supervision for staff, such as in-service training, supervision, individual staff development, accreditation, and promotion. On a practical level, day-to-day issues such as clear communication, availability of help and support, and sufficient time and resources to do their day-to-day work are the basics of demonstrating value to staff. It is notable that all three of these issues are frequently identified as barriers to successful implementation of training interventions and efforts to introduce person-centred care (Barbosa et al. 2017; Fossey et al. 2019; Griffiths et al. 2019; Lawrence et al. 2016).

Third, and of particular importance to maximising person-centred informal learning, staff resources can be maximised by awareness and facilitation of membership of varied and valuable communities of practice in their workplace. Interactions, communications, and interpersonal relationships with colleagues are fundamental to the way that informal learning occurs in the workplace. Latham (2020) showed that the opportunity for and organisation of relationships in a care home had a significant effect on what practice was learned by workers. The variety of colleagues and situations in which they were encountered affected the practice that was learned, with broader variety resulting in more opportunities for learning and therefore more person-centred practice. This means that issues such as how work tasks and teams are organised, the flexibility in areas of responsibility, and opportunities to cross role boundaries are important considerations to creating varied and multiple communities of practice from which to learn.

Following on from this, supporting staff to develop interpersonal abilities that foster positive learning environments – such as communication and coaching skills, giving and receiving feedback, and how to engage in group reflection – will maximise the long-term effectiveness of the community of practice for them and for others. In the evaluation of an educational programme that focused on the use of 'practice educators' (in-house staff who facilitate workplace learning and social learning environments), Grealish et al. (2015) established a positive effect on learning cultures, particularly when the focus of those practice educators was on the organisation rather than solely on the individual.

People directly affected by dementia

The input available from people living with dementia and their supporters is currently the most under-utilised 'resource' available to many services. However, it requires organisations to think beyond familiar 'user-involvement' approaches such as quality assurance, satisfaction surveys, and feedback to genuinely develop partnerships with those who receive their services. This may be challenging and time-consuming, but it is worthwhile and offers gains in terms of truly delivering person-centred care for an organisation in the long term. There are two areas on which to focus to better utilise the input of those directly affected by dementia.

First, the direct influence of people affected by dementia on achieving person-centred outcomes can be fostered by recognising and maximising the many and varied ways that they form part of the learning environment and communities of practice within workplaces. We have discussed in earlier chapters the ways in which people with dementia and their supporters may be involved and their voices and experiences included in formal training programmes. Chapter 3 highlighted the important role they also play in informal learning, suggesting more person-centred outcomes emerge from informal workplace learning when a wider range of people and circumstances are encountered by staff. This is not simply about increasing the frequency of encounters; after all, knowledge of the person and trusting relationships are cornerstones of person-centred dementia care, both of which are potentially diluted by focusing only on frequency. Instead, it is about increasing quality rather than quantity. Someone will learn more and thus be better able to adapt (a core feature of person-centred dementia care) if they have the chance to experience a person in varied circumstances and through a variety of individuals' experiences as well as maximising opportunity to build relationships.

In addition, considering the following factors about day-to-day interactions will help to improve the presence and representation of people directly affected by dementia within those everyday learning environments:

- Actively encourage people living with dementia and their supporters to provide feedback on environments, activities, and interactions.
- Encourage all staff to be responsible for gathering and interpreting feedback.
- Maximise how feedback is gathered and listened to everyday.
- Skill staff in interpreting behaviour as feedback through such methods as observation.
- Ensure a balance between 'static' (e.g. care plans and records) and 'living' (e.g. behaviour) expressions of preferences and feedback.

- Examine team and organisational responses when direct feedback contradicts received wisdom about the 'best' clinical or practice outcomes.

The second area on which to focus to better utilise the input of people directly affected by dementia is to address how they are involved within the process of organisational decision-making and change itself. This is about a shift from seeing people living with dementia not merely as the reason for change, but as influencers and, ultimately, drivers of change themselves. A long-term community project in Canada brought together leadership, staff, and people living with dementia and their supporters to participate in a culture change participatory action research project investigating how to foster positive, relational dementia care in a variety of services. The process of the project was the biggest influence on outcomes because it enabled the following to develop among members of the group (de Witt and Fortune 2019; Dupuis et al. 2016; McKeown et al. 2016):

- the forging of friendships;
- the sharing of common experiences;
- taking time and making time for each other;
- developing trust and feeling appreciated;
- experiencing tensions and boundaries between one another.

Physical resources

The final set of resources available for organisations to utilise are practical, often physical ones. These are likely to change according to setting and over time, and can be easily forgotten as they form part of the background of person-centred care. However, both large- and small-scale changes in these can help to shift culture within a setting and make implementation of learning from training either easier or more challenging. One such practical resource is the way in which a setting uses space and the physical environment. Changes to the physical environment away from institutionalised arrangements towards more home-like provision are important aspects of creating person-centred organisational cultures (Brossard Saxell et al. 2021; Duan et al. 2021; Lima et al. 2020). Whilst some of these can seem costly and beyond the reach of some organisations, it is important to note that smaller changes, such as how chairs are arranged, visibility of staff, decoration, and the availability of personal items, have been identified as enabling a shift towards more person-centred care and increasing motivations of staff to make culture changes (Hermer et al. 2017; Shield et al. 2014). It has also been shown that the use of the environment is more important to positive cultures than the specific design (Killett et al. 2016). Adjacent changes, such as introducing a café into an institutional facility, have been shown to facilitate culture change by providing opportunities for more meaningful relationships and individual choice and control (Andrew and Ritchie 2017).

Moreover, the physical environment is not only important for care but also for learning itself. Where knowledge is physically held, access to people and information and location of interactions with colleagues all affect where, when, how, and what can be learned (Gregory et al. 2014). Therefore, considering the ways learning is helped or hindered by the workplace (such as access to computers, location of information, or where conversations can be conducted) can result in changes that ensure learning takes place frequently and at the right times and place.

A second practical resource is the use of technology. A great many advances have been made in recent decades which have transformed the way we live our lives. These have also provided opportunities to improve care experiences for people as well, such as the use of sensors to reduce risk or internet technology to enhance communication with friends and family. However, technology also has the potential to vastly transform learning in ways that enhance person-centred outcomes. We have touched on this in previous chapters in both general terms (Chapter 2) and more specifically in ways technology is currently being used in different service settings to facilitate training opportunities (Chapters 4–7). Technology is likely to play an increasingly important role in the delivery and implementation of training and person-centred care over coming years.

Summary

This chapter has considered organisational readiness for positive change and provided an overview of three models of implementation and behaviour change that may be used to underpin workforce development through training. These models highlight the need to understand training, its implementation, and barriers and facilitators to this, in a broader context which includes individual, organisational, and wider social, political, and cultural factors. Without this, training as a stand-alone intervention is unlikely to have the desired impact, or certainly any sustained impact. Training is only one of a range of interventions that may be suitable or needed to realise a practice change. It may be training needs to be implemented alongside other interventions to achieve optimal impact and, ultimately, improvements in quality of life for people living with dementia. The next chapter will explore approaches to evaluating training impact.

In this chapter, we have also explored the concept of organisational culture, its theoretical basis, and its relationship with formal training and informal learning. We have emphasised that culture is complex and all-encompassing and strongly affects the outcomes of training and development initiatives, and thus the outcomes that can be achieved for people directly affected by dementia. Starting from an organisational perspective when planning and delivering training will therefore increase effectiveness. Considering interpersonal and operational factors simultaneously will ensure that all aspects are working towards the same end, rather than contradicting or undermining one another.

This chapter has also addressed the ways in which both training and informal learning can be used as means to influence culture change, highlighting that training is an important, but not sufficient component of achieving cultures that support person-centred outcomes for people living with dementia. Other resources in the service setting such as leadership, staff, practical resources, and people directly affected by dementia themselves can be used to facilitate person-centredness and thus the successful implementation of training into practice.

Implications for those delivering dementia training

Those delivering dementia training should:

- Not see training as a stand-alone intervention to change care practice.
- Ensure they consider the range of factors that influence the delivery and implementation of training into practice and address these through developing a training strategy and implementation plan.

- Identify barriers and facilitators to training implementation at an organisational, unit/ward, and individual level and identify ways to build on facilitators and address barriers.
- Recognise when it is, or is not, the right time to embark on a programme of dementia training for an organisation or an individual.
- Encourage an organisational perspective on change, assessing organisational culture prior to designing and delivering training.
- Foster an expansive approach to learning and development in the organisation or setting.
- Ensure training helps key individuals to understand the process of making change happen as well as what a change will look like.

Implications for managers in dementia care settings and services

Leaders and managers in health and social care services should:

- Work alongside those responsible for facilitating training in identifying mechanisms that may support or hinder the implementation of dementia training and in developing a strategy to aid successful implementation.
- Recognise the important role they play in creating and supporting a culture of openness to learning and practice development.
- Provide support to individual staff members who may be struggling with individual barriers to training implementation.
- Adopt non-hierarchical, flexible, and adaptive leadership practices that empower staff and enable diffuse decision-making.
- Be present and involved in day-to-day care to help create trusting and respectful relationships with staff.
- Be thoughtful about the learning process itself; learning and development is a key part of their role.

Implications for staff providing care, services, or support to people living with dementia

Staff working in health and social care settings should:

- Recognise the important role they and others play in the implementation of training into practice, including in setting and supporting a prevailing positive culture towards learning and practice development.
- Share concerns they may have about their own readiness for and ability to implement training in practice, and seek appropriate support.

- Recognise their individual capacity, opportunities, and motivations for implementation of training and modification of individual practices, and engage positively with approaches to reduce any identified individual barriers.
- Identify and build on micro, meso, and macro facilitators to implementation of training.
- Identify, report, and seek to remove or lessen barriers to training implementation at all levels.
- Embrace opportunities to take responsibility and autonomy in their daily work, asking for support when needed.
- Maximise their informal learning through experiencing a wide variety of colleagues, people living with dementia, and different type of situations.
- Take care of their own and others' well-being; value each other.

Implications for those directly affected by dementia

- Recognise the important role people living with dementia and their supporters can play as facilitators of learning and influencers of change. This may be in an active role in delivery of dementia training or through feedback and engagement as users of services.
- Ensure that people directly affected by dementia are engaged and included in change processes so they can inform planned changes and are on board with and supportive of them.
- Engage people directly affected by dementia within the process of organisational decision-making.
- Maximise people's representation in informal learning by facilitating their feedback and involvement on a day-to-day basis.
- Create opportunities for staff to develop relationships with people living with dementia and their supporters outside of specific tasks of care.

10 Measuring and evidencing the impact of training

'Most individuals tasked with responsibility for dementia training within an organisation will be expected to provide some evaluative data to demonstrate impact.'

This chapter will explore practical ways to evidence the impact of dementia training, learning, and development programmes. It will provide an overview of **The Kirkpatrick Model** – Kirkpatrick's four-level model for evaluation of training – as well as revisiting the implementation models from Chapter 9 through an evaluation lens. It will also discuss data collection methods that may be used to gather evidence of training impact, exploring the pros and cons of each. These include methods that are usable in organisations with limited resources through to more well-resourced, formal programmes of research.

Common questions about evaluating dementia training

What should an evaluation of training seek to explore?

An evaluation measures the success of the programme (Kraiger et al. 1993) or the extent to which a training programme meets its intended goals (Alvarez et al. 2004). It can also provide evidence for return on investment – that is, provide a means for demonstrating that the financial and human resources that are invested in developing, delivering, and implementing a programme of dementia training are worth it in terms of benefits. Most individuals tasked with responsibility for dementia training within an organisation will be expected to provide some evaluative data to demonstrate impact. To undertake a thorough evaluation of all the intended outcomes of a training programme requires expertise and resources. Therefore, an individual or team tasked with facilitating training must also determine what it is feasible to evaluate within the skills and resources they have. Deciding what to evaluate, therefore, is the first question for assessing the impact of any training programme. There are many different outcomes that training may seek to impact and choosing which of these are important to assess and ways to practically do this is an essential first step.

Training programmes may offer quite broad content, which could result in a potentially wide range of impacts. For example, training on person-centred dementia care is likely to cover principles around seeing the person and not just their dementia, trying to understand the world from their perspective, and building individualised care based on meeting psychological needs. The way this then impacts on staff knowledge or attitudes and is manifest in terms of staff behaviours in practice, and thus impacts on people living with dementia will be as equally varied.

Likewise, what a training programme consists of can be difficult to define, particularly if it is embedded within a wider programme considering informal learning and readiness for change, as advocated in Chapters 3 and 9. Where does the training itself start and end? What is influencing practice change: the training, the informal learning, or the readiness activities, or a combination of these? In this sense, it may not be appropriate to consider training as a stand-alone intervention that has an impact in its own right. In fact, we have shown in Chapters 4 and 9 that there is widespread evidence that training alone is not enough to change practices in dementia care settings. The Kirkpatrick Model for the evaluation of training we introduce later in this chapter provides a useful guide for considering the different areas or levels of impact that an evaluation of a programme of training may explore. We also provide some examples of specific outcomes and, later in the chapter, data collection methods that may be used to evaluate outcomes.

How do I measure or assess impact?

Choosing the right methods to assess the impact of training on different outcomes is important. Not all outcomes lend themselves readily to measurement, and when they do, there are limitations to what measurable outcomes alone can tell us. For example, if we consider increased staff knowledge as a common expected outcome of training, this may initially seem like something that can be relatively easily measured, and this is to some extent true. We can ask learners questions that reflect factual knowledge they have been taught (e.g. 'Alzheimer's disease is the most common form of dementia – true/false') and assess whether knowledge has improved at all. But what about more complex knowledge that is integral to good person-centred care but is less easy to assess, for example, how best to support a person living with dementia who is distressed? We can ask the learner about which of a range of approaches might be appropriate or not, but this cannot get to the skills staff need to be able to think on the spot and respond in the moment with a particular person living with dementia. This is where knowledge intersects with its application into behaviour in practice.

How do I understand what has led to impacts I have seen?

As we have argued throughout this book, dementia training and workforce development consists of more than learning that occurs within a classroom or via other formal methods of delivery. There are many informal mechanisms that may support or undermine formal learning processes and what these are, and how they operate, may not be readily known. It is, therefore, sometimes difficult to assess whether impacts or lack of them are due solely to a training programme. In most cases, any impacts are likely to reflect a complex influence of a variety of factors. These include broader influencers such as environment and context as well as training-related factors. Therefore, holistic rather than simplistic approaches to evaluating the impacts of dementia training are required when possible, as well as careful presentation of any evaluation findings in the context of known limitations. We consider these issues in further depth later in the chapter.

How do I interpret and draw conclusions from data about impacts of dementia training I have collected?

As discussed above, evaluation of dementia training is complex due to the many potentially influencing factors that may impact outcomes. It can be helpful to think of these factors in terms of those that are closest to the training programme itself (for example, staff reactions to the training and any knowledge gains) and those which are more distant from the influence of training attendance (for example, the impact on quality of life of someone with dementia). We will discuss these further as part of The Kirkpatrick Model. For some programmes of dementia training, where the topic area and thus intended outcomes are very specific, data interpretation and the drawing of conclusions may be more straightforward than for broader training content. For example, training on pain in dementia and the use of a pain assessment tool may include quite specific outcomes such as increased staff knowledge on the causes, assessment, and management of pain in people with dementia. These outcomes may be readily measurable through knowledge tests about pain and its assessment and management, counts of the number of pain assessments conducted, and the resulting actions taken to address identified pain (e.g. seeking medical review, more regular use of pain medications). Programmes of dementia awareness or person-centred care training present greater difficulty in identifying specific expected outcomes and thus in the evaluation being able to draw firm conclusions regarding impact. While it is beyond the remit of this book to provide a detailed account of data analysis and interpretation techniques, we do discuss some of the benefits, challenges, and pitfalls of different data types and their potential contribution to the evaluation of dementia training. We also signpost the reader to useful additional and accessible resources on research design and conduct.

Learning outcomes as the basis for training evaluation

Key criteria underpinning evaluation of dementia training are the learning outcomes. Learning outcomes are statements that set out what the training aims to achieve. They may be cognitive (quantity and type of knowledge), affective (attitudes, motivation, feelings), or skill-based (technical or motor skills) (Kraiger et al. 1993). Learning involves different levels of complexity. Figure 10.1 outlines Bloom's taxonomy of learning, which shows a hierarchy of learning complexity moving from simple memorising and recall of information through to creative synthesis of learning and its application to plan and design. Different types of learning may be appropriate in different circumstances, for different content and different learners. For example, a basic dementia awareness training course might aim to provide learners with knowledge they can remember (e.g. what dementia is, the main types of dementia), understand (e.g. be able to tell a colleague how dementia might affect someone's communication abilities or memory), and apply (e.g. use of communication approaches that can help people with dementia such as giving more time for them to respond). Other programmes, however, might require the full range of learning application. For example, in a programme for care home senior staff addressing how to support people living with dementia who are expressing distress, not only will knowledge, understanding, and application of approaches to distress be required, but also the ability to analyse the individual person's situation, appraise possible approaches, and create an appropriate action plan.

To write learning outcomes it can be helpful to start with some broad statements about the purpose of the training session/programme. For example, the broad aims of a dementia awareness training session might be: *'To understand what dementia is, how it affects people, and ways they can help.'* The next stage is to break this down into a set of specific outcomes. This involves thinking about how whether a learner had met a learning outcome could be assessed – what specifically would the learner know, think, or be able to do? Learning outcomes should reflect knowledge, behaviours, attitudes, or skills that are specific and measurable/demonstrable. They should use specific action words and simple, clear language and be realistic and achievable. Box 10.1 provides example learning outcomes for a dementia awareness training session.

Figure 10.1 Bloom's taxonomy of learning (based on Bloom et al. 1956; Anderson et al. 2001)

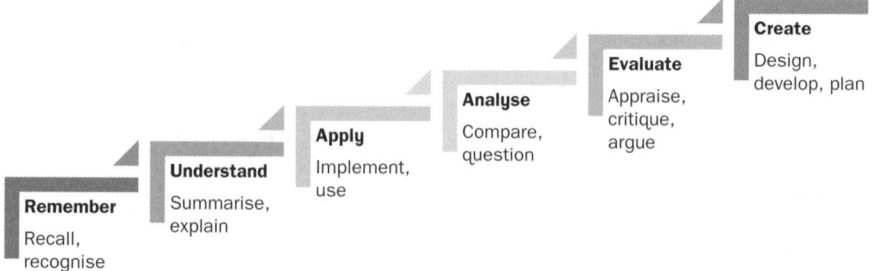

Box 10.1 Example learning outcomes for a dementia awareness training course

At the end of this session, learners should be able to:

- identify the main types of dementia;
- recognise the signs and symptoms associated with dementia;
- explain how living with dementia can affect a person's day-to-day life;
- use appropriate communication strategies to mitigate the communication difficulties that may be experienced by people living with dementia;
- know where to signpost people living with dementia and/or their informal caregivers for advice and support.

Evaluation approaches should then build on learning outcomes to assess whether they have been achieved. This might be a formal process via an assessment of knowledge or competency for individual learners, for example in the format of an assessment or examination. Alternatively, the evaluation might be more focused on whether the training is achieving what it sets out to, or it could offer a combination of both. Learning outcomes apply specifically to the knowledge and behaviour components of Kirkpatrick's model for the evaluation of training, which will be outlined next.

Kirkpatrick's model for the evaluation of dementia training

Donald Kirkpatrick was an academic working in the area of learning and development in the late 1950s. His four-level model of training evaluation – reaction, knowledge, behaviour, results (Kirkpatrick 1979, 1984) – is used widely in education and training to consider the ways in which the impact of education and training can be understood. Here we outline the model and propose ways in which evidence for the impact of dementia training can be gathered to support evaluation at each of the levels.

Level 1: Reaction

How do learners react to the training? How satisfied are they with the programme?

Every training programme should be continually evaluated for learner reaction. This not only shows learners that facilitators value their feedback, but also enables the programme to be developed and improved based on learner feedback (Kirkpatrick and Kirkpatrick 2005). The most traditional method for this is via a standardised, short, written evaluation form that combines numerical or Likert scale (e.g. 'strongly agree' to 'strongly disagree', 'excellent' to 'poor') questions alongside ones with an open text format. Open text allows those completing the questionnaire to expand on their responses and add comments on areas of the training other than those covered by the fixed questions.

In designing a feedback questionnaire, training facilitators should first consider what aspects of the training they wish to evaluate. Examples of useful areas to consider include whether the content meets learners' needs, delivery methods, pace, facilitator approach/skill, and applicability to practice. Avoid asking questions with more than one component to them (e.g. the training content was useful and pitched at the right level) as learners may have different views on each. It may be appropriate to have different evaluation forms for different training programmes, dependent on how it is delivered and what the facilitators most want to capture about learner reactions. Forms should be short and simple to complete – using no more than one or two sides of A4, or taking more than 1–2 minutes to complete electronically. An example training evaluation form for a face-to-face training programme is given in Box 10.2.

Box 10.2 Example training evaluation form

Person-centred care training evaluation form
[Date of training and facilitator names]

Please answer all of the following questions to help us understand what is working well on the training and areas where you feel we could improve it.

	Strongly agree	Agree	Neither agree or disagree	Disagree	Strongly disagree
1. The training content was relevant to my role					
2. I was able to understand the training content					
3. The training was delivered at an appropriate pace for me					
4. The training was enjoyable					
5. The balance between information and practical activities was about right					

6. The training facilitator was knowledgeable					
7. The training facilitator was skilled in supporting my learning needs					
8. The training provided knowledge and skills I will be able to use in my role					

Please provide further information on any of the responses above, particularly if you have answered disagree or strongly disagree to any questions.

One thing I particularly enjoyed about the training was:

One thing I think could be improved about the training is:

Do you feel the training will be useful in your role/duties? Please explain your answer.

Is there anything else you would like to tell us about the training?

Thank you for taking time to complete this form.

The structured, numerical, or Likert scale questions can be analysed by working out an average score per question or presenting responses as a percentage. This then allows each delivery of a training session/programme to be compared with a benchmark standard or with the scores obtained following previous delivery. It is recommended that forms are completed immediately post-training, before learners leave the training environment, to maximise completion rates, and anonymously in order to obtain honest reactions (Kirkpatrick 1967).

However, written evaluation forms do have their limitations. They may not be the most appropriate way to evaluate all types of learning activity, especially informal or less structured programmes. They may also be less suited to certain groups of learners, such as those who have lower literacy levels or low confidence, or who have English as a second or additional language. Completion at the end of a training programme (when most learners are keen to leave!) can mean they may be completed in a hurry and learners may not provide full feedback, particularly for sections asking for written responses. Allowing specific timetabled time at the end of the training to complete evaluations can help with this. Additionally, while immediate completion of the forms ensures a good return rate, it only captures initial reactions rather than those experienced in the days and maybe even weeks after a training course. Therefore, alternative methods of assessing reaction may be appropriate in some cases. These might include, for example, asking managers or mentors to discuss training experiences with learners soon after and then, again, a week or two following completion. These routes may provide a useful mechanism for gaining a more in-depth understanding of individual experiences of training.

Level 2: Learning

To what extent has learning occurred? Has learning impacted on learners' knowledge, skills, and attitudes?

All training programmes would typically aim to increase the knowledge of learners. In the case of many dementia training programmes, increased skills, creation of positive attitudes towards and improved confidence in caring for people with dementia are also a desired outcome. We will examine each of these components in more detail as they can be evaluated in different ways.

Evaluating the impact of training on learners' knowledge can be undertaken through comparing knowledge before and after the training programme, and may be assessed as part of the training itself, or using a combination of the two. To evaluate impact on knowledge, it is important to be clear about what the learning objectives or outcomes of the programme are, and the specific knowledge related to this. One of the most common ways of assessing learning you will see reported in research papers is to use an existing, validated measure, including the Knowledge in Dementia Scale (KIDE; Elvish et al. 2014), the Dementia Knowledge Assessment Scale (DKAS; Annear et al. 2015), the Alzheimer's Disease Knowledge Scale (ADKS; Carpenter et al. 2009), and the DK-20 (Shanahan et al. 2013). These are completed before and after attending the training and the scores compared either descriptively or using statistical methods.

The advantage of these measures is that they have been designed using robust methods, and their properties as a measure have been assessed and confirmed. Disadvantages are that most of them assess broad rather than specific dementia knowledge, and they may cover additional items or miss particular aspects that your training programme addresses. They may also have what is known as a 'ceiling effect'. This is where individuals completing the measure all score highly before training and it is therefore not possible to show any improvement. This does not mean that learners have no need to increase their knowledge but occurs because a measure includes items that reflect too low a level of knowledge or are inappropriate to the staff completing them. Therefore, they might be useful for evaluating the impact on knowledge of a dementia awareness training programme, but might be less useful for a more in-depth or specific programme.

There are alternative ways to assess knowledge gains from training other than standard measures. Examples include surveys asking learners whether and what they have learned, interviews (individual or small/focus group), observation of learners during course activities or when implementing training (for example, if learners are taught to use a pain assessment scale, they could be observed completing it in practice to check they are doing so correctly), formal tests or exams, and knowledge quizzes (Levin-Banchik 2018). We provide an overview of the strengths, limitations, and consideration of different methods of collecting evaluation data later in the chapter. However, a combination of methods might provide the most robust approach to understanding impact on knowledge.

Attitudes and feelings of confidence or competence in caring for people living with dementia are also often measured using standardised measures. Commonly used measures for attitudes include the Approaches to Dementia Questionnaire (Lintern and Woods 1996) and Dementia Attitudes Scale (DAS; O'Connor and McFadden 2010), and for confidence include the Sense of Competence in Dementia Care Staff (SCIDS) scale (Schepers et al. 2012), Confidence in Dementia Scale (CODE; Elvish et al. 2014), and Caring Efficacy Scale (Coates 1997). However, they can also be assessed through a variety of other methods, including: interviews; focus groups; experiential and simulated learning activities and exercises during the training programme; asking people living with dementia about their experiences of care from learners; and by observing learners working in practice. As with assessing the impact of training on knowledge, a combination of methods will probably provide a more holistic picture of the impact on attitudes and feelings of confidence or competence of learners.

Level 3: Behaviour

To what extent has a learner's behaviour in practice changed? Do they do things differently and in line with a person-centred approach?

As discussed in Chapter 9, application of learning into practice is essential for realising any impact of training on outcomes for those directly affected by dementia. What a training facilitator/evaluator might expect to change in practice will be dependent on what the training aims to achieve, determined by the learning outcomes. In some cases, behaviours that might be expected to result from training will be straightforward to identify and to assess; in others, this may be more complex. See Box 10.3 for an example of this.

Box 10.3 Example behavioural outcomes and how they might be evaluated

Sunnyview Care Home has developed a training course for all staff on positive mealtimes and good nutrition and hydration for residents. The outcomes on staff behaviours the training facilitators are hoping to see as a result include:

- all residents being offered a choice of meal and drink at each mealtime;
- accurate recording of daily food and fluid intake in the care records of residents at risk of malnutrition or weight loss;
- the creation of a positive social atmosphere at mealtimes and making mealtimes a pleasurable experience, drawing on each resident's likes, dislikes, and life history.

The first of these outcomes might be evaluated numerically through observing different mealtimes over 7 days with a list of residents and checking whether or not they were offered a choice of meal and drink.

The second outcome might be assessed by undertaking a care plan review and assessing what percentage of residents had an accurate daily recording of food and fluid intake.

The final outcome might be assessed through observation of mealtimes either using a standard observational tool – for example, Dementia Care Mapping (Bradford Dementia Group 2005), Quality of Interactions Schedule (QUIS; Dean et al. 1993) – using a checklist or observation guide developed for the evaluation, or using a more unstructured approach. This might be complemented with interviews and/or informal conversations with residents to ask about their mealtime experiences and interviews with staff to explore how they approach mealtimes and why.

In some cases, it may be appropriate to undertake before and after data collection to see if things have changed; in other cases, it may be sufficient to collect data only after training to see if expected behaviours are present in practice. One thing we know from research into the impact of dementia training on outcomes is that impacts, or effects, often decline over time. Therefore, it may be appropriate to collect data every 3 or 6 months and to offer refresher training or other means of sustaining any impact, should expected behaviours decline.

Level 4: Outcomes

Most often, outcomes will be related to impacts on people living with dementia, or others directly affected by dementia. However, impacts on staff may also be

Figure 10.2 SMART objective-setting approach (Doran 1981)

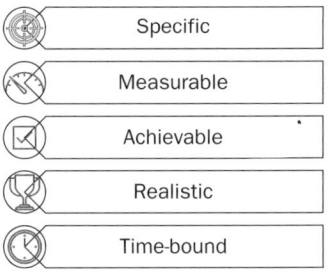

expected and assessed, for example on stress, burnout, turnover, or sickness. The outcomes that might be expected from training for people living with dementia will again be determined by the aims and content of the training. For example, a training programme focused on introducing the theory and principles of person-centred dementia care, and how this can be applied to responding to distressed behaviours, should have different outcomes from a training programme whose focus is pain assessment and management or supporting family caregivers. The outcomes should be determined by the learning outcomes written for a training programme. It may be helpful to use SMART objective-setting approaches (Doran 1981) to determine appropriate outcomes from training initiatives (see Figure 10.2).

Specific: The outcomes need to be clear and precise (e.g. 'Every resident will have a full life history including [list of items] in their care plan, which will have been written with the resident and their family') rather than something vague (e.g. 'Care practices will be improved').

Measurable: The outcomes need to be something that can be measured or assessed through data you can collect.

Achievable and **R**ealistic: It is important to be realistic about what a programme of training might achieve, particularly in the context of the final element of a set timescale. It might, for example, be possible to ensure that mealtime experiences are improved in a hospital setting by having open visiting at mealtimes so family members can support a person living with dementia to eat, or by supporting people with dementia to order/choose their meals or gaining support from a family member to do so. It would not be realistic to expect every person with dementia to eat all the food provided or for there to be no incidents of distress during mealtimes. While these might be desirable, they are beyond the control of individual staff or what a training course might reasonably be expected to achieve.

Time-bound: When do you hope to have achieved the outcomes by? It is important to allow enough time for outcomes to be realised but leaving too long a period after training can result in a decline in impact if implementation is not continually supported or refresher training offered.

Critiques of Kirkpatrick's model

It is important to acknowledge that Kirkpatrick's model has received criticism. For example, it has been challenged for: being too simplistic, particularly in its lack of consideration of how learning is or is not transferred into practice; for seeming to present a hierarchy that suggests results are more important than reactions; and assuming a relationship between the four levels of the model, when evidence has indicated this may not be the case (Surr et al. 2017a). However, despite this, the model provides a useful framework for considering the components that it may be useful to evaluate within dementia training. It is also reasonable to assume that it is unlikely that positive impacts on outcomes for people living with dementia would be realised from training if it has not had a positive impact on staff reaction, knowledge, or behaviours. However, simply because staff have learned something from attending training, or even altered their behaviours in practice as a result, it does not automatically indicate improved outcomes will be realised. As we indicated in Chapter 9, putting training into practice is complex and requires consideration of a range of factors beyond the programme itself. Likewise, the ways training can impact areas such as staff behaviours and outcomes is not linear or influenced only by the training itself. It is important to recognise that training evaluation is complex and imprecise for this very reason. This does not, however, mean evaluations are not worth undertaking, just that we should recognise the limitations of, and boundaries around, any conclusions we might draw from the evaluations we undertake.

Training evaluation

Involving people directly affected by dementia in training evaluation

Involvement of people directly affected by dementia in training evaluation usually occurs in one or more of three ways (NIHR 2021):

1 as *participants*: where users of the service or informal caregivers provide feedback on their experiences of care as a marker of training impact, or
2 through *active involvement*, either:
    a as partners in designing and overseeing training evaluations, for example through sitting on project advisory groups, or
    b as co-evaluators helping to collect data, analyse and interpret it.

We can also *engage* people directly affected by dementia more broadly in training evaluation through: sharing findings with them, for example summaries of findings being sent to those who take part; writing items for organisational newsletters; or presenting at events, workshops, and conferences.

Giving feedback on experiences of care or outcomes

Feedback may be provided on people's experiences of care or outcomes by several routes, including questionnaires/surveys, interviews/informal conversations, and through a range of creative methods, such as the use of pictures or Talking Mats™ to stimulate ideas and responses, writing diaries, walking interviews, and creative or arts-based methods (Phillipson and Hammond 2018). There are a range of resources available that provide excellent guidance in this area (see, for example, Brannelly and Bartlett 2020; Keady et al. 2017; Murphy et al. 2014; Samsi and Manthorpe 2020).

It is important to use methods that are appropriate to the person. Some people living with dementia will be able to fully participate in surveys and interviews, others may need support, and for some these methods will not provide a helpful way to gather their experiences. We need to ensure that we do not exclude the voices, opinions, and experiences of people with more advanced dementia and those least able to communicate with us, simply because it becomes more difficult to find ways to listen effectively to them. It may be that a combination of observation of people's experiences (see below) alongside informal, in-the-moment conversations might work best for some.

As partners in developing approaches to, or content of, evaluations

Gaining input from people living with dementia and their family and friends on training evaluation can provide opportunities to identify innovative and meaningful approaches that are specific and relevant to the training or service. Those evaluating training can consider how people might be involved in identifying evaluation outcomes and approaches for each level of The Kirkpatrick Model, discussed next. For example, they might co-develop a training evaluation form with people directly affected by dementia to understand reactions to training, or ask them about what they would hope to see staff do differently as a result of attending training

In the 'What Works?' study, the expert-by-experience group (people living with or caring for someone with dementia) worked with members of the research team to develop methods for understanding staff knowledge of person-centred care. This included people telling their stories of good and poor experiences of contact within different types of health and social care services. These were turned into written vignettes or case studies (Capstick et al. 2021), with a series of questions about what they saw as good and poor practice in the example and what they thought staff could have done differently. These were designed to be used in focus groups or individual interviews with staff. There are other similar examples reported. For example, Morbey et al. (2019) involved people directly affected by dementia in helping to design a two-round survey that sought to identify outcomes that could be used in research looking at community-based interventions for people living with dementia. This included a variety of methods for consultation with individuals and groups. Those consulted helped to simplify the survey methods, items, and format so the survey was accessible for people living with dementia

As evaluators or co-evaluators

Examples of people living with dementia as co-evaluators or researchers are much more limited than for other levels of involvement. However, this is a growing area of interest. A study exploring the experiences of researchers, key personnel, and people living with dementia who had supported research involving people living with dementia as co-researchers (Waite et al. 2019) identified that there was often scepticism from researchers and others involved about whether people living with dementia would be able to conduct research, largely based on stigma and stereotypes about dementia. This might be mitigated by encouraging a viewpoint that people living with dementia are not a homogeneous group and will have varying degrees of cognitive difficulties alongside different life experiences, skills, and qualities. Researchers and people living with dementia discussed the need to ensure a good fit between the research activities and the people who would undertake them, and the tailoring of activities and provision of appropriate support to enable people to complete their research tasks. For example, this might involve the person living with dementia asking the interview questions, with a researcher taking notes and undertaking transcription and analysis. Ensuring appropriate training, preparation, and ongoing support for co-researchers, and building trusting relationships between the researchers and people living with dementia, were identified as essential in creating a safe environment for the co-research to take place. Practical issues were also a potential barrier, with face-to-face engagement and participation preferred, but this then posed challenges for how the person living with dementia would get to the venue where the research was taking place. The time demands of participation were also identified as a challenge, with those wanting to take part being already busy people. All three groups of participants warned of the dangers of tokenism in involving people living with dementia as co-researchers and the need to ensure involvement was meaningful, beneficial, and empowering for those taking part. These principles are similar to those reported by Mann and Hung (2018), who worked together on a co-researcher project to improve services for people living with dementia within an acute hospital setting. Good communication, trust, respect, understanding, and reciprocity were key to their successful co-working relationship.

Both studies reported personal benefits for the people living with dementia, in taking part in evaluation as a co-researcher. People could gain confidence, a sense of making a difference, and the opportunity to apply existing or learn new skills. The benefits for researchers of conducting co-research with people living with dementia are discussed by Stevenson and Taylor (2017), whose study involved a group of four people with the condition in the analysis of an existing qualitative interview dataset. Of particular note were the new insights into the data that the co-researchers identified, which enhanced Stevenson and Taylor's understanding of the data. The co-researchers were also able to identify findings of practical importance to people living with dementia and ideas for dissemination to lay audiences. Overall, the authors conclude that involvement of people living with dementia improved the quality of the research.

An example of true research empowerment and leadership by people living with dementia is the DEEP Dementia Enquirers programme in the UK (Davies et al. 2021; Dementia Enquirers n.d.). This ground-breaking project supports groups of people living with dementia to apply for project grants to conduct research they are interested in, seeking advice from academics or others as needed. Projects carried out in the initial two rounds of funding are varied but include exploring the impact of urban and rural transport systems on independence (thred CiC 2021), discrimination and dementia (Beth Johnson Foundation 2021), and the impact of community-based groups on people living with dementia (Our Voice Matters 2021). Dementia Enquirers represents an important step forward in how people living with dementia can and should be included in research and evaluation. While those involved in leading and carrying out these projects may not reflect the diversity of people living with dementia, particularly those with moderate to severe dementia, this project and those discussed here, provide a clear challenge for us as evaluators. It is our job to ensure we approach evaluation as being 'with' and 'for' people with dementia and not 'about' and 'on' them. The evidence suggests this needs to be a carefully considered process, one that focuses on building relationships and ensuring the ways we involve, support the participation of, or engage with people living with dementia in the context of training evaluation are appropriate, inclusive, and supportive, so that this is a meaningful process.

Staff as training evaluators

Similar principles to those discussed above around the participation, involvement, and engagement of people directly affected by dementia in training evaluation also apply when considering involving dementia care staff. As evaluators, it is important that we ensure methods for participation and engagement are inclusive and tailored to staff groups and individuals and their needs. As with prior experiences of education and training (see Chapter 9), staff's previous exposure to evaluation and research may be different and not necessarily always positive. While some staff may be open to giving their views on training and its potential impact on them and their practice, others may be suspicious of motivations for collecting data, of being scrutinised, be concerned by what they are being asked, or wary of appearing critical or of being honest if things could be improved. It is therefore important that we are transparent about how evaluation data is being collected, analysed, and used and that people have opportunities to opt in or out of participation, to respond anonymously, and get to see the final findings or outcomes and how they are being used. While there is a body of literature on people living with health conditions and 'service users' as co-researchers (Malterud and Elvbakken 2019) and the benefits of this, there remains a dearth of literature around health and social care staff taking up a similar role, with the exception of studies adopting methodologies where engagement has a practice component, such as action research. We argue that involving staff in the process of evaluating training programmes, either designing the methods and processes used or as co-researchers, would not only enhance the research itself, but may provide a valuable development opportunity for the staff involved. We therefore encourage academics, training providers, and health and social care organisations to consider how they can do this.

Methods for collecting data for the evaluation of training

There are a range of methods for collecting data to support the evaluation of training. We provide an overview of some of these here, which evaluation aspects they may be particularly useful for, and their limitations. It is likely that any evaluation of training will need to use a variety of data collection methods, particularly if evaluation across all the Kirkpatrick levels is planned.

Questionnaires

Questionnaires are one of the most frequently used methods for evaluation of dementia training. As discussed above, questionnaires can take the form of standardised measures, as in the case of knowledge or confidence measures, or they may be designed by the evaluator(s) to be tailored to the training programme being evaluated, or a combination of the two. Questionnaires can include numerical and fixed response questions (e.g. Likert scales as well as space for respondents to write free-text answers; see Box 10.4). They therefore offer a particularly flexible method of data collection that could be used to assess outcomes across all the Kirkpatrick levels.

Box 10.4 Examples of types of questions that can be used in questionnaires

Likert scale

The training will be useful to my day-to-day practice:

| Strongly agree | Agree | Neither agree or disagree | Disagree | Strongly disagree |

The pace of the training was:

| Too fast | | About right | | Too slow |

Dichotomous response

Have you used the pain assessment tool in the last week?

Yes   No

Numerical response
How many times have you used the pain assessment tool in the last month?

_____

Open response
Do you think that the 'Understanding pain in dementia' training has helped to improve care of residents in this care home? Please give examples.

Questionnaires have the benefit of being relatively easy to administer in terms of time and resources and do not need the time for analysis that methods such as interviews or observations require. This allows many responses to identical questions to be collected, which may allow some comparability. They are also relatively straightforward and quick for respondents to complete (if designed correctly) and can be completed anonymously, which can increase return rates.

Questionnaires in the form of a short test or knowledge quiz can be a particularly useful way of understanding if learners have gained the specific knowledge you had hoped from attending training. Knowledge quizzes should be designed to cover the content from the learning outcomes and training content. It is not within the scope of this book to provide detailed guidance on questionnaire or knowledge quiz design and development; there are many textbooks that cover this in detail. We recommend that you design your knowledge quiz carefully and with reference to this literature, so that the items are developed correctly and robustly. For example, you will need to decide between different question formats, such as multiple-choice, Likert scales, or open responses, with different options working better for some types of outcomes than others. Attitudes, for instance, may be more suited to Likert scales, factual or knowledge-based content to multiple-choice responses, while suggestions or explanations might be best gained through open response questions. You will also need to ensure you pilot your quiz and refine it before using it more widely, to ensure that all questions are understood in the same way by respondents, are clear and unambiguous, and that multiple-choice answers provide one clear option for those who know the answer but present equally viable alternatives for those who do not.

There are disadvantages of questionnaires that must also be considered. Self-report is not always accurate. For example, respondents may give the response they feel is more socially acceptable, rather than their actual thoughts or feelings. This might include reporting they felt training was useful or that they have applied it in practice even if this is not the case. Alternatively, their perceptions may influence the answers they give. For example, if they particularly enjoyed a training course and felt they learned a lot from attending, they may be more likely to report this has also impacted positively on care practice or people living with dementia they care for. Questionnaire items can also be understood or interpreted in different ways by different respondents. This can to some extent be avoided through careful design and piloting of a question-naire, but this may not fully eliminate this issue. Fixed response questions (for example, yes/no or Likert scales) can only tell you what people do or think; it is more difficult to assess *why* when using a questionnaire. While open response questions can be helpful to explore the 'why', people will usually only write a small amount on questionnaires and there is no ability to prompt or ask for further information. Questionnaires need to be limited in length for practical reasons, since participants are unlikely to wish to complete a very lengthy questionnaire. In addition, some outcomes do not lend themselves easily to evaluation via a questionnaire format.

These limitations do not mean that questionnaires are not a useful method for evaluation of training, just that anyone undertaking an evaluation should consider these and make a judgement about whether a questionnaire is the most appropriate method of data collection, or whether other approaches might be more useful. If a questionnaire is used, then the limitations should be considered in how the data is analysed and interpreted.

Interviews

Interviews allow you to explore in more detail individuals' experiences and thoughts. They can be conducted individually, in small groups (two to three people), or as focus groups (usually four to eight people). They usually take the form of semi-structured interviews, which is where the interviewer develops a topic guide of questions they wish to cover in the interview, but these are then asked flexibly and with additional prompts and probes depending on the answers the interviewees provide. We recommend piloting the interview topic guide and refining it, if necessary, by carrying out one or two interviews with volunteer colleagues ahead of using it as part of a formal training evaluation.

Interviews with individuals have the benefit of allowing the researcher to explore, in depth, the experiences and views of a single person. They may be easier to arrange in terms of scheduling and can be particularly useful when interviewing people with cognitive or communication difficulties who may need specific support to take part and may fare less well as part of a focus group. Focus groups have the benefit of getting the views of several different people at the same time. While less ground or less depth might be achieved in a focus group than when interviewing a single individual, they do offer the opportunity to give breadth of opinion on a particular topic. This can allow for the raising and exploration of different views and perspectives. One challenge of focus groups is that if there are one or two dominant voices, then quieter individuals may not speak or be heard. There is also a risk that when discussing contentious issues, people may not feel able to share views that are different to those of others. Therefore, facilitation of focus groups requires skill and confidence. It can be helpful to have two facilitators present so they are able to work together to observe the group and ask follow-up questions or prompt responses from quieter individuals. While it can be difficult to find a date and time when multiple people are available to participate in a focus group, they do have the advantage of being more time effective overall given the multiple participants. Interviews and focus groups also allow the evaluator to explore individual differences in the impact of training and reasons for these.

One disadvantage of any kind of interview is that participants may not feel comfortable or able to share their true thoughts or beliefs. They may be inclined to give what they feel is the correct or socially desirable answer. This might be the case, for example, if someone who is responsible for delivering training also conducts interviews with staff that gather their views on that training and its impact. Interviews can also be time-consuming to do well. As well as the time taken to conduct them, the interviews need to be transcribed and analysed appropriately. Thus, while they offer a richer data source than questionnaires, they are more resource-intensive to adopt and can by necessity only include the views of a much smaller group of learners.

Routine data

Routine data refers to data that is routinely collected by health and care services. For example, this might range from data on prescribed medications, health care appointments and other health resource use, to data that might only be available in certain settings such as falls or participation in activities. In the UK, health services have traditionally recorded more items of routine data (and have it available in digital anonymised formats) than social care services. However, technology and electronic care planning systems makes it possible for many social care providers to provide this kind of data as well. Routine data can provide a consistent source of information to evaluate training outcomes, with data available from before and after training programmes and data often available for potentially long periods of time. The data is usually available on many people using a service and if obtained and analysed anonymously, poses fewer ethical issues around consent and permission to use than other types of data.

There are, however, several limitations to routine data that must be considered. Most routine data is collected to support care delivery and for administration purposes, not for research or evaluation (Clarke et al. 2019). Therefore, the quality of the data may be variable, particularly if it is recorded by different individuals and/or if there is not a standardised recording method. There may be missing data, incorrectly inputted data, and data interpreted in different ways (Calanzani et al. 2017). This can mean considerable time may need to be spent 'data cleaning' before it is in a format ready for analysis. In addition, routine data might not be collected on the specific outcomes you are interested in and which you anticipate training might directly impact. Routine data also only helps you to explore group level impacts of training not individual level impacts. It may also be difficult to separate data on people living with dementia only, or specific groups of staff from wider data sets covering all people using or working in a service. Therefore, while routine data can provide a broad dataset collected over a long period of time, the quality of the data and what items are available must be considered when deciding if it will provide a useful source for evaluation of training impact.

Observation

Observation is a commonly used evaluation approach in dementia research, since it can give the researcher an insight into the experiences of a person who is unable to give a detailed account of their experiences in an interview or via a questionnaire due to communication difficulties or problems with recall. Observational methods vary from structured tools such as Dementia Care Mapping (DCM; Bradford Dementia Group 2005, 2014) and the Quality of Interactions Schedule (QUIS; Bowie and Mountain 1993), to more formal semi-structured or unstructured observation using research methodologies such as ethnography (Leverton et al. 2021; Ludwin and Capstick 2017; Scales et al. 2017). Issues to consider when using observation include:

- Whether to be a participant observer, or non-participant observer – observing in the course of daily duties in the care home (participant) or observing 'from the sidelines' (non-participant). There are pros and cons of each approach. Participant observation is easier to carry out over longer and more frequent periods because it is being undertaken while completing usual daily duties. However, this means it can be easy to miss things because the observer's focus is not exclusively on observing. Non-participant observation allows the observer to spend dedicated time observing, although this can be difficult to allocate and protect in busy care services. It may impact how people act because they are aware of being observed. However, our own experiences of conducting observations in a variety of care setting suggests this 'observer impact' is short-lived and people generally do not have the time to think too much about the observer being there, or to noticeably alter what they do from usual practice.
- Where to observe. Non-participant observation should usually be in public areas and should not compromise people's dignity and privacy. For example, the observer should not sit/stand and observe delivery of personal care or people undressing.
- How the observer explains their presence/what they are doing to people in the setting. It is important that people in the care setting/service, including people living with dementia, visitors, and staff, know someone is observing, why they are observing, and what they are going to do with the information.
- Consent. While this is not formal research, it is still important people agree to being observed. This can be obtained by explaining to people what is happening and checking they are okay with this. If anyone expresses concern or says this is okay but later seems upset by the observer's presence, they should not continue to be observed.
- Should an observer interact and engage? A non-participant observer will need to think about how much they engage and interact with other people as

they observe. They might, for example, tell staff members to ignore them, rather than coming to them with questions or asking for help. If people living with dementia or visitors talk to an observer, then it is important that they role-model person-centred care and engage with them. This may mean their presence alters what they observe, so it is then important to be mindful of this in the data recorded.

The strength of observation over other approaches, is that it allows an evaluator to see things they would be unlikely to capture using interviews or other data collection methods. Devoting periods of time to observation allows someone to see things that they would not notice if they were working a busy shift. It can also give a voice to and the perspective of people who might be unable to communicate this for themselves. The challenges of observation are that it can be time-consuming, requires skills and experience to do it well (observing, recording notes, etc.), and sometimes people may act differently while an observer is present or may seek to engage with an observer if there are no staff present.

Documentary analysis

Health and social care services produce a vast array of documents that can be helpful when evaluating the impact of training. These can range from care plans/records and assessment documents, to details of complaints, incidents, or satisfaction with services. The way the documents may contribute to training evaluations will vary depending on the aims and intended outcomes of the training. For example, a training programme on person-centred care and use of life history might have an intended outcome of improved life-history information in care plans. A sample of care plans might be audited before and after the training so see if this is the case.

Documents have the benefit of being an ongoing record, so it is possible to examine if and how any changes occur over time as training programmes are introduced. One of the disadvantages is that standardised formats for and ways of completing documents, especially those that may be subject to more formal or external audit, can mean that there is limited opportunity for or openness to changing how these are written.

Once I have evaluated training, what do I do next?

Evaluation of training should ideally be considered as an ongoing process, conducted in cycles, or as a means of monitoring sustainability of outcomes over time, rather than a one-off activity. After each evaluation, or cycle of evaluation, it is important to feed back findings to people who have taken part, to those with an interest in them, and into the wider training and organisational strategy. Producing reports and summaries of findings suitable for different audiences is an important part of this process. Box 10.5 provides some tips on writing for different audiences.

Box 10.5 Tips on writing for different audiences

- Think about who your audience is: what do they need/want to know about your evaluation? What is the most appropriate format to present it to them in? This might be a written report, one-page summary, a poster, infographics, leaflet, presentation, etc.
- Whoever your audience is, writing in plain English is important. It helps any audience to understand more clearly what you are communicating with them. The Plain English Campaign (2021) has lots of resources and guides on how to do this.
- Avoid using jargon, abbreviations, and technical terms, except if this is for a very specific audience who regularly use these terms and who will all be comfortable with them. Remember, even if your audience is clinicians, different professions may use different terminology and abbreviations, so they are usually best avoided. If you do have to use them, provide a definition or explanation of what they mean.
- Write in short sentences or use bullet points.
- Think about presentation: use headings, pictures, graphs, or tables, and make sure there is white space on the page.
- Ask one or more people from your target audience to read what you have written and to give you feedback on how it might be improved.

It is important that evaluation forms the basis of learning and subsequent action on any findings that indicate ways to improve the content, delivery, or support for application of training programmes into practice. Developing SMART objectives or action points (see Figure 10.2) can be one approach to this.

Summary

This chapter has argued the importance of evaluation of training for measuring the extent to which it has met intended goals as well as for demonstrating a return on investment. It highlighted some of the challenges associated with evaluation of training. Bloom's taxonomy of learning was presented as a model for underpinning the development of learning outcomes for training, which can be used as the basis for its subsequent evaluation. Kirkpatrick's model for the evaluation of training was then presented, including ideas for the type of evidence that can be collected to support evaluation of each level. The chapter highlighted the important role people directly affected by dementia, as well as staff working in dementia care, can play in the evaluation of dementia training. The chapter then provided an overview of a range of methods for collecting data within evaluations of dementia training, including some of their strengths and limitations. Finally, we discussed how training evaluations should be used, including providing ongoing development of the training and its implementation, as well as noting the importance of sharing findings with the various stakeholders, via use of appropriate dissemination methods.

Implications for those delivering dementia training

Those delivering dementia training should:

- Ensure evaluation of training forms a core component of its development, implementation, and ongoing review.
- Aim to conduct evaluation that seeks to explore all four Kirkpatrick levels of training evaluation, recognising that some levels may be more straightforward and less resource-intensive to collect data on.
- Ensure appropriate resources, including time, personnel, and skills, are available to undertake training evaluation.
- Involve people directly affected by dementia appropriately in dementia training evaluation. This may be in one of more of the following roles: participant providing evidence of training impact, supporting the design and delivery of a training evaluation, or as a co-evaluator.
- Ensure findings are shared with the key stakeholders using appropriate dissemination methods.

Implications for managers in dementia care settings and services

Leaders and managers in dementia care settings should:

- Expect the evaluation of training will be undertaken and support this process – for example, through collecting and providing routine data, or encouraging and supporting staff to take part in evaluation activities.
- Read, share, and use the outcomes of training evaluations to support the continued development of dementia training and its application into practice.

Implications for staff providing care, services, or support to people with dementia

Staff working in health and social care settings should:

- Engage with training evaluations through providing feedback or data as requested on their experiences of attending training and implementing it in practice.
- Encourage and support people directly affected by dementia to contribute to the evaluation of training – for example, through providing feedback on their experiences of the service and support received.
- Engage with the findings from training evaluations to identify ways staff can, individually or as a team, sustainably implement dementia training into practice to deliver person-centred dementia care.

Implications for those directly affected by dementia

- People living with dementia and their supporters have an important role to play in dementia training evaluation. This may be as a provider of feedback on care and services received, in supporting the design and delivery of a training evaluation, and/or as a co-evaluator.
- They should be provided with appropriate training, support, and recompense for their time and expertise, for any engagement with training evaluations.

11 The future for dementia training and education

'Dementia training has come a long way in the last 25 years. It still has some way to go to sufficiently address the significant need for a large, skilled, and flexible dementia care workforce that rising numbers of dementia cases globally will require.'

Throughout this book, we have reviewed and summarised theoretical and research evidence to underpin high-quality, impactful dementia training for the dementia workforce. In this chapter, we draw together this evidence and highlight its implications for international practice and research. The chapter will then present our views on the future of learning and development for the dementia care workforce, highlighting some key avenues for innovation. We reflect on the positioning and role of people directly affected by dementia within training and workforce development and the implications of this for delivery of person-centred dementia care.

The current state of play in dementia education and training

Dementia training has become part of the dialogue around good dementia care practice and has advanced significantly in the last 20 years. The World Health Organisation's (WHO) global action plan on the public health response to dementia 2017–2025 (WHO 2017), to which all WHO members states are signatories, was designed to help governments of member states develop and implement their own national dementia plans. Area four of the action plan identifies the requirement for the dementia workforce to be adequately trained and qualified to provide diagnosis, treatment, and support. Thus, dementia training will play a prominent role in international efforts to support good care for people directly affected by dementia.

This book has described approaches to dementia training in different sectors and targeted to different groups of the dementia workforce. In doing so, it has identified some novel approaches for delivering training, which avail of the advancing methods and techniques available to training providers and organisations. For example, the COVID-19 pandemic has meant that technology has played an increasing role in training delivery as health and care providers have turned to online methods to ensure the safety of their staff (and those they support). Finding new ways of working has created opportunities for some providers to explore delivery methods, such as the use of videoconferencing software (described in a case study in Chapter 2), which may enable staff to participate in small group training that may have otherwise been inaccessible or unsafe. Similarly, the adoption of an e-learning CPD programme (pre-COVID-19) delivered for GPs in Australia (Casey et al. 2020) described in Chapter 5 has meant that practitioners living in rural locations have been able to participate in programmes that would have otherwise been impossible. However, the lack of digital infrastructure (phone and internet capacity) in many rural communities, risks of digital exclusion, and the failure of some online interventions in care homes, as discussed in Chapter 4, demonstrate that technological solutions still have limitations and do not always provide a viable solution.

As stated in the sector-specific chapters, there is no 'one-size-fits-all' approach that can be identified as 'good practice' for the delivery of dementia training. Rather, training should be considerate of the nature of the learner, the setting, and the training need that has been identified. There are, however, universal structures and principles that can be followed which enable training providers to be responsive to need and provide overarching guidance that spans sector and workforce. These include:

- Considering the needs of the individual learners, adapting the methods, and using a range of different methods as appropriate.
- Considering the ways in which informal learning is occurring within the organisation and day-to-day conduct of work, and opportunities to promote this.
- Involving people directly affected by dementia and making sure their voice is heard throughout (such as in the development, delivery, and evaluation of training).
- Using frameworks, guidance, benchmark standards, and policies where these exist, or developing in-house frameworks.
- Looking to the evidence base and research (as summarised in this book) for training content and effective delivery methods, as well as additional components that enhance the effectiveness of implementation into practice (such as 'champion' roles, ongoing support, auditing of tools, etc.).
- Evaluating training using structured approaches or models that focus not only on the 'easier' to measure outcomes such as reaction or knowledge, but also examine impact on staff behaviour outcomes for those receiving care.
- Identifying staff or individuals who can take on the role of leaders in championing good dementia training and positive cultures of learning.
- Ensuring that training promotes person-centred approaches and addresses stigmatising attitudes and beliefs concerning dementia.

In summary, whilst this book has demonstrated that dementia training has come a long way in the last 25 years, and certainly since Kitwood's (1997) first conceptualisation of personhood, it still has some way to go to sufficiently address the significant need for a large, skilled, and flexible dementia care workforce that rising numbers of dementia cases globally will require. To equip the workforce to adopt person-centred practices, much more needs to be done to understand successful approaches for the delivery of training in the workforce, and how to overcome barriers to the delivery of such. It will become particularly important to understand if and how approaches developed, implemented, and evaluated in high-income countries translate to low- and middle-income countries.

The future of dementia education and training

Innovation in delivery methods

The evolution of dementia training over the last two decades demonstrates the innovation and creativity that is being applied to the sector. Recent developments, such as the use of arts-based approaches including theatre, film, and poetry to deliver educational content, offer significant promise in bringing creativity to the learning experience and offering non-traditional routes for learning. They may also offer methods and opportunities for learning from and alongside people living with dementia, as described in Chapter 2. Technological advances such as the increasingly accessible virtual reality also offer significant promise for the delivery of impactful dementia training and opportunities for improved realism in simulation-based training. However, the use of creative arts and technology-based training and its formal evaluation remains in its infancy and this, we suggest, should be an area for future research focus.

Alongside the opportunity for innovation brought by new technologies and wider access to those that currently exist, comes increased sophistication in the delivery of online methods of learning. Again, these offer great potential, but will require considerably more formal, large-scale evaluation within different workforces, particularly when compared with the efficacy of more well-evidenced methods such as face-to-face and blended training. Drivers towards online learning innovation such as reduced costs and improved flexibility have been boosted by the necessities of the COVID-19 pandemic, but this alone is not a guarantee of improved quality. It is vitally important not to lose the gains of the last 25 years in all areas of knowledge about dementia training quality. Thorough development and research is required to establish if, when, how, and under what conditions online methods are the most effective route to foster learning of person-centred care.

Recognition and exploration of learning that takes place outside of training

We have highlighted in this book the opportunities presented by properly acknowledging and using the informal learning that takes place within the day-to-day conduct of work in a variety of settings. This book is the first to bring these ideas together with knowledge about traditional approaches to training as applied to dementia care. The next decade offers the chance to capitalise on these in both practice and research.

The current lack of investigations of informal learning within dementia care settings provides an obvious incentive and path for future research. Without a redirection of research focus, the opportunities for improving practice presented by informal learning (and any potential associated benefits of impact and cost-effectiveness) will remain untapped, and the current imbalance in favour of focusing exclusively on formal training will remain. However, it is seemingly easier to conduct a randomised controlled trial to measure the efficacy of a training course than it is to examine the impact of unconscious informal learning mechanisms on staff. This therefore leads to our next core focus for the future – the research design and methods used to evaluate both informal and formal learning.

Evolution in the design and methods to research dementia training and informal learning

This book has highlighted the current state of play regarding research on dementia training and informal learning. We have identified how the majority of research has focused only on the Kirkpatrick levels of reaction and knowledge. Where behaviours and outcomes are explored, it is often in simplistic ways that fail to recognise training's location in a wider context. However, as we have highlighted in Chapters 8, 9, and 10, this is a misleading perspective, and there are in fact many individual, organisational, and societal factors which impact the ability to implement training, affect staff practices, and outcomes for people living with dementia. Evaluation of cause and effect between programmes of training and these outcomes is complex, and the dementia research field is slowly beginning to acknowledge that research designs often considered the 'gold standard' (such as RCTs) may not be appropriate or sensitive enough (as they currently stand) to investigate the complexities of how and why training affects outcomes in dementia care settings. That is not to say that RCTs should be replaced wholesale by other research designs. Rather, we are arguing that creating and sustaining person-centred dementia care, through training or other complex interventions, is not straightforward, and therefore the future role of the researcher should be to explain that complexity rather than to reach for (admittedly more satisfying) simplicity.

However, it is important to note that at least part of the reason for the current research focus is the fit with prevailing preferences for positivist (rooted in the traditional physical sciences) research methodologies and a desire for interventions that can be easily operationalised for such research. Therefore, redirecting research towards informal learning and methods for evaluating formal learning within its wider context will need to address this current preference. The following issues are necessary components of a future research agenda regarding training and informal learning in dementia care:

- Researchers need to better articulate the need for, role, and requirements of research methodologies that are more suited to investigating context-dependent, interaction-, and relationship-based phenomena, especially when examining concepts which may not be understood sufficiently to be operationalised appropriately for an intervention, such as informal learning mechanisms.
- Researchers need to recognise that training alone is unlikely to be sufficient to change practice and that complex, multi-factorial interventions will be required. Research designs need to be able to accommodate such complexity.
- Research is needed to investigate robust methods for understanding and evaluating the manifestation of different informal learning mechanisms within dementia care settings and to build interventions that could influence them.
- Research designs are needed that can scrutinise the complex interplay between, and the relative influence of, informal learning mechanisms compared with training on dementia care practice outcomes and the influence of wider contextual factors.

Improved knowledge transfer from research to practice

Looking at the evidence examined in this book, particularly within Part 2, there is a pressing need to improve knowledge transfer from research. This will require closer working between academics and practitioners and increased awareness of sector needs by research funders. The need for knowledge transfer exists across sectors (there is a notable contrast between the wealth of research into training interventions in the care home field and the lack of it in the community, for example). However, it also exists between academia and practice. For example, dissemination of findings from research once a study is over often lacks coordination and systematic communication, particularly when health and care provider organisations are diverse and diffuse. This means that navigating through the 'evidence base' is a complex task – often requiring specialist skills and resources – beyond the scope of many learning and development roles in the health and social care sector. Increased attention to creating coordinated stores of information and communicating findings in accessible ways (including practical next steps) could help to make better use of the research that already exists in this area. A complementary approach is the investment in leaders and roles within health and care organisations that have the specialist skills to navigate and understand the evidence base as well as the abilities to transfer this knowledge into training and practice.

Involving people directly affected by dementia

It is important that future development continues to expand the involvement and representation of people directly affected by dementia in training and development initiatives. The last decade has seen some promising advances, but there are many more opportunities to be capitalised upon. First, ensuring that training at all levels is directly connected to the experiences of people affected by dementia should move beyond merely representing experiences in content to including first-hand accounts. The gold standard target for this is the introduction of co-trainers and curriculum designers with this direct experience. This will take resources and commitment to ensure success for both learners and those contributing to training. However, developing and sharing evidence as to how to do this well, and engaging with the growing number of self-advocacy organisations dedicated to facilitating people's involvement, will improve training relevance and effectiveness. It will be important that projects which explore techniques for doing this include robust evaluations that consider the complexities of training effectiveness (including, for example, the Kirkpatrick outcome levels) so that this evidence matches the standard now expected of training outcomes more generally.

Second, alongside efforts to increase the involvement of people directly affected by dementia in designing and delivering training, it will also be important to address how to maximise representation across the range of experiences that exist. There is always a danger that 'involvement' can result in representation exclusively of those who are able, willing – and invited – to be involved. Being mindful of how to include experiences of those who are living with advanced dementia, those who experience additional discrimination, those who are living with multiple disabilities, and those who are members of marginalised communities is important, especially where this may challenge conventional and majority views. One reason for acknowledging the complexity of experiences within training is that many health and social care staff will need the insight and skills to engage and work effectively with the diversity of people living with dementia and those who support them. This will require skills in adapting services and support to individual needs, rather than expecting people affected by dementia to accept or adapt to what is on offer. They will also need skills to manage potentially conflicting views and opinions (such as between a person living with dementia and their partner) within the course of their work if it is to be truly person-centred.

A third area where people directly affected by dementia can be more involved in influencing future training and development is through increased understanding and attention to informal ways of learning. Informal learning takes place within day-to-day interactions and relationships. This means those receiving support can be active constituents of that learning alongside colleagues and managers. However, this requires not only recognition and action to utilise informal learning towards person-centred care but also a commitment to maximising the role of people directly affected by dementia within that, so that their status and opportunities are as influential as that of others. We have suggested several ways that this can be achieved elsewhere in this book, such as incorporating their feedback on a daily basis, increasing observation techniques, and increasing opportunities for relationship-building between staff and those they support.

Finally, and building on increasing involvement within informal learning, the best way to secure the representation and interests of people affected by dementia in training and development is for those people to be more fully involved in the commissioning, decision-making, and governance of organisations (and policy-making) overall. It is one thing to incorporate 'real' perspectives into training delivery for staff; it is quite another for the training agenda itself to be set by what skills people directly affected by dementia say their workforce need. Indeed, one might argue that some of the ongoing challenges faced in achieving person-centred care (that we often attempt to fix via training for staff) stem from a fundamental mismatch between the design and purposes of a particular organisation and what people directly affected by dementia want and need. Narrowing this gap is what will ultimately enable us all to achieve person-centred care. This is a lofty goal, but it can begin with simple steps such as involving people directly affected by dementia in training needs analyses and organisational reviews.

The future of person-centred care from a dementia training perspective

It is clear from the projected figures for the coming decades, and the continued need for formal dementia care services in various forms, that there will remain an ongoing need for staff training and development to deliver person-centred care. Most of the dementia training research to date comes from high-income countries. However, the largest growth in numbers of people living with dementia between now and 2050 will be seen in low- and middle-income countries. These countries, too, will need to develop services and a workforce that is knowledgeable and skilled to deliver person-centred care. They will need an evidence base to underpin this, and we cannot assume that the research conducted to date will transfer to these contexts. It will be the role of researchers working in dementia training, education, and workforce development to ensure that this need is met.

In addition, currently most of the training evidence comes from the complex care settings of hospitals and care homes. As the number of people living with dementia rises more people will need support in the community, and it is hoped we will see more innovation in personalised, community solutions. The challenges of working with and providing training for organisations operating in the community were outlined in Chapter 7, namely: the range of professionals, paraprofessionals, and informal caregivers providing support in the community; geographical issues; and diversity of services and people receiving support. The complexities and scarcity of research in this field mean that we need much more evidence about what works with regards to dementia training for these organisations and staff, who are working in diverse ways and with different structures around them.

Summary

Dementia training and workforce development will continue to have a central role in driving forward the delivery of person-centred care to people living with dementia for many years to come. We cannot have a workforce that can deliver good dementia care without them also being well trained. Training is not a one-off event but should provide a continual programme of development throughout a career. There is broad scope for our understanding of what constitutes effective learning in both informal and formal contexts to grow, for our methods of evaluation and our understanding of how learning occurs and is implemented to become more refined and nuanced, and for technological solutions to play an ever greater role in training delivery. What is clear is the importance of the voice of people directly affected by dementia in impactful learning, and the absolute necessity for this to remain at the core of any national or local workforce development programme.

References

Abley, C., et al. 2019. Training interventions to improve general hospital care for older people with cognitive impairment: Systematic review. *British Journal of Psychiatry*, 214(4), 201–212.

Abraham, J., et al. 2019. Implementation of a multicomponent intervention to prevent physical restraints in nursing homes (IMPRINT): A pragmatic cluster randomized controlled trial. *International Journal of Nursing Studies*, 96, 27–34.

Abraham, J., et al. 2020. Interventions to reduce physical restraints in general hospital settings: A scoping review of components and characteristics. *Journal of Clinical Nursing*, 29(17–18), 3183–3200.

Aerts, L., et al. 2019. Why deprescribing antipsychotics in older people with dementia in long-term care is not always successful: Insights from the HALT study. *International Journal of Geriatric Psychiatry*, 34(11), 1572–1581.

Aged Care Quality and Safety Commission (ACQSC). 2018. *Enhanced Safety Standards*. ACQSC, Australian Government.

Aged Care Workforce Strategy Taskforce. 2018. *A Matter of Care: Australia's Aged Care Workforce Strategy. Report of the Aged Care Workforce Strategy Taskforce* [online]. Available from: https://www.health.gov.au/resources/publications/a-matter-of-care -australias-aged-care-workforce-strategy.

Ahmad, S., et al. 2010. GPs' attitudes, awareness, and practice regarding early diagnosis of dementia. *British Journal of General Practice*, 60(578), e360–e365.

Ajjawi, R. and Higgs, J. 2008. Learning to reason: A journey of professional socialisation. *Advances in Health Sciences Education*, 13(2), 133–150.

All Party Parliamentary Group (APPG). 2013. *Dementia Does Not Discriminate: The experiences of black, Asian and minority ethnic communities*. London: All Party Parliamentary Group on Dementia [online]. Available from: https://www.alzheimers. org.uk/sites/default/files/migrate/downloads/appg_2013_bame_report.pdf.

All Party Parliamentary Group (APPG). 2021. *Housing for People with Dementia – Are we ready?* London: All Party Parliamentary Group on Housing and Care for Older People [online]. Available from: https://www.housinglin.org.uk/_assets/Resources/ Housing/Support_materials/Reports/HCOP_APPG_Dementia_Housing_and_Care_ Inquiry-LowRes.pdf.

Allen, J., Mahamed, F. and Williams, K. 2020. Disparities in education: E-Learning and COVID-19, who matters? *Child and Youth Services*, 41(3), 208–210.

Alushi, L., Hammond, J. and Wood, J. 2015. Evaluation of dementia education programs for pre-registration healthcare students: A review of the literature. *Nurse Education Today*, 35(9), 992–998.

Alvarez, K., Salas, E. and Garofano, C. 2004. An integrated model of training evaluation and effectiveness. *Human Resource Development Review*, 3(4), 385–416.

Alzheimer's Association. 2020. 2020 Alzheimer's disease facts and figures. *Alzheimer's and Dementia*, 16(3), 391–460 [online]. Available from: https://alz-journals.onlineli-brary.wiley.com/doi/full/10.1002/alz.12068.

Alzheimer's Disease International (ADI). n.d. *Accreditation*. London: ADI [online]. Available from: https://www.alzint.org/what-we-do/accreditation/ [Accessed 6 June 2022].

Alzheimer's Disease International (ADI). 2019. *World Alzheimer Report 2019: Attitudes to dementia*. London: ADI [online]. Available from: https://www.alzint.org/resource/world-alzheimer-report-2019/.

Alzheimer's Disease International (ADI). 2021. *Dementia Statistics*. London: ADI [online]. Available from: https://www.alzint.org/about/dementia-facts-figures/dementia-statistics/.

Alzheimer's Society. 2009. *Counting the Cost: Caring for people with dementia on hospital wards*. London: Alzheimer's Society.

Alzheimer's Society. 2016. *Fix Demenia Care: Hospitals*. London: Alzheimer's Society [online]. Available from: https://www.alzheimers.org.uk/sites/default/files/migrate/downloads/fix_dementia_care_-_hospitals.pdf.

Alzheimer's Society. 2021. *This is Me*. London: Alzheimer's Society.

Amjad, H., et al. 2018. Underdiagnosis of dementia: An observational study of patterns in diagnosis and awareness in US older adults. *Journal of General Internal Medicine*, 33(7), 1131–1138.

Anderson, L., et al. 2001. *A Taxonomy for Learning, Teaching, and Assessing: A revision of Bloom's Taxonomy of Educational Objectives*. New York: Longman.

Andrew, A. and Ritchie, L. 2017. Culture change in aged-care facilities: A café's contribution to transforming the physical and social environment. *Journal of Housing for the Elderly*, 31(1), 34–46.

Annear, M., et al. 2015. Dementia Knowledge Assessment Scale: Development and preliminary psychometric properties. *Journal of the American Geriatrics Society*, 63(11), 2375–2381.

Anon. 2022. *Liberty Protection Safeguards*. England.

Atkins, L., et al. 2017. A guide to using the Theoretical Domains Framework of behaviour change to investigate implementation problems. *Implementation Science*, 12, 77. https://doi.org/10.1186/s13012-017-0605-9.

Attard, R., Sammut, R. and Scerri, A. 2020. Exploring the knowledge, attitudes and perceived learning needs of formal carers of people with dementia. *Nursing Older People*, 32(3), 25–31.

Avby, G. 2015. Professional practice as processes of muddling through: A study of learning and sense making in social work. *Vocations and Learning*, 8(1), 95–113.

Baillie, L. and Sills, E. 2015. The use of ethnodrama with healthcare staff to prompt empathy for people with dementia. *In:* Wain, V. and Pimomo, P., eds. *Encountering Empathy: Interrogating the past, envisioning the future*. Oxford: Inter-disciplinary Press.

Baillie, L., Sills, E. and Thomas, N. 2016. Educating a health service workforce about dementia: A qualitative study. *Quality in Ageing and Older Adults*, 17(2), 119–130.

Baker, C. 2021. *NHS Staff from Overseas: Statistics*. London: House of Commons Library [online]. Available from: https://commonslibrary.parliament.uk/research-briefings/cbp-7783/.

Ballard, C. and Corbett, A. 2020. Reducing psychotropic drug use in people with dementia living in nursing homes. *International Psychogeriatrics*, 32(3), 291–294.

Ballard, C., et al. 2018. Impact of person-centred care training and person-centred activities on quality of life, agitation, and antipsychotic use in people with dementia living in nursing homes: A cluster-randomised controlled trial. *PLoS Medicine*, 15, e1002500. https://doi.org/10.1371/journal.pmed.1002500.

Ballard, C., et al. 2020. Improving mental health and reducing antipsychotic use in people with dementia in care homes: The WHELD research programme including two RCTs. *Programme Grants for Applied Research*, 8(6), 1–98.

Bandura, A. 1986. *Social Foundations of Thought and Action: A social cognitive theory.* Englewood Cliffs, NJ: Prentice Hall.

Bandura, A. 2018. Toward a psychology of human agency: Pathways and reflections. *Perspectives on Psychological Science,* 13(2), 130–136.

Banerjee, S. 2015. Multimorbidity – older adults need health care that can count past one. *Lancet,* 385(9968), 587–589.

Banerjee, S., et al. 2017. How do we enhance undergraduate healthcare education in dementia? A review of the role of innovative approaches and development of the Time for Dementia Programme. *International Journal of Geriatric Psychiatry,* 32(1), 68–75.

Barbosa, A., et al. 2017. Implementing a psycho-educational intervention for care assistants working with people with dementia in aged-care facilities: Facilitators and barriers. *Scandinavian Journal of Caring Sciences,* 31(2), 222–231.

Barrett, J., Evans, S. and Pritchard-Wilkes, V. 2020. Understanding and supporting safe walking with purpose among people living with dementia in extra care, retirement and domestic housing. *Housing, Care and Support,* 23(2), 37–48.

Bartlett, R. 2022. Inclusive (social) citizenship and persons with dementia. *Disability and Society,* 37(7), 1129–1145.

Bauer, M., et al. 2015. An introduction to implementation science for the non-specialist. *BMC Psychology,* 3, 32. https://doi.org/10.1186/s40359-015-0089-9.

Bauer, M., et al. 2018. The impact of nurse and care staff education on the functional ability and quality of life of people living with dementia in aged care: A systematic review. *Nurse Education Today,* 67, 27–45.

Bentley, M., et al. 2019. Behavioural change in primary care professionals undertaking online education in dementia care in general practice. *Australian Journal of Primary Health,* 25(3), 244–249.

Berings, M., Poell, R. and Gelissen, J. 2008. On-the-job learning in the nursing profession – developing and validating a classification of learning activities and learning themes. *Personnel Review,* 37(4), 442–459.

Berridge, C., Tyler, D. and Miller, S. 2018. Staff empowerment practices and CNA retention: Findings from a nationally representative nursing home culture change survey. *Journal of Applied Gerontology,* 37(4), 419–434.

Beth Johnson Foundation. 2021. *Does Class, Ethnicity or Intellect Affect the Dementia Pathway?* Dementia Enquirers Report [online]. Available from: https://dementiaenquirers.org.uk/wp-content/uploads/2021/05/beth_johnson_foundation_in_stoke-on-trent_report.pdf.

Beville, P. 2002. Virtual Dementia Tour© helps sensitize health care providers. *American Journal of Alzheimer's Disease and Other Dementias,* 17(3), 183–190.

Bickford, B., et al. 2019. Understanding compassion for people with dementia in medical and nursing students. *BMC Medical Education,* 19, 35. https://doi.org/10.1186/s12909-019-1460-y.

Billett, S. 2006. Constituting the workplace curriculum. *Journal of Curriculum Studies,* 38(1), 31–48.

Billett, S. 2014a. Mimesis: Learning through everyday activities and interactions at work. *Human Resource Development Review,* 13(4), 462–482.

Billett, S. 2014b. Securing intersubjectivity through interprofessional workplace learning experiences. *Journal of Interprofessional Care,* 28(3), 206–211.

Billett, S. 2015. Work, discretion and learning: Processes of life learning and development at work. *International Journal of Training Research,* 13(3), 214–230.

Billett, S., Fenwick, T. and Somerville, M. 2006. *Work, Subjectivity and Learning.* Dordrecht: Springer.

Bligh, J. 2016. A mainstream social housing response to dementia. *Working with Older People*, 20(3), 144–150.

Bloom, B., et al. 1956. *Taxonomy of Educational Objectives: The classification of educational goals*. London: Longman.

Bolt, S., et al. 2020. Nursing staff needs in providing palliative care for persons with dementia at home or in nursing homes: A survey. *Journal of Nursing Scholarship*, 52(2), 164–173.

Boud, H. and Middleton, H. 2003. Learning from others at work: Communities of practice and informal learning. *Journal of Workplace Learning*, 15(5), 194–202.

Bowie, P. and Mountain, G. 1993. Using direct observation to record the behaviour of long stay patients with dementia. *International Journal of Geriatric Psychiatry*, 8(10), 857–864.

Bradbury, N. 2016. Attention span during lectures: 8 seconds, 10 minutes, or more? *Advances in Physiology Education*, 40(4), 509–513.

Bradford Dementia Group. 2005. *DCM 8 User's Manual*. Bradford: University of Bradford.

Bradford Dementia Group. 2014. *Dementia Care Mapping: Process and application*. Bradford: University of Bradford.

Brannelly, T. and Bartlett, R. 2020. Using walking interviews to enhance research relations with people with dementia: Methodological insights from an empirical study conducted in England. *Ethics and Social Welfare*, 14(4), 432–442.

Bridges, J. and Fuller, A. 2015. Creating learning environments for compassionate care: A programme to promote compassionate care by health and social care teams. *International Journal of Older People Nursing*, 10(1), 48–58.

Brodaty, H., et al. 2013a. Dementia: 14 essentials of assessment and care planning. *Medicine Today*, 14(8), 18–27.

Brodaty, H., et al. 2013b. Dementia: 14 essentials of management. *Medicine Today*, 14(9), 29–41.

Brooke, J. and Ojo, O. 2018. Elements of a sustainable, competent, and empathetic workforce to support patients with dementia during an acute hospital stay: A comprehensive literature review. *International Journal of Health Planning and Management*, 33(1), e10–e25.

Brooker, D. 2004. What is person-centred care in dementia? *Reviews in Clinical Gerontology*, 13(3), 215–222.

Brooker, D. 2007. *Person-centred Dementia Care: Making services better*. London: Jessica Kinglsey.

Brooker, D. and Latham, I. 2016. *Person-centred Dementia Care: Making services better with the VIPS framework*, 2nd edition. London: Jesscia Kingsley.

Brooker, D. and Woolley, R. 2007. Enriching opportunities for people living with dementia: The development of a blueprint for a sustainable activity-based model. *Aging and Mental Health*, 11(4), 371–383.

Brooker, D., Woolley, R. and Lee, D. 2007. Enriching opportunities for people living with dementia in nursing homes: An evaluation of a multi-level activity-based model of care. *Aging and Mental Health*, 11(4), 361–370.

Brooker, D., et al. 2014. Public health guidance to facilitate timely diagnosis of dementia: ALzheimer's COoperative Valuation in Europe recommendations. *International Journal of Geriatric Psychiatry*, 29(7), 682–693.

Brooker, D., et al. 2015. FITS into practice: Translating research into practice in reducing the use of anti-psychotic medication for people with dementia living in care homes. *Aging and Mental Health*, 20(7), 709–718.

Brookfield, S. 1984. Self-directed adult learning: A critical paradigm. *Adult Education Quarterly*, 35(2), 59–71.

Brossard Saxell, T., Ingvert, M. and Lethin, C. 2021. Facilitators for person-centred care of inpatients with dementia: A meta-synthesis of registered nurses' experiences. *Dementia*, 20(1), 188–212.

Brown Wilson, C., et al. 2013. The senses in practice: Enhancing the quality of care for residents with dementia in care homes. *Journal of Advanced Nursing*, 69(1), 77–90.

Browne, J., et al. 2017. Association of comorbidity and health service usage among patients with dementia in the UK: A population-based study. *BMJ Open*, 7, e012546. https://doi.org/10.1136/bmjopen-2016-012546.

Brunkert, T., et al. 2019. Pain management in nursing home residents: Findings from a pilot effectiveness-implementation study. *Journal of the American Geriatrics Society*, 67(12), 2574–2580.

Bull, D., et al. 2014. *Supporting Good Health: The role of the charity sector*. London: NPC [online]. Available from: https://www.thinknpc.org/wp-content/uploads/2018/07/NPC_Supporting-good-health.pdf.

Burke, G. and Orlowski, G. 2015a. *Training to Serve People with Dementia: Is our health care system ready? Paper 2: A review of dementia training standards across health care settings*. Washington, DC: Justice in Aging [online]. Available from: https://www.justiceinaging.org/wp-content/uploads/2015/08/Training-to-serve-people-with-dementia-Alz2FINAL.pdf.

Burke, G. and Orlowski, G. 2015b. *Training to Serve People with Dementia: Is our health care system ready? Paper 3: A review of dementia training standards across professional licensure*. Washington, DC: Justice in Aging [online]. Available from: . https://www.justiceinaging.org/wp-content/uploads/2015/08/Training-to-serve-people-with-dementia-Alz3_FINAL.pdf.

Burton, A., Ogden, M. and Cooper, C. 2019. Planning and enabling meaningful patient and public involvement in dementia research. *Current Opinion in Psychiatry*, 32(6), 557–562.

Butler, K. and Gregorc, A. 1988. *It's All in Your Mind: A student's guide to learning style*. Columbia, CT: Learner's Dimension.

Calanzani, N., et al. 2017. *Exploring Challenges and Strategies when Using Routine Data in Research: A systematic review. Final report*. Edinburgh: University of Edinburgh.

Cameron, K. and Freeman, S. 1991. Cultural congruence, strength, and type: Relationships to effectiveness. *Research in Organizational Change and Development*, 5, 23–58.

Cameron, K. and Quinn, R. 2011. *Diagnosing and Changing Organizational Culture*, 3rd edition. San Francisco, CA: Jossey-Bass.

Cane, J., O'Connor, D. and Michie, S. 2012. Validation of the theoretical domains framework for use in behaviour change and implementation research. *Implementation Science*, 7, 37. https://doi.org/10.1186/1748-5908-7-37.

Cant, R. and Cooper, S. 2017. Use of simulation-based learning in undergraduate nurse education: An umbrella systematic review. *Nurse Education Today*, 49, 63–71.

Capstick, A., et al. 2021. Drawn from life: Cocreating narrative and graphic vignettes of lived experience with people affected by dementia. *Health Expectations*, 24(5), 1890–1900.

Care Council for Wales (CCW). 2016. *Good Work: A dementia learning and development framework for Wales*. Cardiff: CCW [online]. Available from: https://socialcare.wales/cms_assets/file-uploads/Good-Work-Dementia-Learning-And-Development-Framework.pdf.

Care Quality Commission (CQC). 2015. *Guidance for Providers on Meeting the Regulations*. London: CQC [online]. Available from: https://www.cqc.org.uk/sites/default/files/2015024%20Guidance%20for%20providers%20on%20meeting%20the%20regulations.pdf.

Care Quality Commission (CQC). 2017. *The Fundamental Standards* [online]. Available from: https://www.cqc.org.uk/what-we-do/how-we-do-our-job/fundamental-standards [Accessed 15 February 2021].

Carpenter, B., et al. 2009. The Alzheimer's Disease Knowledge Scale: Development and psychometric properties. *The Gerontologist*, 49(2), 236–247.

Carter, D. 2016. *Fix Dementia Care: Homecare*. London: Alzheimer's Society [online]. Available from: https://www.alzheimers.org.uk/sites/default/files/migrate/downloads/fix_dementia_care_homecare_report.pdf.

Casey, A.-N., et al. 2020. GP awareness, practice, knowledge and confidence: Evaluation of the first nation-wide dementia-focused continuing medical education program in Australia. *BMC Family Practice*, 21, 104. https://doi.org/10.1186/s12875-020-01178-x.

Cashin, Z., et al. 2019. Involving people with dementia and their carers in dementia education for undergraduate healthcare professionals: A qualitative study of motivation to participate and experience. *International Psychogeriatrics*, 31(6), 869–876.

Cavendish, C. 2013. *The Cavendish Review: An independent review into healthcare assistants and support workers in the NHS and social care settings*. London: Department of Health and Social Care [online]. Available from: https://assets.publishing.service.gov.uk/government/uploads/system/uploads/attachment_data/file/236212/Cavendish_Review.pdf.

Chan, S. 2015. The contribution of observation to apprentices' learning. *Journal of Vocational Education and Training*, 67(4), 442–459.

Chatterjee, A., Pereira, A. and Bates, R. 2018. Impact of individual perception of organizational culture on the learning transfer environment. *International Journal of Training and Development*, 22(1), 15–33.

Chenoweth, L., et al. 2018. Critical contextual elements in facilitating and achieving success with a person-centred care intervention to support antipsychotic deprescribing for older people in long-term care. *BioMed Research International*, 2018: 7148515. https://doi.org/10.1155/2018/7148515.

City and Guilds. 2016. *Level 5 Diploma in Leadership for Health and Social Care*, 2nd edition. London: Hodder Education.

Clague, F., et al. 2017. Comorbidity and polypharmacy in people with dementia: Insights from a large, population-based cross-sectional analysis of primary care data. *Age and Ageing*, 46(1), 33–39.

Clark, M., et al. 2017. Sporting memories, dementia care and training staff in care homes. *Journal of Mental Health Training, Education and Practice*, 12(1), 55–66.

Clarke, G., et al. 2019. Evaluating the impact of healthcare interventions using routine data. *British Medical Journal*, 365, l2239 [online]. Available from: https://www.bmj.com/content/365/bmj.l2239.

Coates, C. 1997. The Caring Efficacy Scale: Nurses' self-reports of caring in practice settings. *Advanced Practice Nursing Quarterly*, 3(1), 53–59.

Collis, B. and Winnips, K. 2002. Two scenarios for productive learning environments in the workplace. *British Journal of Educational Technology*, 33(2), 133–148.

Colón-Emeric, C. et al. 2016. Sustaining complex interventions in long-term care: A qualitative study of direct care staff and managers. *Implementation Science*, 11, 94. https://doi.org/10.1186/s13012-016-0454-y.

Cooper, E., et al. 2017. Priorities for the professional development of registered nurses in nursing homes: A Delphi study. *Age and Ageing*, 46(1), 39–45.

Corazzini, K., et al. 2015. Implementing culture change in nursing homes: An adaptive leadership framework. *The Gerontologist*, 55(4), 616–627.

Cornelison, L. 2016. The culture change movement in long-term care: Is person-centered care a possibility for the looming age wave? *NAELA Journal*, 12(2), 121–131.

Cuevas, J. 2015. Is learning styles-based instruction effective? A comprehensive analysis of recent research on learning styles. *Theory and Research in Education*, 13(3), 308–333.

Cunningham, N., et al. 2020. Understanding the training and education needs of home-care workers supporting people with dementia and cancer: A systematic review of reviews. *Dementia*, 19(8), 2780–2803.

Dahl, H., et al. 2018. Facilitation of a workplace learning intervention in a fluctuating context: An ethnographic, participatory research project in a nursing home in Norway. *International Practice Development Journal*, 8(2), 1–17.

Daley, S., et al. 2019. A feasibility study of the effects of implementing a staff-level recovery-oriented training intervention in older people's mental health services. *Aging and Mental Health*, 24(11), 1926–1934.

Daley, S., et al. 2020. A qualitative evaluation of the effect of a longitudinal dementia education programme on healthcare student knowledge and attitudes. *Age and Ageing*, 49(6), 1080–1086.

Darbyshire, P. 1993. In defence of pedagogy: A critique of the notion of andragogy. *Nurse Education Today*, 13, 328–335.

Davies, T., et al. 2021. Dementia Enquirers: Pioneering approaches to dementia research in UK. *Disability and Society*, 37(1), 129–147.

de Witt, L. and Fortune, D. 2019. Relationship-centered dementia care: Insights from a community-based culture change coalition. *Dementia*, 18(3), 1146–1165.

Dean, R., Proudfoot, R. and Lindesay, J. 1993. The Quality of Interactions Schedule (QUIS): Development, reliability and use in the evaluation of two domus units. *International Journal of Geriatric Psychiatry*, 8(10), 819–826.

DEEP, n.d. *Involving People with Dementia* [online]. Available from: https://www.dementiavoices.org.uk/deep-resources/involving-people-with-dementia/ [Accessed 30 September 2021].

Dementia Alliance International, 3 Nations Dementia Working Group and Alzheimer's Society. 2019. *Supporting Dementia Self Advocates: A directory of resources* [online]. Available from: https://www.dementiaallianceinternational.org/wp-content/uploads/2019/07/Directory-of-Dementia-Self-Advocacy-Resources_July-2019_1st-Edition.pdf.

Dementia Enquirers. n.d. *Innovations in Dementia* [online]. Available from: https://dementiaenquirers.org.uk/ [Accessed 5 November 2021].

Department for Education (DfE). n.d. *Teaching for Neurodiversity: A guide to specific learning difficulties*. London: DfE [online]. Available from: https://dyspraxiafoundation.org.uk/wp-content/uploads/2016/09/P16-A_Guide_to_SpLD_copy_2.pdf.

Department of Health (DoH). 2005. *Mental Capacity Act*. London: HMSO.

Department of Health (DoH). 2009. *Living Well with Dementia: A national dementia strategy*. London: DoH [online]. Available from: https://assets.publishing.service.gov.uk/government/uploads/system/uploads/attachment_data/file/168220/dh_094051.pdf.

Department of Health (DoH). 2013. *Delivering High Quality, Effective, Compassionate Care: Developing the right people with the right skills and the right values. A mandate from the Government to Health Education England: April 2013 to March 2015*. London: DoH [online]. Available from: https://assets.publishing.service.gov.uk/

government/uploads/system/uploads/attachment_data/file/203332/29257_2900971
_Delivering_Accessible.pdf.

Department of Health (DoH). 2014. *Delivering high quality, effective, compassionate care: Developing the right people with the right skills and the right values. A mandate from the Government to Health Education England: April 2014 to March 2015.* London: DoH [online]. Available from: https://assets.publishing.service.gov.uk/government/uploads/system/uploads/attachment_data/file/310170/DH_HEE_Mandate.pdf.

Department of Health (DoH). 2015. *Delivering High Quality, Effective, Compassionate Care: Developing the right people with the right skills and the right values. A mandate from the Government to Health Education England: April 2015 to March 2016.* London: DoH [online]. Available from: https://assets.publishing.service.gov.uk/government/uploads/system/uploads/attachment_data/file/411200/HEE_Mandate.pdf.

Department of Health and Social Care (DHSC). 2012. *The Prime Minister's 'Dementia Challenge': Delivering major improvements in dementia care and research by 2015.* London: DHSC [online]. Available from: https://assets.publishing.service.gov.uk/government/uploads/system/uploads/attachment_data/file/215101/dh_133176.pdf.

DeSouza, K., Pit, S. and Moehead, A. 2020. Translating facilitated multimodal online learning into effective person-centred practice for the person living with dementia among health care staff in Australia: An observational study. *BMC Geriatrics*, 20, 33. https://doi.org/10.1186/s12877-020-1417-3.

Deutsch, A., et al. 2017. A pilot study on the feasibility of training nurses to formulate multicomponent oral health interventions in a residential aged care facility. *Gerodontology*, 34(4), 469–478.

Dewar, B. and Nolan, M. 2013. Caring about caring: Developing a model to implement compassionate relationship centred care in an older people care setting. *International Journal of Nursing Studies*, 50(9), 1247–1258.

Di Giulio, P., et al. 2019. The impact of nursing homes staff education on end-of-life care in residents with advanced dementia: A quality improvement study. *Journal of Pain and Symptom Management*, 57(1), 93–99.

Di Lorito, C., et al. 2020. Adding to the knowledge on patient and public involvement: Reflections from an experience of co-research with carers of people with dementia. *Health Expectations*, 23(3), 691–706.

Dobbs, D., et al. 2018. Certified nursing assistants' perspectives of the CARES® activities of daily living dementia care program. *Applied Nursing Research*, 39, 244–248.

Dodds, P. 2003. Involving the recipients of dementia care in training for staff. *Mental Health Practice*, 6(10), 34–37.

Doll, G. et al. 2017. Actualizing culture change: The Promoting Excellent Alternatives in Kansas Nursing Homes (PEAK 2.0) program. *Psychological Services*, 14(3), 307–315.

Doran, G. 1981. There's a S.M.A.R.T. way to write management's goal and objectives. *Management Review*, 70(11), 35–36.

Duan, Y., et al. 2021. An empirical typology of nursing home culture change implementation. *Journal of Applied Gerontology*, 40(9), 1039–1050.

Dunn, R. and Dunn, K. 1992. *Teaching Elementary Students Through Their Individual Learning Styles: Practical approaches for grades 3–6.* Boston, MA: Allyn & Bacon.

Dunn, R. and Dunn, K., 1993. *Teaching Secondary Students Through Their Individual Learning Styles.* Boston, MA: Allyn & Bacon.

Dupuis, S., et al. 2016. Theoretical foundations guiding culture change: The work of the Partnerships in Dementia Care Alliance. *Dementia*, 15(1), 85–105.

Dutton, R. 2010. People with dementia living in extra care housing: Learning from the evidence. *Working with Older People*, 14(1), 8–11.

Eastman, C., Charlesworth, S. and Hill, E. 2019. *Factsheet 1: Migrant workers in front-line care*. Melbourne: RMIT University.

Eliopoulos, C. 2013. Affecting culture change and performance improvement in Medicaid nursing homes: The Promote Understanding, Leadership, and Learning (PULL) Program. *Geriatric Nursing*, 34(3), 218–223.

Ellström, E. and Ellström, P. 2018. Two modes of learning-oriented leadership: A study of first-line managers. *Journal of Workplace Learning*, 30(7), 545–561.

Ellström, E., Ekholm, B. and Ellström, P. 2008. Two types of learning environment: Enabling and constraining a study of care work. *Journal of Workplace Learning*, 20(2), 84–97.

Elpers, K., et al. 2017. Effectiveness of a psycho-educational staff training program on attitudes of staff in a long-term care facility: A pilot study and framework. *Educational Gerontology*, 43(9), 431–439.

Elvish, R., et al. 2014. 'Getting to Know Me': The development and evaluation of a training programme for enhancing skills in the care of people with dementia in general hospital settings. *Aging and Mental Health*, 18(4), 481–488.

Eraut, M. 2004. Informal learning in the workplace. *Studies in Continuing Education*, 26(2), 247–273.

Eraut, M. 2007. Learning from other people in the workplace. *Oxford Review of Education*, 33(4), 403–422.

Etherton-Beer, C., et al. 2021. Development of a toolkit to support sustainable culture change in residential aged care. *Australasian Journal on Ageing*, 40(1), 77–83.

Evans, K., et al. 2006. *Improving Workplace Learning*. London: Routledge.

Evans, S., et al. 2020. Can extra care housing support the changing needs of older people living with dementia? *Dementia*, 19(5), 1492–1508.

Fallahpour, M., et al. 2020. Dementia care education targeting job strain and organizational climate among dementia care specialists in Swedish home care services. *Journal of Multidisciplinary Healthcare*, 13, 85–97.

Faraday, J., Salis, C. and Barrett, A. 2019. Equipping nurses and care staff to manage mealtime difficulties in people with dementia: A systematic scoping review of training needs and interventions. *American Journal of Speech-Language Pathology*, 28(2), 717–742.

Farina, L., et al. 2021. Getting to know you but also to know me: Changes in self-perceptions of aging among aged care workers after a Virtual Dementia Tour. *International Psychogeriatrics*, 33(1), 97–98.

Fazio, S., et al. 2018. The fundamentals of person-centered care for individuals with dementia. *The Gerontologist*, 58(suppl. 1), S10–S19.

Fejes, A. and Nicholl, K. 2011. Activating the worker in elderly care: A technique and tactics of invitation. *Studies in Continuing Education*, 33(3), 235–249.

Flavin, T. and Sinclair, C. 2019. Reflections on involving people living with dementia in research in the Australian context. *Australasian Journal on Ageing*, 38(2), 6–8.

Fogg, C., et al. 2017. The relationship between cognitive impairment, mortality and discharge characteristics in a large cohort of older adults with unscheduled admissions to an acute hospital: A retrospective observational study. *Age and Ageing*, 46(5), 794–801.

Foley, T., et al. 2017. 'We're certainly not in our comfort zone': A qualitative study of GPs' dementia-care educational needs. *BMC Family Practice*, 18, 66. https://doi.org/10.1186/s12875-017-0639-8.

Foley, T., et al. 2018. The development and evaluation of peer-facilitated dementia workshops in general practice. *Education for Primary Care*, 29(1), 27–34.

Fossey, J., et al. 2019. What influences the sustainability of an effective psychosocial intervention for people with dementia living in care homes? A 9 to 12-month follow-up of the perceptions of staff in care homes involved in the WHELD randomised controlled trial. *International Journal of Geriatric Psychiatry*, 34(5), 674–682.

Fossey, J., et al. 2020. A qualitative analysis of trainer/coach experiences of changing care home practice in the Well-being and Health in Dementia randomised control trial. *Dementia*, 19(2), 237–252.

Fowler, J. 2008. Experiential learning and its facilitation. *Nurse Education Today*, 28, 427–433.

Fukuda, K., et al. 2018. Effectiveness of educational program using printed educational material on care burden distress among staff of residential aged care facilities without medical specialists and/or registered nurses: Cluster quasi-randomization study. *Geriatrics and Gerontology International*, 18(3), 487–494.

Fuller, A., et al. 2005. Learning as peripheral participation in communities of practice: A reassessment of key concepts in workplace learning. *British Educational Research Journal*, 31(1), 49–68.

Fuller, A., et al. 2007. Creating and using knowledge: An analysis of the differentiated nature of workplace learning environments. *British Educational Research Journal*, 33(5), 743–759.

Garrison, D. 1997. Self-directed learning: Toward a comprehensive model. *Adult Education Quarterly*, 48(1), 18–33.

Gartmeier, M., Gruber, H. and Heid, H. 2010. Tracing error-related knowledge in interview data: Negative knowledge in elder care nursing. *Educational Gerontology*, 36(9), 733–752.

Gauthier, S., et al. 2021. *World Alzheimer Report 2021: Journey through the diagnosis of dementia*. London: Alzheimer's Disease International [online]. Available from: https://www.alzint.org/u/World-Alzheimer-Report-2021.pdf.

George, D., Stuckey, H. and Whitehead, M. 2013. An arts-based intervention at a nursing home to improve medical students' attitudes toward persons with dementia. *Academic Medicine*, 88(6), 837–842.

Gerritsen, D., et al. 2021. Implementing a multidisciplinary psychotropic medication review among nursing home residents with dementia: A process evaluation. *International Psychogeriatrics*, 33(9), 933–945.

Gibbs, G. 1988. *Learning by Doing: A guide to teaching and learning methods*. Oxford: Further Education Unit, Oxford Polytechnic.

Gibson, S., et al. 2019. Clinical educators' skills and qualities in allied health: A systematic review. *Medical Education*, 53(5), 432–442.

Gilmartin-Thomas, J. et al. 2018. Qualitative evaluation of how a virtual dementia experience impacts medical and pharmacy students' self-reported knowledge and attitudes towards people with dementia. *Dementia*, 19(2), 205–220.

Gilster, S., Boltz, M. and Dalessandro, J. 2018. Long-term care workforce issues: Practice principles for quality dementia care. *The Gerontologist*, 58(suppl. 1), S103–S113.

Gkioka, M., et al. 2020. Evaluation and effectiveness of dementia staff training programs in general hospital settings: A narrative synthesis with Holton's three-level model applied. *Journal of Alzheimer's Disease*, 78(3), 1089–1108.

Gleason, L., et al. 2019. An innovative model using telementoring to provide geriatrics education for nurses and social workers at skilled nursing facilities. *Geriatric Nursing*, 40(5), 517–521.

Godfrey, M., et al. 2018. The Person, Interactions and Environment Programme to improve care of people with dementia in hospital: A multisite study. *Health Services and Delivery Research*, 6, 23. https://doi.org/10.3310/hsdr06230.

Goeman, D., et al. 2019. Partnering with people with dementia and their care partners, aged care service experts, policymakers and academics: A co-design process. *Australasian Journal on Ageing*, 38(2), 53–58.

Goossen, C. and Austin, M. 2017. Service user involvement in UK social service agencies and social work education. *Journal of Social Work Education*, 53(1), 37–51.

Goossens, B., et al. 2019. 'We DECide optimized' – training nursing home staff in shared decision-making skills for advance care planning conversations in dementia care: Protocol of a pretest-posttest cluster randomized trial. *BMC Geriatrics*, 19, 33. https://doi.org/10.1186/s12877-019-1044-z.

GOV.UK. 2021. *NHS Workforce* [online]. Available from: https://www.ethnicity-facts-figures.service.gov.uk/workforce-and-business/workforce-diversity/nhs-workforce/latest [Accessed 6 December 2021].

Gove, D., et al. 2016. Stigma and GPs' perceptions of dementia. *Ageing and Mental Health*, 20(4), 391–400.

Gove, D., et al. 2018. Alzheimer Europe's position on involving people with dementia in research through PPI (patient and public involvement). *Aging and Mental Health*, 22(6), 723–729.

Grant, S., et al. 2014. A meta-ethnography of organisational culture in primary care medical practice. *Journal of Health, Organisation and Management*, 28(1), 21–40.

Grealish, L., et al. 2015. The significance of 'facilitator as a change agent' – organisational learning culture in aged care home settings. *Journal of Clinical Nursing*, 24(7–8), 961–969.

Greenwood, D. 2015. Using a drama-based education programme to develop a 'relational' approach to care for those working with people living with dementia. *Research in Drama Education: The Journal of Applied Theatre and Performance*, 20(2), 225–236.

Gregory, L., Hopwood, N. and Boud, D. 2014. Interprofessional learning at work: What spatial theory can tell us about workplace learning in an acute care ward. *Journal of Interprofessional Care*, 28(3), 200–205.

Griffiths, A., et al. 2019. Barriers and facilitators to implementing dementia care mapping in care homes: Results from the DCM™ EPIC trial process evaluation. *BMC Geriatrics*, 19, 37. https://doi.org/10.1186/s12877-019-1045-y.

Griffiths, A., et al. 2021. Staff experiences of implementing Dementia Care Mapping to improve the quality of dementia care in care homes: A qualitative process evaluation. *BMC Health Services Research*, 21, 138. https://doi.org/10.1186/s12913-021-06152-6.

Guy's and St. Thomas' NHS Foundation Trust (dir.). 2014. *Barbara, the Whole Story*. White Boat TV.

Guzmán, A., et al. 2017a. Evaluation of a Staff Training Programme using Positive Psychology coaching with film and theatre elements in care homes: Views and attitudes of residents, staff and relatives. *International Journal of Older People Nursing*, 12(1), e12126. https://doi.org/10.1111/opn.12126.

Guzmán, A., et al. 2017b. Evaluation of the 'Ladder to the Moon, Culture Change Studio Engagement Programme' staff training: Two quasi-experimental case studies. *International Journal of Older People Nursing*, 12(3), e12147. https://doi.org/10.1111/opn.12147.

Gwernan-Jones, R., et al. 2020a. The experiences of hospital staff who provide care for people living with dementia: A systematic review and synthesis of qualitative studies.

International Journal of Older People Nursing, 15(4), e12325. https://doi.org/10.1111/opn.12325.

Gwernan-Jones, R., et al. 2020b. Understanding and improving experiences of care in hospital for people living with dementia, their carers and staff: Three systematic reviews. *Health Services and Delivery Research*, 8(43), 1–248.

Haemer, H., Borges-Andrade, J. and Cassiano, S. 2017. Learning strategies at work and professional development. *Journal of Workplace Learning*, 29(6), 490–506.

Hager, P. 2000. Know-how and workplace practical judgement. *Journal of Philosophy of Education*, 34(2), 281–296.

Hallberg, I., et al. 2016. Professional care providers in dementia care in eight European countries: Their training and involvement in early dementia stage and in home care. *Dementia*, 15(5), 931–957.

Hamiduzzaman, M., et al. 2020. Towards personalized care: Factors associated with the quality of life of residents with dementia in Australian rural aged care homes. *PLoS One*, 15(5), e0233450. https://doi.org/10.1371/journal.pone.0233450.

Han, A., Kunik, M. and Richardson, A. 2020. Compassionate Touch® delivered by long-term care staff for residents with dementia: Preliminary results. *Journal of Social Service Research*, 46(5), 685–692.

Handley, M., Bunn, F. and Goodman, C. 2019. Supporting general hospital staff to provide dementia sensitive care: A realist evaluation. *International Journal of Nursing Studies*, 96, 61–71.

Hansen, J. 2014. *How Much should Charities Expect from Their Volunteers?* ThirdSector [online]. Available from: https://www.thirdsector.co.uk/charities-expect-volunteers/volunteering/article/1231054 [Accessed 10 June 2022].

Hanshaw, S. and Dickerson, S. 2020. High fidelity simulation evaluation studies in nursing education: A review of the literature. *Nurse Education in Practice*, 46, 102818. https://doi.org/10.1016/j.nepr.2020.102818.

Hanson, G., et al. 2015. Workplace violence against homecare workers and its relationship with workers health outcomes: A cross-sectional study. *BMC Public Health*, 15, 11. https://doi.org/10.1186/s12889-014-1340-7.

Harvey, G. and Kitson, A. 2016. PARIHS revisited: From heuristic to integrated framework for the successful implementation of knowledge into practice. *Implementation Science*, 11, 33. https://doi.org/10.1186/s13012-016-0398-2.

Harwood, R., et al. 2018. A staff training intervention to improve communication between people living with dementia and health-care professionals in hospital: The VOICE mixed-methods development and evaluation study. *Health Services and Delivery Research*, 6(41). https://doi.org/10.3310/hsdr06410.

Haugland, V. and Reime, M. 2018. Scenario-based simulation training as a method to increase nursing students' competence in demanding situations in dementia care: A mixed method study. *Nurse Education in Practice*, 33, 164–171.

Health Education England (HEE). 2014 (revised 2020). *The Care Certificate Framework: Assessor document* [online]. Available from: https://www.skillsforhealth.org.uk/wp-content/uploads/2020/11/Care-Certificate-Framework-Assessor.pdf.

Health and Social Care Board (HSCB). 2016. *The Dementia Learning and Development Framework*. Belfast: HSCB.

Hendriks, S., et al. 2021. Global prevalence of young-onset dementia: A systematic review and meta-analysis. *JAMA Neurology*, 78(9), 1080–1090.

Hermer, L., et al. 2017. Does comprehensive culture change adoption via the household model enhance nursing home residents' psychosocial well-being? *Innovation in Aging*, 1(2), igx033. https://doi.org/10.1093/geroni/igx033.

Herrmann, L., et al. 2019. A new curriculum to address dementia-related stigma: Preliminary experience with Alzheimer's Association staff. *Dementia*, 18(7–8), 2609–2619.

Hetzner, S., Heid, H. and Gruber, H. 2015. Using workplace changes as learning opportunities: Antecedents to reflection in professional work. *Journal of Workplace Learning*, 27(1), 34–50.

Heward, M., et al. 2021a. Barriers and enablers to implementing 'DEALTS2' simulation-based train-the-trainer dementia training programme in hospital settings across England: A qualitative study. *BMC Health Services Research*, 21, 946. https://doi.org/10.1186/s12913-021-06977-1.

Heward, M., et al. 2021b. Impact of 'DEALTS2' education intervention on trainer dementia knowledge and confidence to utilise innovative training approaches: A national pre-test–post-test survey. *Nurse Education Today*, 97, 104694. https://doi.org/10.1016/j.nedt.2020.104694.

Hirt, J. and Beer, T. 2020. Use and impact of virtual reality simulation in dementia care education: A scoping review. *Nurse Education Today*, 84, 104207. https://doi.org/10.1016/j.nedt.2019.104207.

Hobday, J., et al. 2010. Feasibility of Internet training for care staff of residents with dementia: The CARES program. *Journal of Gerontological Nursing*, 36(4), 13–21.

Honey, P. and Mumford, A. 1986. *The Manual of Learning Styles*. Maidenhead: Peter Honey.

Horgan, A., et al. 2020. Expert by experience involvement in mental health nursing education: The co-production of standards between experts by experience and academics in mental health nursing. *Journal of Psychiatric and Mental Health Nursing*, 27(5), 553–562.

Howe, D., et al. 2021. Health professions faculty experiences teaching online during the COVID-19 pandemic. *ABNF Journal*, 32(1), 6–11.

Howie, P. and Bagnall, R. 2013. A beautiful metaphor: Transformative learning theory. *International Journal of Lifelong Education*, 32(6), 816–836.

Hucker, D. 2013. Preparing for the housing needs of people with dementia. *Mental Health Today*, September [online]. Available from: https://www.mentalhealthtoday.co.uk/preparing-for-the-housing-needs-of-people-with-dementia.

Huijg, J., et al. 2014. Measuring determinants of implementation behavior: Psychometric properties of a questionnaire based on the theoretical domains framework. *Implementation Science*, 9, 33. https://doi.org/10.1186/1748-5908-9-33.

Hung, L., Son, C. and Hung, R. 2019. The experience of hospital staff in applying the Gentle Persuasive Approaches to dementia care. *Journal of Psychiatric and Mental Health Nursing*, 26(1–2), 19–28.

Hunter, C., et al. 2008. Learning how we learn: An ethnographic study in a neonatal intensive care unit. *Journal of Advanced Nursing*, 62(6), 657–664.

Hurley, M., et al. 2020. The feasibility of increasing physical activity in care home residents: Active Residents in Care Homes (ARCH) programme. *Physiotherapy (UK)*, 107, 50–57.

Hussein, S. and Manthorpe, J. 2012. The dementia social care workforce in England: Secondary analysis of a national workforce dataset. *Aging and Mental Health*, 16(1), 110–118.

Hyde, J., Perez, R. and Forester, B. 2007. Dementia and assisted living. *The Gerontologist*, 47(suppl. 1), 51–67. https://doi.org/10.1093/geront/47.Supplement_1.51.

Iliffe, S. and Wilcock, J. 2005. The identification of barriers to the recognition of, and response to, dementia in primary care using a modified focus group approach. *Dementia*, 4(1), 73–85.

Iliffe, S., McGrath, T. and Mitchell, D. 2013. The impact of patient and public involvement in the work of the Dementias & Neurodegenerative Diseases Research Network (DeNDRoN): Case studies. *Health Expectations*, 16(4), 351–361.

Illeris, K. 2003. Workplace learning and learning theory. *Journal of Workplace Learning*, 15(4), 167–178.

Inker, J., et al. 2020. Implementing microlearning in nursing homes: Implications for policy and practice in person-centered dementia care. *Journal of Applied Gerontology*, 40(9), 1062–1070.

Jack-Waugh, A., Ritchie, L. and MacRae, R. 2018. Assessing the educational impact of the dementia champions programme in Scotland: Implications for evaluating professional dementia education. *Nurse Education Today*, 71, 205–210.

Jackson, T., et al. 2017. Challenges and opportunities in understanding dementia and delirium in the acute hospital. *PLoS Medicine*, 14(3), e1002247. https://doi.org/10.1371/journal.pmed.1002247.

Jacobsen, F., et al. 2017. A mixed method study of an education intervention to reduce use of restraint and implement person-centered dementia care in nursing homes. *BMC Nursing*, 16, 55. https://doi.org/10.1186/s12912-017-0244-0.

Jennings, A., et al. 2019. Development and evaluation of a primary care interprofessional education intervention to support people with dementia. *Journal of Interprofessional Care*, 33(5), 579–582.

Jessop, T., et al. 2017. Halting Antipsychotic Use in Long-Term care (HALT): A single-arm longitudinal study aiming to reduce inappropriate antipsychotic use in long-term care residents with behavioral and psychological symptoms of dementia. *International Psychogeriatrics*, 29(8), 1391–1403.

John's Campaign, n.d. *John's Campaign* [online]. Available from: https://johnscampaign.org.uk/ [Accessed 4 October 2021].

Johns, C. 1995. Framing learning through reflection within Carper's fundamental ways of knowing in nursing. *Journal of Advanced Nursing*, 22, 226–234.

Johns, C. 2017. *Becoming a Reflective Practitioner*, 5th edition. Chichester: Wiley.

Johnston, K., et al. 2020. Understandings of dementia in low and middle income countries and amongst indigenous peoples: A systematic review and qualitative meta-synthesis. *Aging and Mental Health*, 24(8), 1183–1195.

Jones, D., et al. 2020. Investigating cancer symptoms in older people: What are the issues and where is the evidence? *British Journal of General Practice*, 70(696), 321–322.

Kaasalainen, S., et al. 2019. Launching 'Namaste Care' in Canada: Findings from training sessions and initial perceptions of an end-of-life programme for people with advanced dementia. *Journal of Research in Nursing*, 24(6), 403–417.

Kadri, A., et al. 2018. Care workers, the unacknowledged persons in person-centred care: A secondary qualitative analysis of UK care home staff interviews. *PLoS One*, 13(7), e0200031. https://doi.org/10.1371/journal.pone.0200031.

Kaduszkiewicz, H., Wiese, B. and van den Bussche, H. 2008. Self-reported competence, attitude and approach of physicians towards patients with dementia in ambulatory care: Results of a postal survey. *BMC Health Services Research*, 8, 54. https://doi.org/10.1186/1472-6963-8-54.

Karlin, B., Young, D. and Dash, K. 2017. Empowering the dementia care workforce to manage behavioral symptoms of dementia: Development and training outcomes from the VOICE Dementia Care Program. *Gerontology and Geriatrics Education*, 38(4), 375–391.

Karrer, M., et al. 2020. What hinders and facilitates the implementation of nurse-led interventions in dementia care? A scoping review. *BMC Geriatrics*, 20, 127. https://doi.org/10.1186/s12877-020-01520-z.

Katwa, A., et al. 2020. Improving advance care planning for care home residents with dementia: Evaluation of simulation training for care home workers. *Dementia*, 19(3), 822–829.

Keady, J. and Elvish, R. 2019. Requirements of a caregiver: Commentary. *In:* Kitwood, T. *Dementia Reconsidered, Revisited*, ed. D. Brooker. London: Open University Press.

Keady, J., et al. 2017. *Social Research Methods in Dementia Studies: Inclusion and innovation*. London: Routledge.

Keane, J., Franklin, N. and Vaughan, B. 2020. Simulation to educate healthcare providers working within residential age care settings: A scoping review. *Nurse Education Today*, 85, 104228. https://doi.org/10.1016/j.nedt.2019.104228.

Keenan, J., et al. 2020. Implementing e-learning and e-tools for care home staff supporting residents with dementia and challenging behaviour: A process evaluation of the ResCare study using normalisation process theory. *Dementia*, 19(5), 1604–1620.

Kelley, R., et al. 2020. The influence of care home managers on the implementation of a complex intervention: Findings from the process evaluation of a randomised controlled trial of dementia care mapping. *BMC Geriatrics*, 20, 303. https://doi.org/10.1186/s12877-020-01706-5.

Kenny, J., et al. 2016. Facilitating an evolving service user involvement group for people with dementia: What can we learn? *Journal of Mental Health Training, Education and Practice*, 11(2), 81–90.

Killett, A., et al. 2016. Digging deep: How organisational culture affects care home residents' experiences. *Ageing and Society*, 36(1), 160–188.

Kimzey, M., Patterson, J. and Mastel-Smith, B. 2021. Effects of simulation on nursing students' dementia knowledge and empathy: A mixed method study. *Issues in Mental Health Nursing*, 42(3), 274–279.

Kirkley, C., et al. 2011. The impact of organisational culture on the delivery of person-centred care in services providing respite care and short breaks for people with dementia. *Health and Social Care in the Community*, 19(4), 438–448.

Kirkpatrick, D. 1967. Evaluation of training. *In:* Craig, R. and Bittel, L. eds. *Training and Development Handbook*. New York: McGraw-Hill.

Kirkpatrick, D. 1979. Techniques for evaluating training programmes. *Training and Development Journal*, 33(6), 78–92.

Kirkpatrick, D. 1984. *Evaluating Training Programs: The four levels*. San Francisco, CA: Berrett-Koehler.

Kirkpatrick, D. and Kirkpatrick, J. 2005. *Transferring Learning to Behavior: Using the four levels to improve performance*. Oakland, CA: Berrett-Koehler.

Kitchenham, A. 2008. The evolution of John Mezirow's transformative learning theory. *Journal of Transformative Education*, 6(2), 104–123.

Kitwood, T. 1995. Cultures of care: Traditions and change. *In:* Kitwood, T. and Benson, S., eds. *The New Culture of Dementia Care*. London: Hawker Publications.

Kitwood, T. 1997. *Dementia Reconsidered: The person comes first*. Buckingham: Open University Press.

Kitwood, T. 2019. *Dementia Reconsidered, Revisited: The person still comes first*, ed. D. Brooker. London: Open University Press.

Knowles, M. 1970. *The Modern Practice of Adult Education: Andragogy versus pedagogy*. New York: Association Press.

Kolb, A. and Kolb, D. 2008. Experiential learning theory: A dynamic, holistic approach to management, learning and education. *In:* Armstrong, S. and Fukami, C., eds. *The SAGE Handbook of Management Learning, Education and Development*. London: Sage.

Kolb, D. 1984. *Experiential Learning: Experience as a source of learning and development*. Englewood Cliffs, NJ: Prentice Hall.

Kolb, D. 1985. *Learning Style Inventory*. Boston, MA: McBer.

Kong, E., Song, E. and Evans, L. 2017. Effects of a multicomponent restraint reduction program for Korean nursing home staff. *Journal of Nursing Scholarship*, 49(3), 325–335.

Kosteniuk, J., et al. 2016. Focus on dementia care: Continuing education preferences, challenges, and catalysts among rural home care providers. *Educational Gerontology*, 42(9), 608–620.

Kraiger, K., Ford, J. and Salas, E. 1993. Application of cognitive, skill-based and affective theories of learning outcomes to new methods of training evaluation. *Journal of Applied Psychology*, 78(2), 311–328.

Kubiak, C. and Sandberg, F. 2011. Paraprofessionals and caring practice: Negotiating the use of self. *Scandinavian Journal of Caring Sciences*, 25(4), 653–660.

Kutschar, P., et al. 2020. Nursing education intervention effects on pain intensity of nursing home residents with different levels of cognitive impairment: A cluster-randomized controlled trial. *Journal of Pain Research*, 13, 633–648.

Kyndt, E., Vermeire, E. and Cabus, S. 2016. Informal workplace learning among nurses: Organisational learning conditions and personal characteristics that predict learning outcomes. *Journal of Workplace Learning*, 28(7), 435–450.

Latham, I. 2020. *What Works is What Matters: An ethnographic study of how care workers in care homes learn to care for people living with dementia*. PhD thesis, University of Worcester [online]. Available from: http://eprints.worc.ac.uk/10392/.

Latham, I. and Brooker, D. 2017. Reducing anti-psychotic presecribing for care home residents with dementia. *Nurse Prescriber*, 15(10), 504–511.

Lave, J. and Wenger, E. 1991. *Situated Learning*. Cambridge: Cambridge University Press.

Lawrence, V., et al. 2016. Helping staff to implement psychosocial interventions in care homes: Augmenting existing practices and meeting needs for support. *International Journal of Geriatric Psychiatry*, 31(3), 284–293.

Lee, L., Kasperski, M. and Weston, W. 2011. Building capacity for dementia care. *Canadian Family Physician*, 57(7), e249–e252.

Lee, L., Weston, W. and Hillier, L. 2013. Developing memory clinics in primary care: An evidence-based interprofessional program of continuing professional development. *Journal of Continuing Education in the Health Professions*, 33(1), 24–32.

Leeds Beckett University. n.d. *'What Works' in Dementia Education and Training?* [online]. Leeds: Leeds Beckett University. Available from: https://www.leedsbeckett.ac.uk/research/centre-for-dementia-research/what-works/ [Accessed 20 September 2021].

Leicher, V. and Mulder, R. 2016. Team learning, team performance and safe team climate in elder care nursing. *Team Performance Management*, 22(7–8), 399–414.

Leicher, V., Mulder, R. and Bauer, J. 2013. Learning from errors at work: A replication study in elder care nursing. *Vocations and Learning*, 6(2), 207–220.

Lepore, M., Lima, J. and Miller, S. 2020. Nursing home culture change practices and survey deficiencies: A national longitudinal panel study. *The Gerontologist*, 60(8), 1411–1423.

Leung, C., et al. 2020. Early detection of dementia: The knowledge and attitudes of primary care physicians in Hong Kong. *Dementia (London)*, 19(3), 830–846.

Leverton, M., et al. 2021. 'You can't just put somebody in a situation with no armour': An ethnographic exploration of the training and support needs of homecare workers caring for people living with dementia. *Dementia*, 20(8), 2982–3005.

Levin-Banchik, L. 2018. Assessing knowledge retention, with and without simulations. *Journal of Political Science Education*, 14(3), 341–359.

Lichtwarck, B., et al. 2019a. Experiences of nursing home staff using the targeted interdisciplinary model for evaluation and treatment of neuropsychiatric symptoms (TIME) – a qualitative study. *Aging and Mental Health*, 23(8), 966–975.

Lichtwarck, B., et al. 2019b. TIME to reduce agitation in persons with dementia in nursing homes: A process evaluation of a complex intervention. *BMC Health Services Research*, 19, 349. https://doi.org/10.1186/s12913-019-4168-0.

Lima, J., et al. 2020. The changing adoption of culture change practices in U.S. nursing homes. *Innovation in Aging*, 4(3), igaa012. https://doi.org/10.1093/geroni/igaa012.

Lintern, T. and Woods, B. 1996. *Approaches to Dementia Questionnaire*. Bangor: University of Wales, Bangor.

Lipman, V. and Manthorpe, G. 2017. Social housing provision for minority ethnic older people with dementia: Findings from a qualitative study. *Dementia*, 16(6), 750–765.

Liveng, A. 2010. Learning and recognition in health and care work: An inter-subjective perspective. *Journal of Workplace Learning*, 22(1), 41–52.

Ludwin, K. and Capstick, A. 2015. Using participatory video to understand diversity among people with dementia in long-term care. *Journal of Psychological Issues in Organizational Culture*, 5(4), 30–38.

Ludwin, K. and Capstick, A. 2017. *Ethnography in Dementia Care Research: Observations on ability and capacity*. London: Sage.

Malcolm, J., Hodkinson, P. and Colley, H. 2003. The interrelationships between informal and formal learning. *Journal of Workplace Learning*, 15(7–8), 313–318.

Malterud, K. and Elvbakken, K. 2019. Patients participating as co-researchers in health research: A systematic review of outcomes and experiences. *Scandinavian Journal of Public Health*, 48(6), 617–628.

Man Chui, K. C. and Lam, C. M. 2019. P4-618: 'Dementitude' from the voice of dementia: Promoting proper caring attitude to the person with dementia in Chinese society. *Alzheimer's and Dementia*, 15(7S, Part 30), P1562–P1563. https://doi.org/10.1016/j.jalz.2019.08.166.

Mann, J. and Hung, L. 2018. Co-research with people living with dementia for change. *Action Research*, 17(4), 573–590.

Manuti, A., et al. 2015. Formal and informal learning in the workplace: A research review. *International Journal of Training and Development*, 19(1), 1–17.

Maran, N. and Glavin, R. 2003. Low- to high-fidelity simulation – a continuum of medical education? *Medical Education*, 37(suppl. 1), 22–28.

Marsick, V., et al. 2009. Informal and incidental learning in the workplace. *In:* Smith, M. and DeFrates-Densch, N., eds. *Handbook of Research on Adult Learning and Development*. Abingdon: Routledge.

Mash, R., De Sa, A. and Christodoulou, M. 2016. How to change organisational culture: Action research in a South African public sector primary care facility. *African Journal of Primary Health Care and Family Medicine*, 8(1), e1–e9.

Massoth, C., et al. 2019. High-fidelity is not superior to low-fidelity simulation but leads to overconfidence in medical students. *BMC Medical Education*, 19, 29. https://doi.org/10.1186/s12909-019-1464-7.

Matthews, F., et al. 2013. A two-decade comparison of prevalence of dementia in individuals aged 65 years and older from three geographical areas of England: Results of the Cognitive Function and Ageing Study I and II. *The Lancet*, 382(9902), 1405–1412.

Mavromaras, K., et al. 2017. *The Aged Care Workforce, 2016*. Canberra: Australian Government Department of Health [online]. Available from: https://www.gen-agedcare-data.gov.au/www_aihwgen/media/Workforce/The-Aged-Care-Workforce-2016.pdf.

McCabe, M. 2019. *Report to the Royal Commission on Aged Care Quality and Safety.*

McDermid, J., et al. 2018. O4-03-06: A randomized controlled trial evaluating the impact of an e-learning intervention based on the improving well-being and health for people with dementia (WHELD) person-centred care training programme. *Alzheimer's and Dementia*, 14(7S, Part 26), P1406. https://doi.org/10.1016/j.jalz.2018.06.2926.

McKay, M., et al. 2021. Comparing occupational adaptation-based and traditional training programs for dementia care teams: An embedded mixed-methods study. *The Gerontologist*, 61(4), 582–594.

McKeown, J., Fortune, D. and Dupuis, S. 2016. 'It is like stepping into another world': Exploring the possibilities of using appreciative participatory action research to guide culture change work in community and long-term care. *Action Research*, 14(3), 318–334.

Meirink, J., et al. 2009. How do teachers learn in the workplace? An examination of teacher learning activities. *European Journal of Teacher Education*, 32(3), 209–224.

Merizzi, A. 2018. Virtual Dementia Tour®: Limitations and ethics. *Quality in Ageing and Older Adults*, 19(2), 146–155.

Merriam, S. 2001. Andragogy and self-directed learning: Pillars of adult learning theory. *In:* Merriam, S., ed. *The New Update on Adult Learning Theory: New Directions for Adult and Continuing Education.* Hoboken, NJ: Wiley.

Merriam, S. 2018. Adult learning theory: Evolution and future directions. *In:* Illeris, K., ed. *Contemporary Theories of Learning: Learning theorists … in their own words,* 2nd edition. London: Routledge.

Meyer, K., et al. 2022. Simulation learning to train healthcare students in person-centered dementia care. *Gerontology and Geriatrics Education*, 43(2), 209–224.

Mezirow, J. 1978. Perspective transformation. *Adult Education*, 28, 100–110.

Mezirow, J. 1997. Transformative learning: Theory to practice. *In:* Cranton, P., ed. *Transformative Learning in Action: Insights from practice.* San Francisco, CA: Jossey-Bass.

Michie, S., et al. 2005. Making psychological theory useful for implementing evidence based practice: A consensus approach. *Quality and Safety in Health Care*, 14(1), 26–33.

Michie, S., van Stralen, M. and West, R. 2011. The behaviour change wheel: A new method for characterising and designing behaviour change interventions. *Implementation Science*, 6, 42. https://doi.org/10.1186/1748-5908-6-42.

Mikkonen, K., et al. 2018. Competence areas of health science teachers – a systematic review of quantitative studies. *Nurse Education Today*, 70, 77–86.

Miles, S. and Pritchard-Wilkes, V. 2018. Dementia-friendly housing charter. *Working with Older People*, 22(2), 76–82.

Miller, G. 1990. The assessment of clinical skills/competence/performance. *Academic Medicine*, 65(9), S63–S67.

Moehead, A., et al. 2020. A web-based dementia education program and its application to an Australian web-based dementia care competency and training network: Integrative systematic review. *Journal of Medical Internet Research*, 22(1), e16808. https://doi.org/10.2196/16808.

Moniz-Cook, E., et al. 2017. Challenge Demcare: Management of challenging behaviour in dementia at home and in care homes – development, evaluation and implementation of an online individualised intervention for care homes; and a cohort study of specialist community mental health car. *Programme Grants for Applied Research*, 5(15), 1–290.

Morbey, H., et al. 2019. Involving people living with dementia in research: An accessible modified Delphi survey for core outcome set development. *Trials*, 20, 12. https://doi.org/10.1186/s13063-018-3069-6.

Morgan, D., et al. 2016. Dementia-related work activities of home care nurses and aides: Frequency, perceived competence, and continuing education priorities. *Educational Gerontology*, 42(2), 120–135.

Mornata, C. and Cassar, I. 2018. The role of insiders and organizational support in the learning process of newcomers during organizational socialization. *Journal of Workplace Learning*, 30(7), 562–575.

Mukadam, N., et al. 2015. What would encourage help-seeking for memory problems among UK-based South Asians? A qualitative study. *BMJ Open*, 5, e007990. https://doi.org/10.1136/bmjopen-2015-007990.

Murphy, K., et al. 2014. Articulating the strategies for maximising the inclusion of people with dementia in qualitative research studies. *Dementia*, 14(6), 800–824.

Murray, M., et al. 2019. Impact of the Dementia Care in Hospitals Program on acute hospital staff satisfaction. *BMC Health Services Research*, 19, 680. https://doi.org/10.1186/s12913-019-4489-z.

Nakanishi, M., et al. 2018. Dementia behaviour management programme at home: Impact of a palliative care approach on care managers and professional caregivers of home care services. *Aging and Mental Health*, 22(8), 1057–1062.

National Center for Education Statistics (NCES). 2017. *Highlights of PIAAC 2017 U.S. Results* [online]. Available from: https://nces.ed.gov/surveys/piaac/national_results.asp [Accessed 3 December 2021].

National Collaborating Centre for Mental Health (NCCMH). 2018. *The Dementia Care Pathway: Full implementation guidance* [online]. Available from: https://www.rcpsych.ac.uk/docs/default-source/improving-care/nccmh/dementia/nccmh-dementia-care-pathway-full-implementation-guidance.pdf?sfvrsn=cdef189d_8.

National Dementia Action Alliance (NDAA). 2020. *Dementia-Friendly Hospital Charter Revised 2020: COVID-19 recommendations*. London: NDAA.

National Institute for Health and Care Research (NIHR). 2021. *Briefing Notes for Researchers – public involvement in NHS, health and social care research* [online]. Available from: https://www.nihr.ac.uk/documents/briefing-notes-for-researchers-public-involvement-in-nhs-health-and-social-care-research/27371.

National Literacy Trust (NLT). 2012. *Adult Literacy* [online]. Available from: https://literacytrust.org.uk/parents-and-families/adult-literacy/ [Accessed 3 December 2021].

Naughton, C., et al. 2018. A dementia communication training intervention based on the VERA framework for pre-registration nurses: Part I developing and testing an implementation strategy. *Nurse Education Today*, 63, 94–100.

Naylor, C., et al., 2016. *Physical and Mental Health: A new frontier for integrated care*. London: The King's Fund.

Negin, J., et al. 2013. Foreign-born health workers in Australia: An analysis of census data. *Human Resources for Health*, 11, 69. https://doi.org/10.1186/1478-4491-11-69.

NHS Digital. 2021. *Recorded Dementia Diagnose Data August 2021* [online]. Available from: https://digital.nhs.uk/data-and-information/publications/statistical/recorded-dementia-diagnoses/august-2021.

NHS Education for Scotland and the Scottish Social Services Council. 2011. *Promoting Excellence: A framework for all health and social services staff working with people with dementia, their families and carers*. Edinburgh: The Scottish Government [online]. Available from: https://www.gov.scot/publications/promoting-excellence-framework-health-social-services-staff-working-people-dementia-families-carers/.

NHS England. 2021. *Quality and Outcomes Framework Guidance for 2021/22* [online]. Available from: https://www.england.nhs.uk/wp-content/uploads/2021/03/B0456-update-on-quality-outcomes-framework-changes-for-21-22-.pdf.

NICE. 2018. *Dementia: Assessment, management and support for people living with dementia and their carers.* NICE Guideline NG97 [online]. Available from: https://www.nice.org.uk/guidance/ng97.

NICE/SCIE. 2011. *Dementia: A NICE–SCIE Guideline on supporting people with dementia and their carers in health and social care.* National Clinical Practice Guideline No. 42. Leicester: British Psychological Society and Gaskell [on;ine]. Available from: https://www.scie.org.uk/publications/misc/dementia/dementia-fullguideline.pdf?res=true.

Nolan, M., et al. 2004. Beyond 'person-centred' care: A new vision for gerontological nursing. *Journal of Clinical Nursing*, 13(3a), 45–53.

Nolan, M., et al. 2006. *The Senses Framework: Improving care for older people through a relationship-centred approach.* Getting Research into Practice (GRIP) Report No. 2. Sheffield: University of Sheffield [online]. Available from: http://shura.shu.ac.uk/280/.

Norris, T., et al. 2009. Longitudinal integrated clerkships for medical students: An innovation adopted by medical schools in Australia, Canada, South Africa, and the United States. *Academic Medicine*, 84(7), 902–907.

Northern Ireland Health and Social Care Board. 2016. *The Dementia Learning and Development Framework.* Belfast: Health and Social Care Board [online]. Available from: https://hscboard.hscni.net/dementia/learning-development-framework/.

O'Brien, R., et al. 2018. The VOICE study – a before and after study of a dementia communication skills training course. *PLoS One*, 13(6), e0198567. https://doi.org/10.1371/journal.pone.0198567.

O'Connor, M. and McFadden, S. 2010. Development and psychometric validation of the Dementia Attitudes Scale. *International Journal of Alzheimer's Disease*, 2010, 454218. https://doi.org/10.4061/2010/454218.

O'Shea, E., et al. 2017. Key stakeholders' experiences of respite services for people with dementia and their perspectives on respite service development: A qualitative systematic review. *BMC Geriatrics*, 17, 282. https://doi.org/10.1186/s12877-017-0676-0.

OECD. 2016. *Skills Matter: Further results from the survey of adult skills.* Paris: OECD Publishing [online]. Available from: https://www.oecd.org/skills/skills-matter-9789264258051-en.htm.

Oliveira, M. and Sousa, L. 2020. VᴬᴸIDA: A Validation Therapy-training program for staff of a residential care facility. *International Journal of Aging and Human Development*, 93(2), 786–802.

Our Voice Matters. 2021. *We Have Dementia! Our research is your future.* Dementia Enquirers.

Paré, A. and Le Maistre, C. 2006. Active learning in the workplace: Transforming individuals and institutions. *Journal of Education and Work*, 19(4), 363–381.

Parveen, S., et al. 2018. Involving minority ethnic communities and diverse experts by experience in dementia research: The Caregiving HOPE Study. *Dementia*, 17(8), 990–1000.

Parveen, S., et al. 2021. The impact of dementia education and training on health and social care staff knowledge, attitudes and confidence: A cross-sectional study. *BMJ Open*, 11, e039939. https://doi.org/10.1136/bmjopen-2020-039939.

Pashler, H., et al. 2008. Learning styles: Concepts and evidence. *Psychological Science in the Public Interest*, 9(3), 105–119.

Pearce, J., et al. 2012. The most effective way of delivering a Train-the-Trainers program: A systematic review. *Journal of Continuing Education in the Health Professions*, 32(3), 215–226.

Peng, X., et al. 2020. Impact of Virtual Dementia Tour on empathy level of nursing students: A quasi-experimental study. *International Journal of Nursing Sciences*, 7(3), 258–261.

Peri, K., et al. 2015. Is psychotropic medication use related to organisational and treatment culture in residential care. *Journal of Health, Organisation and Management*, 29(7), 1065–1079.

Perry, M. 2011. O3-02-01: Training family physicians and primary care nurses improves diagnostic assessment of dementia: Results of a randomized controlled trial. *Alzheimer's and Dementia*, 7(4S, Part 14), S498. https://doi.org/10.1016/j.jalz.2011.05.2393.

Petyaeva, A., et al. 2018. Feasibility of a staff training and support programme to improve pain assessment and management in people with dementia living in care homes. *International Journal of Geriatric Psychiatry*, 33(1), 221–231.

Pfeifer, P., et al. 2018. The impact of education on certified nursing assistants' identification of strategies to manage behaviors associated with dementia. *Journal for Nurses in Professional Development*, 24(1), 26–30.

Phillips, C., et al. 2015. Experiences of using the Theoretical Domains Framework across diverse clinical environments: A qualitative study. *Journal of Multidisciplinary Healthcare*, 8, 139–146.

Phillipson, L. and Hammond, A. 2018. More than talking: A scoping review of innovative approaches to qualitative research involving people with dementia. *International Journal of Qualitative Methods*, 17(1), 1609406918782784. https://doi.org/10.1177/1609406918782784.

Plain English Campaign, 2021. *Plain English Campaign: Free guides* [online]. Available from: http://www.plainenglish.co.uk/free-guides.html [Accessed 19 November 2021].

Polacsek, M., et al. 2020. 'I know they are not trained in dementia': Addressing the need for specialist dementia training for home care workers. *Health and Social Care in the Community*, 28(2), 475–484.

Pollak, D. 2009. Introduction. *In:* Pollak, D., ed. *Neurodiversity in Higher Education: Positive responses to particular learning differences*. Chichester: Wiley.

Pollard, C., et al. 2007. Clinical education: A review of the literature. *Nurse Education in Practice*, 7(5), 315–322.

Pool, I., et al. 2015. Strategies for continuing professional development among younger, middle-aged, and older nurses: A biographical approach. *International Journal of Nursing Studies*, 52(5), 939–950.

Power, G. 2010. *Dementia Beyond Drugs; Changing the culture of care*. Baltimore, MD: Healthcare Professions Press.

Prince, M., et al. 2014. *Dementia UK: Update*. London: Alzheimer's Society [online]. Available from: https://www.alzheimers.org.uk/sites/default/files/migrate/downloads/dementia_uk_update.pdf.

Public Health England (PHE). 2018. *Statistical Commentary: Dementia profile (March 2018 update)* [online]. Available from: https://www.gov.uk/government/statistics/dementia-profile-updates/statistical-commentary-dementia-profile-march-2018-update.

Pulsford, D., Hope, K. and Thompson, R. 2007. Higher education provision for professionals working with people with dementia: A scoping exercise. *Nurse Education Today*, 27(1), 5–13.

Puts, M., et al. 2010. Does frailty predict hospitalization, emergency department visits, and visits to the general practitioner in older newly-diagnosed cancer patients? Results of a prospective pilot study. *Critical Reviews in Oncology/Hematology*, 76(2), 142–151.

Queen's Nursing Institute (QNI). 2021. *Standards of Education and Practice for Nurses New to Care Home Nursing* [online]. Available from: https://www.qni.org.uk/wp-content/uploads/2021/01/Standards-of-Education-and-Practice-for-Nurses-New-to-Care-Home-Nursing-2021.pdf.

Quinn, R. and Rohrbaugh, J. 1981. A competing values approach to organizational effectiveness. *Public Productivity Review*, 5(2), 122–140.

Rausch, A., Seifried, J. and Harteis, C. 2017. Emotions, coping and learning in error situations in the workplace. *Journal of Workplace Learning*, 29(5), 370–389.

Redmond, B. 1997. *Reflection in Action: Developing reflective practice*. London: Routledge.

Reece, I. and Walker, S., 2007. *Teaching, Training and Learning: A practical guide*. Tyne & Wear: Business Education Publishers.

Reinhardt, J., et al. 2020. Dementia-focused person-directed care training with direct care workers in nursing homes: Effect on symptom reduction. *Journal of Gerontological Nursing*, 46(8), 7–11.

Rentenbach, B., Prislovsky, L. and Gabriel, R. 2017. Valuing differences: Neurodiversity in the classroom. *Phi Delta Kappan*, 98(8), 59–63.

Reynish, E., et al. 2017. Epidemiology and outcomes of people with dementia, delirium, and unspecified cognitive impairment in the general hospital: Prospective cohort study of 10,014 admissions. *BMC Medicine*, 15, 140. https://doi.org/10.1186/s12916-017-0899-0.

Riener, C. and Willingham, D. 2010. The myth of learning styles. *Change: The Magazine of Higher Learning*, 42(5), 32–35.

Riesch, J., et al. 2018. Dementia-specific training for nursing home staff. *Zeitschrift für Gerontologie und Geriatrie*, 51(5), 523–529.

Roberts, H. and Noble, J. 2015. Education research: Changing medical student perceptions of dementia: An arts-centered experience. *Neurology*, 85(8), 739–741.

Rogers, A. 2003. *What is the Difference? A new critique of learning and teaching*. Leicester: NIACE.

Rohrer, D. and Pashler, H. 2012. Learning styles: Where's the evidence? *Medical Education*, 46(7), 634–635.

Rokstad, A., et al. 2013. The effect of person-centred dementia care to prevent agitation and other neuropsychiatric symptoms and enhance quality of life in nursing home patients: A 10-month randomized controlled trial. *Dementia and Geriatric Cognitive Disorders*, 36(5–6), 340–353.

Rokstad, A., et al. 2015. The role of leadership in the implementation of person-centred care using Dementia Care Mapping: A study in three nursing homes. *Journal of Nursing Management*, 23(1), 15–26.

Rokstad, A., et al. 2017. The impact of the Dementia ABC educational programme on competence in person-centred dementia care and job satisfaction of care staff. *International Journal of Older People Nursing*, 12(2), 1–10.

Rolewicz, L. and Palmer, B. 2020. *The NHS Workforce in Numbers*. London: Nuffield Trust [online]. Available from: https://www.nuffieldtrust.org.uk/resource/the-nhs-workforce-in-numbers [Accessed 21 April 2021].

Rooney, D., Manidis, M. and Scheeres, H. 2016. Making space for consuming practices. *Vocations and Learning*, 9(2), 167–184.

Røsvik, J., et al. 2011. A model for using the VIPS framework for person-centred care for persons with dementia in nursing homes: A qualitative evaluative study. *International Journal of Older People Nursing*, 6(3), 227–236.

Røsvik, J. and Mjørud, M. 2021. 'We must have a new VIPS meeting soon!' Barriers and facilitators for implementing the VIPS practice model in primary health care. *Dementia (London)*, 20(8), 2649–2667.

Royal College of Psychiatrists (RCP). 2019a. *National Audit of Dementia Care in General Hospitals 2018–2019: Round four audit report*. London: RCP [online]. Available from: https://www.rcpsych.ac.uk/docs/default-source/improving-care/ccqi/national-clinical-audits/national-audit-of-dementia/r4-resources/reports---core-audit/national-audit-of-dementia-round-4-report-online.pdf.

Royal College of Psychiatrists (RCP). 2019b. *The Role of Liaison Psychiatry in Integrated Physical and Mental Healthcare: Position statement*. London: RCP [online]. Available from: https://www.rcpsych.ac.uk/docs/default-source/improving-care/better-mh-policy/position-statements/ps07_19.pdf?sfvrsn=563a6bab_2.

Ryan, A., et al. 2018. The 'My Home Life' Leadership support and community development programme. *Innovation in Aging*, 2(suppl. 1), 187.

Ryding, J., Sorbring, E. and Wernersson, I. 2018. The understanding and use of reflection in family support social work. *Journal of Social Service Research*, 44(4), 494–508.

Sævareid, T., et al. 2018. Implementing advance care planning in nursing homes – study protocol of a cluster-randomized clinical trial. *BMC Geriatrics*, 18, 180. https://doi.org/10.1186/s12877-018-0869-1.

Sævareid, T., et al. 2019. Improved patient participation through advance care planning in nursing homes – a cluster randomized clinical trial. *Patient Education and Counseling*, 102(12), 2183–2191.

Sagbakken, M., Spilker, R. and Nielsen, T. 2018. Dementia and immigrant groups: A qualitative study of challenges related to identifying, assessing, and diagnosing dementia. *BMC Health Services Research*, 18, 910. https://doi.org/10.1186/s12913-018-3720-7.

Salsberg, E., et al. 2021. Estimation and comparison of current and future racial/ethnic representation in the US health care workforce. *JAMA Network Open*, 4(3), e213789. https://doi.org/10.1001/jamanetworkopen.2021.3789.

Sampson, E., et al. 2017. Improving the care of people with dementia in general hospitals: Evaluation of a whole-system train-the-trainer model. *International Psychogeriatrics*, 29(4), 605–614.

Samsi, K. and Manthorpe, J., 2020. *Interviewing People Living with Dementia in Social Care Research: Methods review*. London: NIHR School for Social Care Research [online]. Available from: https://www.sscr.nihr.ac.uk/wp-content/uploads/SSCR-methods-review_MR022.pdf.

Sass, C., et al. 2019. Factors associated with successful dementia education for practitioners in primary care: An in-depth case study. *BMC Medical Education*, 19, 393. https://doi.org/10.1186/s12909-019-1833-2.

Sawan, M., Jeon, Y.-H. and Chen, T. 2018. Shaping the use of psychotropic medicines in nursing homes: A qualitative study on organisational culture. *Social Science and Medicine*, 202, 70–78.

Scales, K., et al. 2017. Power, empowerment, and person-centred care: Using ethnography to examine the everyday practice of unregistered dementia care staff. *Sociology of Health and Illness*, 39(2), 227–243.

Scammell, J., Heaslip, V. and Crowley, E. 2016. Service user involvement in preregistration general nurse education: A systematic review. *Journal of Clinical Nursing*, 25(1–2), 53–69.

Scerri, A. and Scerri, C. 2019. Outcomes in knowledge, attitudes and confidence of nursing staff working in nursing and residential care homes following a dementia training programme. *Aging and Mental Health*, 23(8), 919–928.

Scerri, A., Innes, A. and Scerri, C. 2017. Dementia training programmes for staff working in general hospital settings – a systematic review of the literature. *Aging and Mental Health*, 21(8), 783–796.

Schein, E. 2017. *Organizational Culture and Leadership*, 5th edition. New York: Wiley.

Schepers, A., et al. 2012. Sense of Competence in Dementia Care Staff (SCIDS) scale: Development, reliability and validity. *International Psychogeriatrics*, 24(7), 1153–1162.

Schick, D. 2017. Culture change within the long-term care setting as envisioned by the concepts of the Eden Alternative®. *Canadian Nursing Home*, 28(1), 21–23.

Schneider, J. 2017. Evaluation of the impact on audiences of Inside Out of Mind, research-based theatre for dementia carers. *Arts and Health*, 9(3), 238–250.

Schneider, J., et al. 2019. Expectations of nursing personnel and physicians on dementia training: A descriptive survey in general hospitals in Germany and Greece. *Zeitschrift für Gerontologie und Geriatrie*, 52(suppl. 4), S249–S257.

Schnelli, A., et al. 2020. Aggressive behaviour of persons with dementia towards professional caregivers in the home care setting – a scoping review. *Journal of Clinical Nursing*. https://doi.org/10.1111/jocn.15363.

Schön, D. 1983. *The Reflective Practitioner: How professionals think in action*. New York: Basic Books.

Schön, D. 1987. *Educating the Reflective Practitioner*. San Fransisco, CA: Jossey-Bass.

Schön, D. 1992. *The Reflective Practitioner: How professionals think in action*. London: Routledge.

Scott, T., Kugelman, M. and Tulloch, K. 2019. How medical professional students view older people with dementia: Implications for education and practice. *PLoS One*, 14(11), e0225329. https://doi.org/10.1371/journal.pone.0225329.

Shanahan, N., et al. 2013. The development and evaluation of the DK-20: A knowledge of dementia measure. *International Psychogeriatrics*, 25(11), 1899–1907.

Sharp, E., et al. 2021. Optimizing synchronous online teaching sessions: A guide to the 'new normal' in medical education. *Academic Pediatrics*, 21(1), 11–15.

Sheaff, R., Sherriff, I. and Hennessy, C. 2018. Evaluating a dementia learning community: Exploratory study and research implications. *BMC Health Services Research*, 18, 83. https://doi.org/10.1186/s12913-018-2894-3.

Shield, R., et al. 2014. 'Would you do that in your home?' Making nursing homes home-like in culture change implementation. *Journal of Housing for the Elderly*, 28(4), 383–398.

Singh, S., et al. 2013. Qualities of an effective teacher: What do medical teachers think? *BMC Medical Education*, 13, 128. https://doi.org/10.1186/1472-6920-13-128.

Skaalvik, M., Normann, K. and Henriksen, N. 2012. Nursing homes as learning environments: The impact of professional dialogue. *Nurse Education Today*, 32(4), 412–416.

Skar, R. 2010. How nurses experience their work as a learning environment. *Vocations and Learning*, 3(1), 1–18.

Skills for Care. 2021. *The State of the Adult Social Care Sector and Workforce in England 2021*. Leeds: Skills for Care [online]. Available from: https://www.skillsforcare.org.uk/adult-social-care-workforce-data/Workforce-intelligence/publications/national-information/The-state-of-the-adult-social-care-sector-and-workforce-in-England.aspx.

Skills for Health. 2018. *Dementia Training Standards Framework*. London: Skills for Health [online]. Available from: https://www.skillsforhealth.org.uk/wp-content/uploads/2021/01/Dementia-Core-Skills-Education-and-Training-Framework.pdf.

Slater, P., Hasson, F. and Gillen, P. 2017. *A Research Evaluation of an Interactive Training Experience: The Virtual Dementia Tour® (VDT®)*. Ballyshannon, Co. Donegal: Health Service Executive.

Smith, S., et al. 2019. An audit of dementia education and training in UK health and social care: A comparison with national benchmark standards. *BMC Health Services Research*, 19, 711. https://doi.org/10.1186/s12913-019-4510-6.

Smythe, A., et al. 2013. Evaluation of dementia training for staff in acute hospital settings. *Nursing Older People*, 26(2), 18–24.

Smythe, A., et al. 2017. A qualitative study investigating training requirements of nurses working with people with dementia in nursing homes. *Nurse Education Today*, 50, 119–123.

Smythe, A., et al. 2020. A qualitative study exploring nursing home nurses' experiences of training in person centred dementia care on burnout. *Nurse Education in Practice*, 44, 102745. https://doi.org/10.1016/j.nepr.2020.102745.

Snyder, C., et al. 2015. *Facilitating Racial and Ethnic Diversity in the Health Workforce*. Washington: Center for Health Workforce Studies, University of Washington [online]. Available from: https://depts.washington.edu/uwrhrc/uploads/FINALREPORT_Facilitating%20Diversity%20in%20the%20Health%20Workforce_7.8.2015.pdf.

Soklaridis, S., et al. 2016. Relationship-centred care in health: A 20-year scoping review. *Patient Experience Journal*, 3(1), 130–145.

Somerville, M., 2006. Subjected bodies or embodied subjects: Subjectivity and learning safety at work. *In:* Billett, S., Fenwick, T. and Somerville, M., eds. *Work, Subjectivity and Learning*. Dordrecht: Springer.

Sparr, J., Knipfer, K. and Willems, F. 2017. How leaders can get the most out of formal training: The significance of feedback-seeking and reflection as informal learning behaviours. *Human Resource Development Quarterly*, 28(1), 29–54.

St. Clair, R. 2002. *Andragogy Revisited: Theory for the 21st century?* Columbus, OH: ERIC [online]. Available from: https://files.eric.ed.gov/fulltext/ED468612.pdf.

Stevenson, M. and Taylor, B. 2017. Involving individuals with dementia as co-researchers in analysis of findings from a qualitative study. *Dementia*, 18(2), 701–712.

Streater, A., et al. 2017. Staff training and outreach support for Cognitive Stimulation Therapy and its implementation in practice: A cluster randomised trial. *International Journal of Geriatric Psychiatry*, 32(12), e64–e71.

Su, H.-F., et al. 2021. A dementia care training using mobile e-learning with mentoring support for home care workers: A controlled study. *BMC Geriatrics*, 21, 126. https://doi.org/10.1186/s12877-021-02075-3.

Surr, C. 2019. The task of cultural transformation: A critical commentary. *In:* Brooker, D., ed. *Dementia Reconsidered Revisited: The person still comes first*. Buckingham: Open University Press.

Surr, C. and Gates, C. 2017. What works in delivering dementia education or training to hospital staff? A critical synthesis of the evidence. *International Journal Nursing Studies*, 75, 172-188.

Surr, C., et al. 2017a. Effective dementia education and training for the health and social care workforce: A systematic review of the literature. *Review of Educational Research*, 87(5), 966–1002.

Surr, C., et al. 2017b. *Dementia Training Design and Delivery Audit Tool (DeTDAT) v4.0*. Leeds: Leeds Beckett University [online]. Available from: https://www.leeds-beckett.ac.uk/-/media/files/research/dementia/dementia-training-design-and-delivery-audit-tool-manual-v4_0.pdf.

Surr, C., Griffiths, A. and Kelley, R. 2018a. Implementing Dementia Care Mapping as a practice development tool in dementia care services: A systematic review. *Clinical Interventions in Aging*, 13, 165–177.

Surr, C., et al. 2018b. O3-08-06: Results of a pragmatic cluster randomised controlled trial of the effectiveness and cost effectiveness of dementia care mapping (DCM) in UK care homes (DCM EPIC trial). *Alzheimer's and Dementia*, 14(7S, Part 19), P1035. https://doi.org/10.1016/j.jalz.2018.06.2817.

Surr, C., et al. 2018c. Components of impactful dementia training for general hospital staff: A collective case study. *Aging and Mental Health*, 24(3), 511–521.

Surr, C., et al. 2019a. The implementation of Dementia Care Mapping™ in a randomised controlled trial in long-term care: Results of a process evaluation *American Journal of Alzheimer's Disease and Other Dementias*, 34(6), 390–398.

Surr, C., et al. 2019b. A collective case study of the features of impactful dementia training for care home staff. *BMC Geriatrics*, 19, 175. https://doi.org/10.1186/s12877-019-1186-z.

Surr, C., et al. 2020. The barriers and facilitators to implementing dementia education and training in health and social care services: A mixed-methods study. *BMC Health Services Research*, 20, 512. https://doi.org/10.1186/s12913-020-05382-4.

Surr, C., et al. 2021. Effectiveness of Dementia Care Mapping™ to reduce agitation in care home residents with dementia: An open-cohort cluster randomised controlled trial. *Aging and Mental Health*, 25(8), 1410–1423.

Sutcliffe, D., et al. 2012. NICE and the Quality and Outcomes Framework (QOF) 2009–2011. *Quality in Primary Care*, 20(1), 47–55.

Sutkin, G., et al. 2008. What makes a good clinical teacher in medicine? A review of the literature. *Academic Medicine*, 83(5), 452–466.

Swaffer, K. 2018. Human rights, disability and dementia. *Australian Journal of Dementia Care*, 7(1), 25–28.

Takase, M., et al. 2015. The relationship between workplace learning and midwives' and nurses' self-reported competence: A cross-sectional survey. *International Journal of Nursing Studies*, 52(12), 1804–1815.

Takase, M., Yamamoto, M. and Sato, Y. 2018. Effects of nurses' personality traits and their environmental characteristics on their workplace learning and nursing competence. *Japan Journal of Nursing Science*, 15(2), 167–180.

Taylor, D. and Hamdy, H. 2013. Adult learning theories: Implications for learning and teaching in medical education: AMEE Guide No. 83. *Medical Teacher*, 35, e1561–e1572.

Taylor, N., et al. 2013. Development and initial validation of the Influences on Patient Safety Behaviours Questionnaire. *Implementation Science*, 8, 81. https://doi.org/10.1186/1748-5908-8-81.

Testad, I., et al. 2016. Modeling and evaluating evidence-based continuing education program in nursing home dementia care (MEDCED) – training of care home staff to reduce use of restraint in care home residents with dementia. A cluster randomized controlled trial. *International Journal of Geriatric Psychiatry*, 31(1), 24–32.

Teunissen, P. 2015. Experience, trajectories, and reifications: An emerging framework of practice-based learning in healthcare workplaces. *Advances in Health Sciences Education*, 20(4), 843–856.

Thomas, W. 2004. *What Are Old People For? How elders will save the world*. Acton, MA: VanderWyk & Burnham.

Thomson, L., et al. 2018. *Evaluating the Care Certificate (ECCert): A cross-sector solution to assuring fundamental skills in caring*. Department of Health Policy Research Programme Project (PR-R14-0915-12004) [online]. Available from: https://nottingham-repository.worktribe.com/output/1065017/evaluating-the-care-certificate-eccert-a-cross-sector-solution-to-assuring-fundamental-skills-in-caring.

thred CiC. 2021. *How Can Urban and Rural Transport Systems Help People Diagnosed with Dementia Live Independently for Longer?* Dementia Enquirers [online]. Available from: https://dementiaenquirers.org.uk/wp-content/uploads/2021/05/thred-in-liverpool_report.pdf.

Thyrian, R. and Hoffmann, W. 2012. Dementia care and general physicians – a survey on prevalence, means, attitudes and recommendations. *Central European Journal of Public Health*, 20(4), 270–275.

Tompkins, C., et al. 2020. A web-based training program for direct care workers in long-term care communities: Providing knowledge and skills to implement a music and memory intervention. *Gerontology and Geriatrics Education*, 41(3), 367–379.

Travers, C., et al. 2020. Using a reflective diary method to investigate the experiences of paid home care workers caring for people with dementia. *Home Health Care Management and Practice*, 32(1), 10–21.

Triliva, S., et al. 2020. Healthcare professionals' perspectives on mental health service provision: A pilot focus group study in six European countries. *International Journal of Mental Health Systems*, 14, 16. https://doi.org/10.1186/s13033-020-00350-1.

Tullo, E. and Gordon, A. 2013. Teaching and learning about dementia in UK medical schools: A national survey. *BMC Geriatrics*, 13, 29. https://doi.org/10.1186/1471-2318-13-29.

Venturato, L., Moyle, W. and Steel, A. 2011. Exploring the gap between rhetoric and reality in dementia care in Australia: Could practice documents help bridge the great divide? *Dementia*, 12(2), 251–267.

Venturato, L., Horner, B. and Etherton-Beer, C. 2020. Development and evaluation of an organisational culture change intervention in residential aged care facilities. *Australasian Journal on Ageing*, 39(1), 56–63.

Verreault, R., et al. 2018. Quasi-experimental evaluation of a multifaceted intervention to improve quality of end-of-life care and quality of dying for patients with advanced dementia in long-term care institutions. *Palliative Medicine*, 32(3), 613–621.

Waite, J., Poland, F. and Charlesworth, G. 2019. Facilitators and barriers to co-research by people with dementia and academic researchers: Findings from a qualitative study. *Health Expectations*, 22(4), 761–771.

Waldemar, G., et al. 2007. Access to diagnostic evaluation and treatment for dementia in Europe. *International Journal of Geriatric Psychiatry*, 22(1), 47–54.

Waller, S., Masterson, A. and Finn, H. 2013. *Improving the Patient Experience. Developing supportive design for people with dementia: The King's Fund's Enhancing the Healing Environment Programme 2009–2012*. London: The King's Fund [online]. Available from: https://www.kingsfund.org.uk/publications/developing-supportive-design-people-dementia.

Wells, C. and Smith, S. 2017. Diagnostic care pathways in dementia. *Journal of Primary Care and Community Health*, 8(2), 103–111.

Wenger, E. 2009. A social theory of learning. *In:* Illeris, K., ed. *Contemporary Theories of Learning*. Abingdon: Routledge.

Wilcock, J., et al. 2013. Tailored educational intervention for primary care to improve the management of dementia: The EVIDEM-ED cluster randomized controlled trial. *Trials*, 14, 397. https://doi.org/10.1186/1745-6215-14-397.

Wilesmith, K. and Major, R. 2020. Evaluation of a course to prepare volunteers to support individuals with dementia in the community. *Nurse Education in Practice*, 48, 102862. https://doi.org/10.1016/j.nepr.2020.102862.

Wilkinson, T. 2017. Kolb, integration and the messiness of workplace learning. *Perspectives on Medical Education*, 6(3), 144–145.

Williams, C. 2010. Understanding the essential elements of work-based learning and its relevance to everyday clinical practice. *Journal of Nursing Management*, 18(6), 624–632.

Williams, K., et al. 2017. A communication intervention to reduce resistiveness in dementia care: A cluster randomized controlled trial. *The Gerontologist*, 57(4), 707–718.

Williams, K., et al. 2020. Moving online: A pilot clinical trial of the changing talk online (CHATO) communication education for nursing home staff. *The Gerontologist*, 61(8), 1338–1345.

Williams, M. and Daley, S. 2021. Innovation in dementia education within undergraduate healthcare programmes: A scoping review. *Nurse Education Today*, 98, 104742. https://doi.org/10.1016/j.nedt.2020.104742.

Wimo, A., Gauthier, S. and Prince, M. 2018. *Global Estimates of Informal Care*. London: Alzheimer's Disease International (ADI). Available from: https://www.alzint.org/u/global-estimates-of-informal-care.pdf.

Windle, G., et al. 2020. Enhancing communication between dementia care staff and their residents: An arts-inspired intervention. *Aging and Mental Health*, 24(8), 1306–1315.

Wittenberg, R., et al. 2019a. *Projections of Older People with Dementia and Costs of Dementia Care in the United Kingdom, 2019–2040*. London: The London School of Economics and Political Science [online]. Available from: https://www.alzheimers.org.uk/sites/default/files/2019-11/cpec_report_november_2019.pdf.

Wittenberg, R., et al. 2019b. The costs of dementia in England. *International Journal of Geriatric Psychiatry*, 34(7), 1095–1103.

World Health Organisation (WHO). 2017. *Global Action Plan on the Public Health Response to Dementia 2017–2025*. Geneva: WHO [online]. Available from: https://www.who.int/publications/i/item/global-action-plan-on-the-public-health-response-to-dementia-2017--2025.

World Health Organisation (WHO). 2021. *Global Status Report on the Public Health Response to Dementia*. Geneva: WHO [online]. Available from: https://www.who.int/publications/i/item/9789240033245.

Yasuda, M. and Sakakibara, H. 2017. Care staff training based on person-centered care and dementia care mapping, and its effects on the quality of life of nursing home residents with dementia. *Aging and Mental Health*, 21(9), 991–996.

Yen, M., Trede, F. and Patterson, C. 2016. Learning in the workplace: The role of nurse managers. *Australian Health Review*, 40(3), 286–291.

Yorkshire and Humber Clinical Network (YHCN). 2018. *Guidance for the Consideration of the Wider Application of Diagnosing Advanced Dementia Mandate (DiADeM)* [online]. Available from: http://yhscn.nhs.uk.213-171-198-252.cubecreativegroup.com/media/PDFs/mhdn/Dementia/Dementia%20Diagnosis/2018/DiADeM/DiADeM%20guidance%20paper%20Draftv1.pdf.

Zeilig, H., et al. 2015. The arts in dementia care education: A developmental study. *Journal of Public Mental Health*, 14(1), 18–23.

Zimmerman, S., Sloane, P. and Reed, D. 2014. Dementia prevalence and care in assisted living. *Health Affairs*, 33(4), 658–666.

Zukas, M., et al. 2010. Conceptual challenges. *In:* Bradbury, H., Frost, N., Kilminster, S. and Zukas, M., eds. *Beyond Reflective Practice: New approaches to professional lifelong learning*. London: Routledge.

Index

Page numbers with 'b' and 't' indicate boxes and tables respectively.